DANCING THROUGH AND BEYOND CANCER

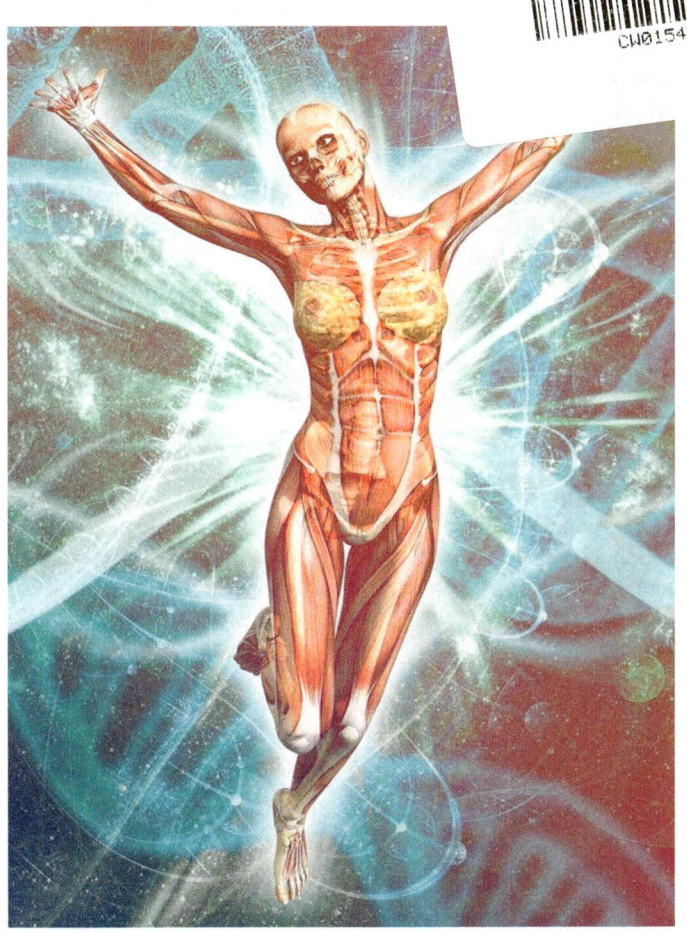

An informative guide to the use of dance and nutrition to prevent, augment the treatment of, and survive cancer

Editors: *Fenella J Barker, Dr. Dee Bhakta and Prof. Chris Palmer*

Forward by Conchita del Campo

Contributors

Afshan Aghili Senior Lecturer in Human Nutrition, London Metropolitan University. Fellow of Higher Education Academy.

Eliz Arter Senior Instructor, Eastern Mediterranean University. Visiting researcher and Doctoral student, London Metropolitan University. BSc (Hons) Biochemistry, BSc Nutrition and Dietetics, MSc Nutrition and Food Science, Associate Registered Nutritionist by The Association for Nutrition, Registered Dietitian by the Turkish Cypriot Dietitians Union.

Dr Ebru Aydar Neurophysiologist, DPhil in Neurobiology, Senior lecturer at Roehampton University, Lecturer at University of West London, Diploma in Modern dance, Fellow of Higher Education Academy, Artistic Director of Random Transformations Dance Company.

Fenella J Barker Lecturer in Ballet, Flamenco & Spanish Dance, Morley College London; Performer & Choreographer with Flamenco y Danza and Grupo Flamenco de Londres; BA (Hons) in Dance, MA in Performing Arts, Instructor de Baile 2 (Category A) with Spanish Dance Society, RSL Diploma in Dance Teaching, Royal Academy of Dance Registered Teacher & Silver Swans' Licensee, Associate of International Dance Teachers' Association (Ballet) and Society for Education & Training, Certified Teacher of Progressing Ballet Technique, Recognised Teacher with Council for Dance & Musical Theatre

Dr Dee Bhakta Reader in Nutrition and Health in School of Human Sciences, London Metropolitan University; Course Leader MSc Human Nutrition; Registered Dietitian UK, Registered Nutritionist (Public Health); Fellow of Higher Education Academy

Conchita del Campo Maestro de Baile, Director and International examiner for the Spanish Dance Society; Pilates Foundation examiner; Member of education team for the Body Control Pilates Association; RAD teacher and a Craniosacral Therapist. Ex-professional dancer with Ballet Rambert, Scottish Ballet, London City Ballet and Ballet International. Emeritus teacher at London studio centre for 29 years. Member of Society for Education and Training, Lifelong member of Equity. PdB Spanish Dance Society, ARAD dip PDTC.

Krisztina Kerek Student of Flamenco, Spanish Dance and Ballet at Morley College London

Sarah Menser Registered dance movement therapist (American Dance Therapy Association (ADTA), Choreographer and dance Instructor, Ohio, Cleveland. BSc Psychology, MA in Clinical Health counselling with a specialization in dance/movement therapy

Dorrie Orchard Student of Flamenco and Spanish Dance at Morley College London

Prof Chris Palmer Professor of Health Sciences and cellular signalling, London Metropolitan University; Evening School Lecturer - "The body in sickness and Health", Imperial College; Instructor de Baile, Spanish Dance Society. BSc (Hons) Applied Biology, Ph.D. Molecular virology/biology, IdB1 Spanish dance society, PGCert Education, Fellow of Higher education Academy.

Marlena Sakala Student of Flamenco and Spanish Dance at Morley College London

Dr Justin Webb Associate Professor of Public Health, School of Human Sciences and Professions, London Metropolitan University, Fellow of the Royal Society of Public Health, and Fellow of the Higher Education Academy

Declarations

Edition one

First published in 2023 by the Vibrant Dancer

www.the-vibrant-dancer.co.uk

ISBN: 9798847389044

This is a not for profit publication.

This book and the individual contributions contained in it are protected under copyright. Permissions are given to transmit this publication in its original and entire unchanged form as a pdf file.

If you have a medical condition please consult with your medical practitioner before making changes to your nutrition or physical activity.

Copyright © 2023

Acknowledgements

This has been a collaborative project. I would like to thank all the scientists, teachers, dancers, artists, and students who contributed to this endeavour.

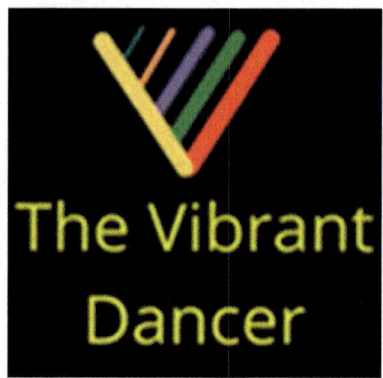

What or who is the Vibrant Dancer?

The Vibrant Dancer is the feeling or sensation you get after a dance class. Dance is not only a medium of artistic expression but also a great form of exercise with physical, mental, and social benefits. By dancing, eating well and looking after ourselves we can extend that sensation to the whole of our life, improve our physical and mental wellbeing, become more creative and prevent injury and illness – Be Vibrant!

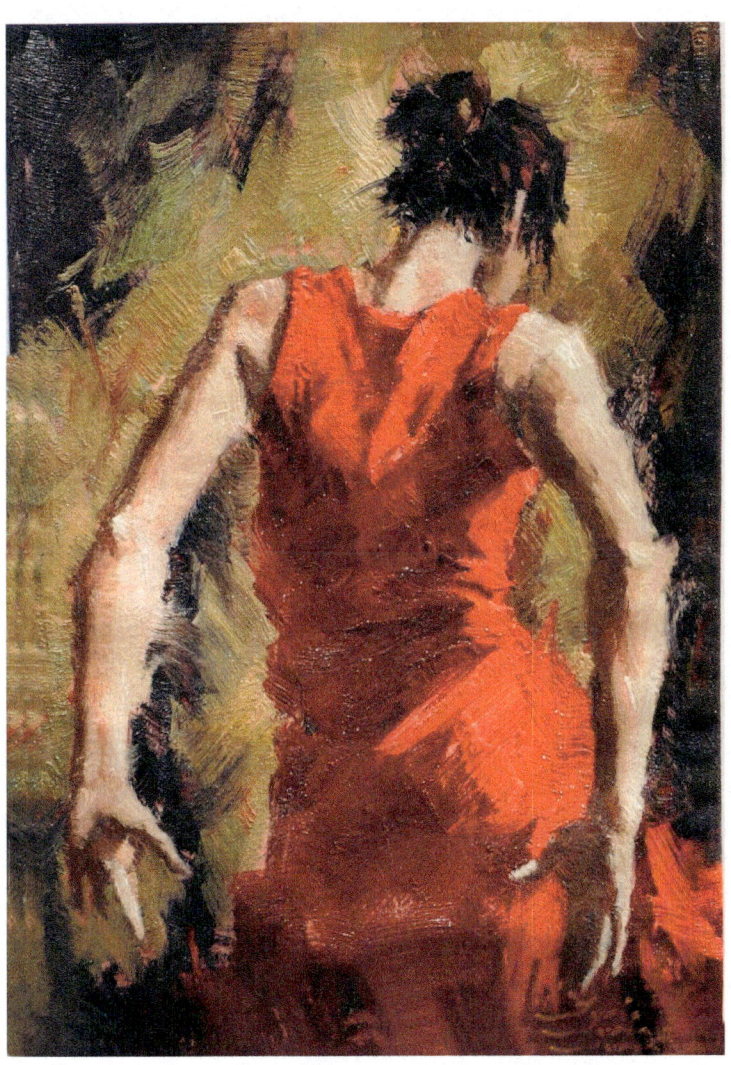

Forward by Conchita del Campo

I trained as a dancer from the age of four and successfully became a professional contemporary and classical ballet dancer performing in the UK and Internationally for twelve years, followed by over 36 years of teaching Pilates, classical ballet, and Spanish dancing. My other great interests have been yoga, nutrition, and health. I am also a director of the Spanish Dance Society providing a methodical programme of study and examination to dance teachers worldwide. I have known Professor Chris Palmer and Dr Ebru Aydar since 2010 when they joined my Spanish Dance classes in London, UK. I have known Fenella J Barker since 1997 when she also came to my classes to learn the Spanish Dance Society syllabus.

In this book "Dancing Through and Beyond Cancer" the authors clearly introduce to a non-scientific audience the technical terminology related to cancer and offer us some very interesting insights. including clarifying the different causes and types of cancer, plus the benefits of dance for preventing cancer and for people undergoing cancer treatment. I think this book is also very useful for all people as it offers a way to "self-check" to see if they have a propensity towards a particular lifestyle which could lead to the occurrence of cancer. Chris explains thoroughly the many factors that affect the development of cancer which leads into later chapters which describe how those factors can be modified by dance and nutrition to favour a better outcome in terms of treatment, progression, and survival. I personally have taught Pilates to several cancer patients in their different stages of remission and agree wholeheartedly that reducing mental stress, can help people recover and return to a cancer-free life. Dr Justin Webb outlines a very safe and useful plan clearly guiding the reader into setting realistic SMART goals to help make the necessary lifestyle changes to sensibly include and maintain more achievable healthy activities in their daily life. Fenella J Barker is a very accomplished dance teacher with over thirty years of experience teaching dance and offers useful advice for individuals who wish to begin taking dance classes. The testimonials from her dance students who used dance to help them through their cancer therapy are very touching, inspiring, and encouraging. Sara Menser includes a very useful and personal account of her cancer recovery and the importance of maintaining physical and mental health during this process. Writing in this book nutritionists and dieticians offer sound nutritional advice and describe in detail the effects of micronutrients on cognitive function, the gut microbiome, mental health, sleep, and the immune system which can all affect the progression of cancer.

Overall, I find it a very informative book explaining the benefits of dance and how dancing reduces hypertension, aids circulation, improves bone density, strengthens ligaments and muscles, improves balance and coordination plus how dancing in groups can help to combat isolation, stress, and loneliness. Thereby this increases happiness, elation, and euphoria, and helps to ultimately energise, relax and calm the nervous system by reducing anxiety. This book is a compilation of wisdom aimed to provide information on using dance and nutrition to augment the prevention and treatment of cancer holistically in parallel to targeted medical treatments. It attempts to bring about a synergy of information to help and inform the reader and bring hope to those who wish to improve their lifestyle for a cancer-free future. I highly recommend this book to anyone interested in recovering from cancer, and also to everyone who wants to learn how to optimise their general health and wellbeing.

CONTENTS

Introduction	9
What is cancer?	13
Factors that affect cancer	18
Epigenetics	29
Cancer and physical activity	31
Making a change when change is hard	39
The benefits of dance	44
Tips for taking up dancing	59
Mental health and cancer	63
What was lost?	65
Dancing with cancer	73
The Tao Te Ching of Vibrant nutrition	79
Microbiome, Nutrition, Cancer and Mental Health	83
Nutrition and cancer	92
Plant based diet and cancer prevention	109
Effect of nutrition on mental health and sleep	116
Nutrition and the immune system	123

INTRODUCTION

Over the last one hundred years amazing developments in science and medicine have extended our expected lifespans. However, modern lifestyles have broken the connection between the natural world and ourselves. The result is that while many people are living longer, we are living those later years with poorer health. Diseases such as cardiovascular disease, dementia, diabetes, and cancer are increasing. Many people are content to rely on quick fixes from modern medicine often treating the symptoms of a disease rather than its root causes. However, the root causes are often our nutrient-poor diets and physical activity-deficient lifestyles. The easy answer is to take a pill provided by pharmaceutical companies with ever-increasing profits to treat those symptoms. The more sustainable way is to remodel our lives placing our body's health as the number one priority. This does not mean that we should reject the advances in modern medicine which have improved our everyday life's but that we should find a balance between modern medicine and traditional ways to maintain our health and treat disease. The result of a modern lifestyle is that the incidence of cancer has increased, although the chances of surviving many kinds of cancer have also increased. Cancer is an umbrella term which often strikes fear in people and families. In many cases, cancer can be prevented or successfully treated. Both cancer prevention and treatment can be augmented through natural means by altering our lifestyles to include more nutritious food and including more physical activity. This does not mean we need to go on an extreme diet or begin running ultra-marathons. Balance is the key to implementing changes in our lifestyle. Additionally, for cancer, the importance of treating the whole person - including body, mind and spirit is essential to surviving cancer and reducing the risk of reoccurrence. The natural processes in the body such as the immune system, the nervous system, and the digestive system which are all important in treating and surviving cancer can be augmented by improving our lifestyles with better nutrition, increased physical activity and by treating the whole body.

The therapeutic benefits of dance

Our ancestors danced to celebrate life's events, attract a partner, and increase fitness for daily activities and for social bonding and communication. The psychotherapeutic use of group movement is ancient with the circle dance being one of the oldest known dances and is a ritual that has been practised across many different cultures. In modern society we have in many ways lost that connection but it still waits to be rediscovered with dance movement giving us access to improved physical and mental well-being. Additionally, dance represents an opportunity to express ourselves through dance movement and enhance our social and spiritual awareness. Sufism is a practice incorporating dance that involves individual turning or 'whirling' to music as a core part of the act of worship. As well as having a deep transforming effect on the turners, the whole ceremony has profound inner symbolism, which represents humankind's inner journey back to the realisation of their essential oneness with nature and the unity of all creation. Dance therapy and therapeutic dance lie at the intersection of science and art. It is a psychotherapeutic use of body movements on music that produces transformations in emotional, mental, and physical states. Examples of its benefits include Parkinson's patients enjoying dance and in so doing, improving their balance and coordination. Additionally, people living with dementia unable to express themselves verbally can enjoy communication through movement and dance. It should be noted that there are some cross-overs and differences between dance therapy and therapeutic dance. Both can help a person achieve emotional, cognitive, physical, and social integration. Additionally, both can produce improvements in physical and mental health, stress reduction, disease prevention, disease management and mood management as well as increased muscular strength, coordination, mobility, and decreased muscular tension. However, dance therapy goes one step further by providing guided, structured and targeted therapy by a professional therapist in a safe space. Dance therapy is a versatile form of therapy founded on the idea that motion and emotion are interconnected. The creative expression of dance therapy and therapeutic dance can bolster communication skills and inspire dynamic relationships. It is commonly used to treat physical, psychological, cognitive, and social issues.

Healing foods

Processed low-variety and nutritionally poor foods which many people consume are convenient and flavoursome but in the long-term are detrimental to our health both physical and mental. In modern life, we have lost the connection between the cultivation and preparation of food and the eventual consumption of food. As a result, food consumption has become dysfunctional, and we no longer reap the many benefits which are associated with these activities. Hippocrates who is thought to be the founder of rational modern medicine stated, "Let food be thy medicine and medicine be thy food". The concept of "functional foods" which supply both nutritional and therapeutic value dates back 4000 years to China. In the early Zhou dynasty (1100-221 BC) the imperial palace court appointed a nutritionist to examine the medicinal properties of food. More recently the Functional Food Science in Europe project, stated that: "A food can be regarded as functional if it is satisfactorily demonstrated to affect beneficially one or more target functions in the body, beyond adequate nutritional effects, thus either improving general physical conditions or/and decreasing the risk of the generation of diseases". Plants contain thousands of chemicals (Phytochemicals) that can be found as bioactive components in foods, additionally, the cooking and processing of foods can provide new subsets of dietary phytochemicals by the formation of new conjugates and intermediates. However, there is a multitude of misinformation concerning nutrition as an outcome of a "frenzy" of alternative diets and a plethora of internet "health" gurus propounding the benefits of different diets. The fact is that no one food can be used to prevent or aid the treatment of cancer. Cancer is a disease involving multiple processes and interactions with the human body as such no one food can be successful in the treatment or prevention of cancer. Additionally, some phytochemicals, in particular in supplement form, may have detrimental effects when consumed at higher concentrations than normally found in natural food. The concept of cancer "superfoods" is a concept that has limitations. Therefore, it is necessary to eat a wide variety of plant-based products.

The rationale for this book

Although there have been many studies on the effects of physical activity or dance and nutrition on the prevention and treatment of cancer many of these studies have been of small scale leading to inconclusive outcomes or contradictory claims as such it is advantageous to investigate a wide range of research articles and sources to obtain wisdom. In terms of cancer treatment, it is important to realise the interconnectivity of the physical body and mental state of a person in overcoming this disease. In effect, the body can affect the mind and *vice-versa* the mind can affect the body. Thus when overcoming cancer it is vital to sustain both using physical activity and nutrition to improve both physical and mental health. Fear, anxiety and depression can affect the progression of cancer and we often look for hope from outside ourselves. However, the fact is that hope to combat fear and anxiety can be found from within ourselves and enhanced by improving our mental state through physical activity and nutrition. Due to advances in cancer treatment more and more people are surviving cancer. One thing that is important for many people is a feeling of being in control of their life. A cancer diagnosis can cause that feeling to spiral into chaos. However, we can regain that control by continuing to do things that we enjoy or to take up new activities to enhance our enjoyment of life.

Dance has some particular benefits which are unique in nature compared to other forms of physical activity. In effect, dance is more than a physical activity but also a social, emotional and spiritual activity. Therefore, this book is a compilation of wisdom from nutritionists, dancers, dance teachers, dance therapists, public health practitioners, cancer survivors, neurobiologists, and biologists, aimed to provide information on using dance and nutrition to augment the prevention and treatment of cancer holistically using both modern medicine and traditional knowledge. In particular, a person who is diagnosed with cancer and undergoing treatment can take control of their health and recovery positively by treating themselves as a whole of their physical, mental and spiritual parts.

Ultimately, this book brings together information and wisdom from multiple sources. The interconnectivity of processes within the human body which are separated by science in order to study them effectively are often ignored. Our mind can have a powerful influence on our bodily processes - in both a positive and negative way. Emotions such as fear, anxiety, hope, happiness, and joy can all influence our body. Therefore, this book attempts to bring about a synergy of information to help and inform the reader and bring hope to those who are on this path.

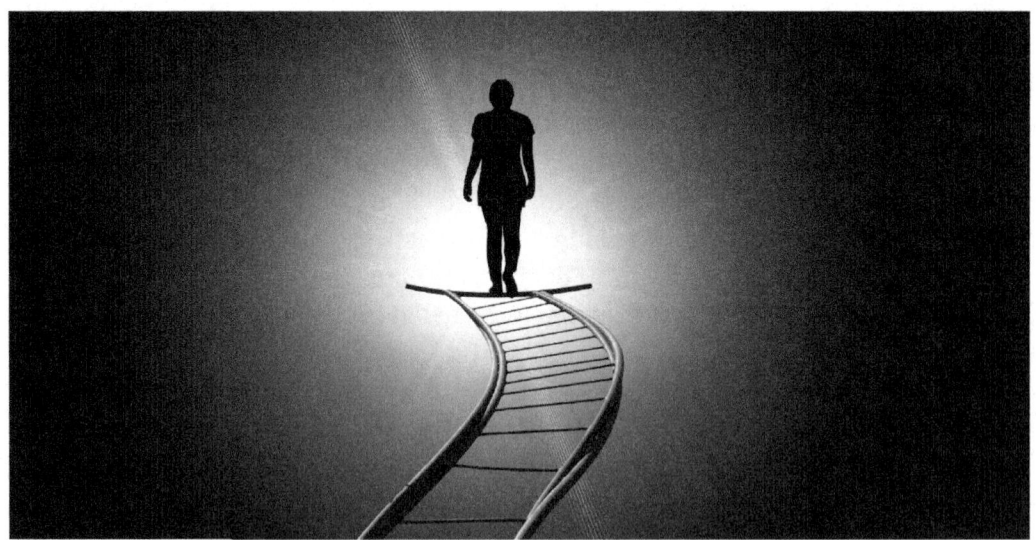

The pathway to hope?

CANCER

What is it?

Prof Christopher Palmer and Dr Ebru Aydar

A diagnosis of cancer may provoke anxiety and fear. This is in part due to a feeling of uncertainty. These feelings are common and not due to weakness but a process of adjustment. These feelings will normally subside which can be helped along the way by understanding what is happening to your body. Cells are the building blocks of your body. Within your body, there are millions of cells. Each cell is more complex than any man-made machine. Cells group together to form a tissue and different tissues form an organ within your body which performs your body's functions (see the picture below). Some cells are free-floating for example the cells within your blood. Each living cell within your body contains genetic information stored in the biological molecule DNA which is contained within a central structure termed the nucleus.

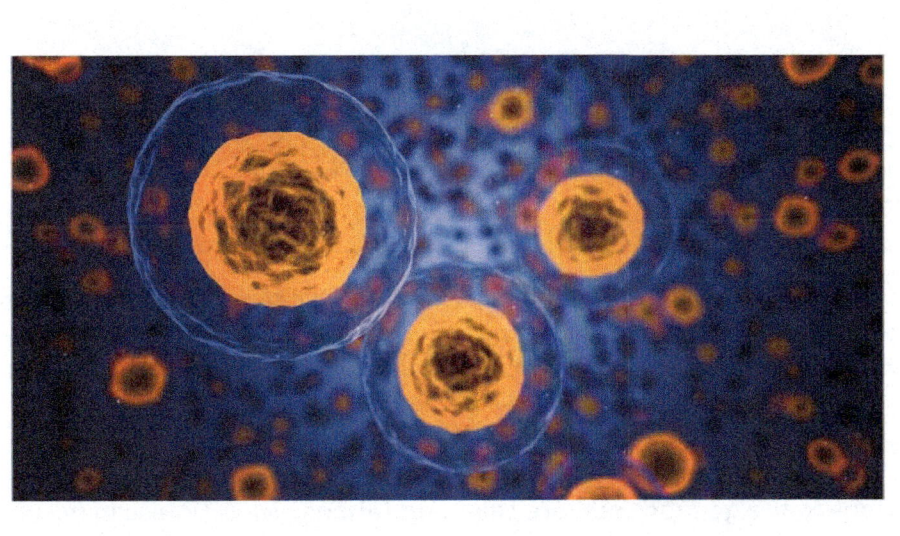

Cells are the building blocks of our tissues and organs. Shown are cells with a central nucleus containing DNA surrounded by a lipid membrane

DNA (deoxyribonucleic acid) is a linear molecule containing information that acts as the blueprint for instructing your cells how to perform their function. Long strings of DNA are found within the nucleus packaged up with protein to form chromosomes. Chemical bases within the DNA molecule provide information in a sequence termed a gene. A gene is a specific section of DNA which encodes the information to synthesize a protein (see the picture below). There are thousands of proteins within a cell which are coded by different genes. Genes encoded by the molecule DNA on your chromosomes control the production of proteins within a cell and therefore determine how the cell functions. Cancer begins with a change in the genetic code of your DNA within a few of the cells in your body. If the genetic material encoded within DNA is changed then cells can have altered proteins and functions which can cause them to behave abnormally.

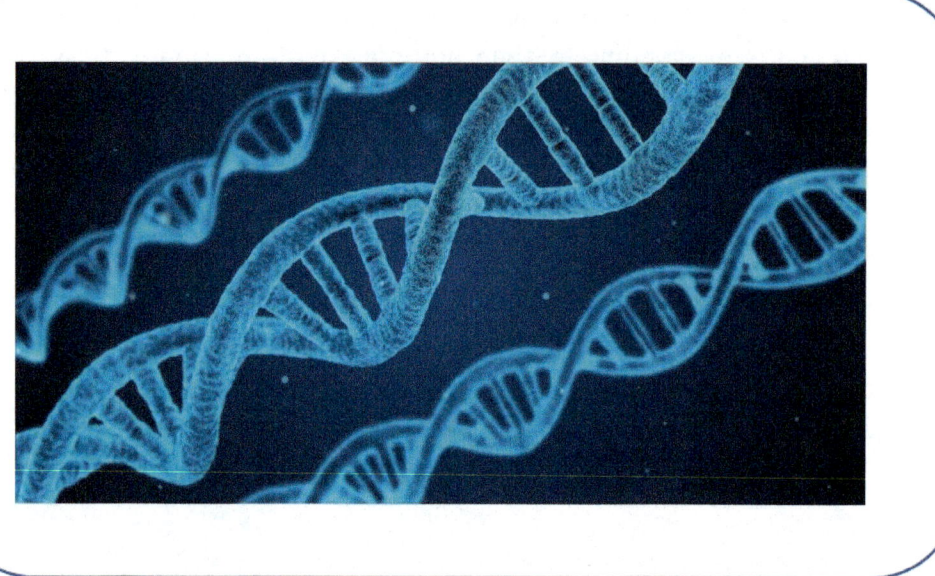

Our genetic material is made of the linear molecular DNA which encodes the information to make a cell. Each piece of DNA contains individual genes which provide specific instructions to make different proteins. Proteins form structural components and control all the chemical reactions in our cells

Alterations to the genetic code are called mutations. Mutations can occur in a variety of ways:

- By chance when a cell divides
- By reactions and processes within the cell
- External factors – chemicals in tobacco, UV light, alcohol
- Inherited mutations

At the beginning of cancer as the result of changes in the genetic code of genes involved in cell growth a few cells begin to divide more frequently. These cells form what we call a tumour or a growth (see the figure below). So a tumour is a small mass of cells which have divided in an uncontrolled manner. This tumour is not cancer but has the potential to transform into cancer if left untreated.

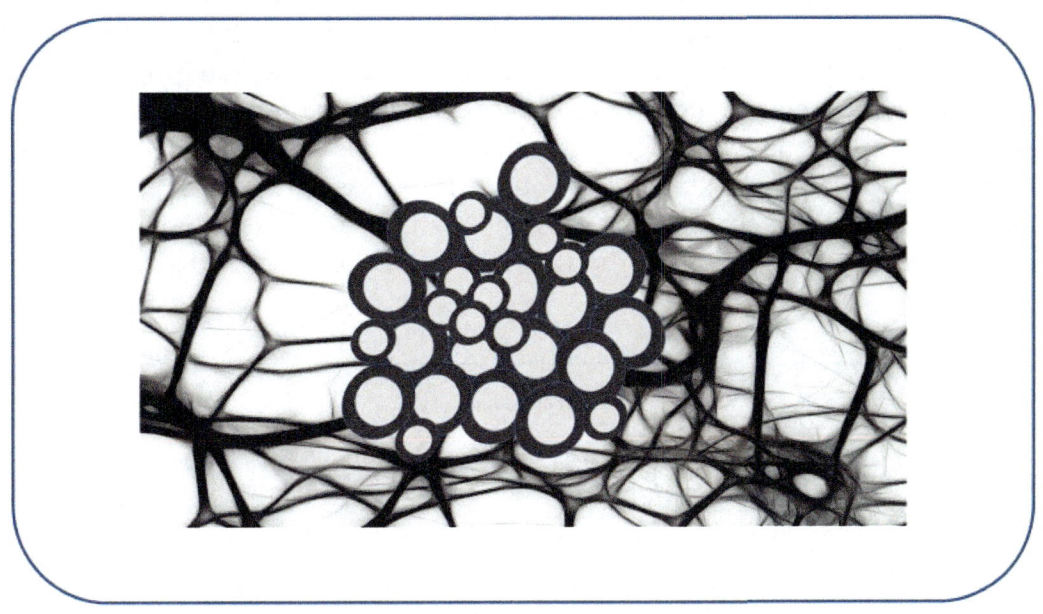

A tumour can develop from an abnormal cell which forms a mass of unorganised cells

Cells within a tissue will under normal conditions only divide if they receive signals such as growth factors to divide. However, cancer cells as a result of a mutation can acquire the ability to divide without requiring external signals. Generally, there is a loss of communication where cancer cells resist signals to die leading to disorganized growth and forming a mass of disorganized cells. Additionally, cancer cells can ignore signals from neighbouring cells when they start to get too crowded. If the cells are left untreated then they can acquire further mutations in their DNA causing them to transform from normal cells into cancer cells. Properties of tumour cells include:

- Uncontrolled cell division
- Loss of cell communication (ignoring growth suppressors)
- Resistance to dying (ignoring death signals)
- Irregular cell size and shape
- Genetic instability (the DNA code varies from cell to cell)
- Altered cell functions
- Ignoring signals from neighbouring cells when overcrowding occurs

There are different types of cancer, some cancers occur in solid tissues and some occur in cells which do not form solid tissues such as leukaemia (blood cell cancer). Additionally, cancers can be subdivided into tissue types. The most common types of cancer are breast cancer, skin cancer, lung cancer, prostate cancer, colon cancer, pancreatic cancer, testicular cancer, blood cancer (leukaemia), brain cancer, and liver cancer. This cancer subtype refers to the location where cancer first occurs. If cancer cells remain untreated then there is a possibility that they will acquire further mutations transforming them into metastatic cells. Metastatic cells derived from solid tissues can detach themselves from the surrounding cells and material holding them in place and migrate to other parts of the body forming secondary growths (see figure below).

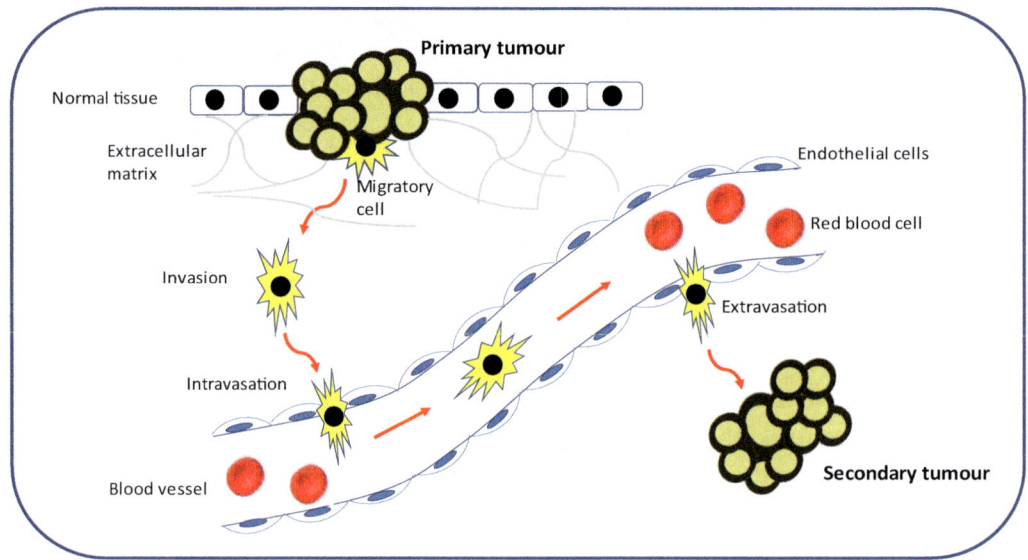

The spread of cancer (metastasis)

Ultimately these secondary growths (metastases) can disrupt body function, cause pain and eventually death. Metastasis is when cancer cells break away from the original tumour and travel via the bloodstream or lymphatic system to other parts of the body. Whether a tumour spreads depends on several factors including the type of cancer and how fast the tumour cells are growing. Some types of cancer can spread to particular parts of the body. For example:

- Breast cancer spreads to bones, liver, lungs, chest wall, and the brain
- Lung cancer spreads to the brain, bones, liver and adrenal glands
- Prostate cancer spread to the bones

- Colon and rectal cancers spread to the liver and lungs

Treatment of cancer

Cancer treatment of solid tumours may involve surgery to remove the primary tumour. Additionally, radiotherapy may be used to kill cancer cells. These treatments are usually used in combination with chemotherapy using chemicals which target rapidly growing cells or prevent cells from receiving or reacting to growth or hormonal signals. Due to advances in treatment, there may be more selective chemotherapeutic agents which target selective processes within cancer cells. Additionally, some cancer treatments augment the immune system to attack cancer cells leading to better outcomes. Generally, the prognosis for the person is far better if the cancer is detected early. Therefore screening is very important to detect primary tumours at an early stage. Finally, it should be noted that personal therapy can play a big role in the progression and reoccurrence of cancer. Personal therapy includes physical activity, nutrition and stress-reducing activities (see below).

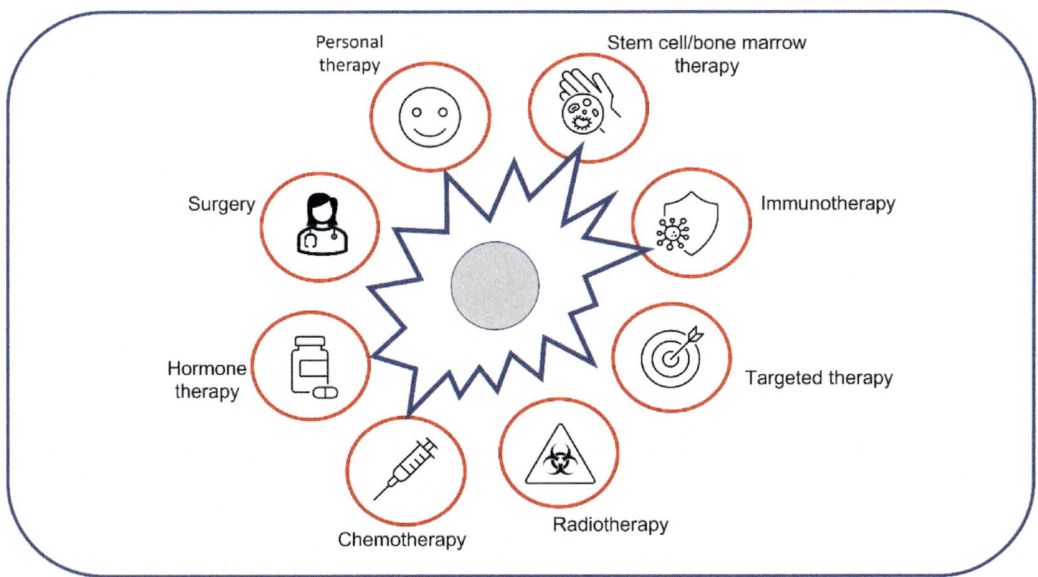

There are many ways to treat cancer and personal therapy including physical activity, nutrition and stress reduction can augment your therapy with other medical treatments

Side effects of cancer treatment

Cancer treatments may adversely affect the body. Some of these lessen in a short time, and others may take months or years to completely recover from. Side effects will vary depending on the type of cancer, treatment and the individual. Common side effects include anorexia, cachexia, depression, fatigue, anxiety, neuropathic pain, cognitive impairment, sleep disorders and confusion.

FACTORS THAT AFFECT CANCER

Prof Christopher Palmer

Approximately 10% of cancers are associated with inherited genes [Pomerantz and Freedman, 2011]. There are also lifestyle risk factors which can increase our risk of getting cancer. In the UK it is estimated that at least a third of cancers can be attributed to a poor lifestyle. This means that approximately 100,000 cancer cases per year in the UK could have been avoided by adopting a healthier lifestyle [www.cancerresearchuk.org]. We are still learning about how these risk factors increase the occurrence of cancer. Some of these risk factors can be avoided or reduced but it can be difficult to change our life habits. However, some factors will have an effect within a few weeks on the metabolism and DNA of our cells so change even in later life can be beneficial. Note these risk factors may have accumulative effects. Additionally, some of these factors can affect the reoccurrence of cancer.

UV light exposure

UV light from the sun or a sunbed is a major factor in the occurrence of skin cancer [Narayanan et al., 2010]. UV light is capable of altering the DNA in your skin cells making it more likely for a mutation to occur which can lead to cancer. Skin cancer if caught early can be effectively treated and the prognosis is far better for early-stage cancers It is advised to take preventative action by staying out of intense sunlight and using suncream on exposed areas. Additionally, self-surveillance of the skin is a helpful practice.

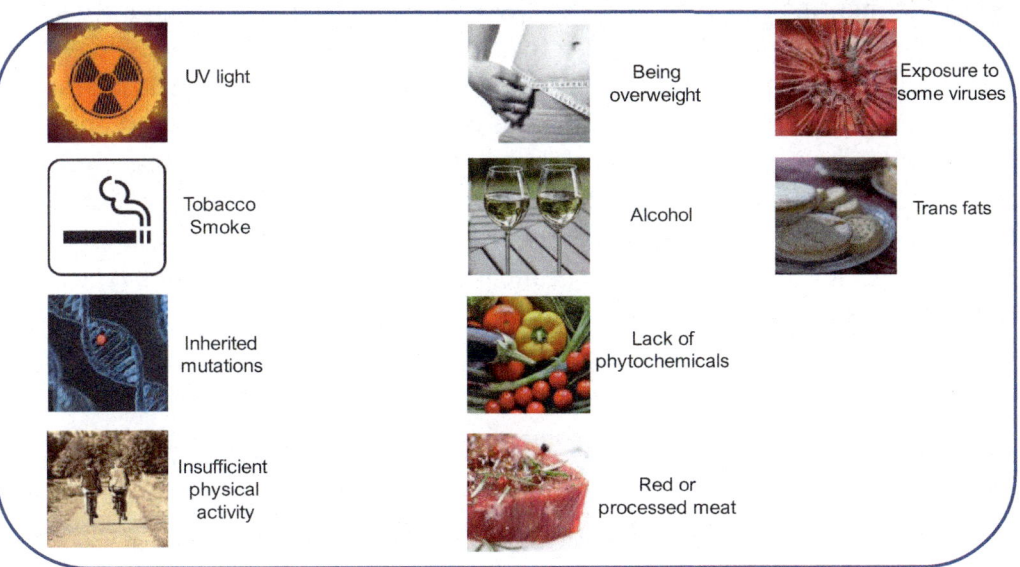

Risk factors that affect the incidence of cancer

Smoking

Cigarette smoking can cause cancer almost anywhere in the body. Cigarette smoking causes cancer of the mouth and throat, oesophagus, stomach, colon, rectum, liver, pancreas, voice box (larynx), trachea, bronchus, kidney and renal pelvis, urinary bladder, and cervix, and causes acute myeloid leukaemia. Additionally secondary smoke is a significant cause of cancer in adults and children [Jacob et al., 2018]. Note also that poor air quality is linked to an increased risk of lung cancer [Huang et al., 2022].

Inherited mutations

Approximately 10% of cancers are linked to the inheritance of a gene that does not function correctly [Pomerantz and Freedman, 2011]. This does not mean that you will definitely get cancer but it makes it more likely to get cancer and also more likely to develop cancer at a younger age. This is called a genetic predisposition for cancer. For cancer to occur further mutations need to happen which generally occur over many years.

Insufficient physical activity

Lack of physical activity is associated with a higher risk of developing many types of cancer. For example a 14% higher risk for colon cancer and an 11% higher risk of post-menopausal breast cancers [www.cancer.gov]. The mechanisms are still being investigated but being inactive contributes to weight gain which can lead to being overweight and obesity which are risk factors for cancer. Growth factors such as insulin-growth factor and oestrogen are regulated by physical activity which can cause tumour cells to grow faster. Additionally, exercise speeds up bowel movements reducing contact with carcinogens in our diet. Maintaining bone density, muscle mass and reducing stress are also important factors, especially when undertaking cancer treatment. Please refer to the later chapter on physical activity and cancer.

Being overweight

Being overweight is the third highest risk factor for cancer [Renehan and Soerjomataram, 2016]. It is unclear how being overweight contributes to an increase in cancer occurrence but one mechanism may be that excess visceral fat cells become starved for oxygen which leads to inflammation which is associated with cancer development. Additionally, additional fat in our body affects how we deal with hormones which are also important in the development of cancer.

Alcohol

Alcohol can damage our DNA and also can cause inflammation which results in a higher risk of cancer. Alcohol is a toxin and is rapidly detoxified by your body's cells and in particular your liver. The issue is that while alcohol is being detoxified your cells metabolism can produce dangerous side products which can damage your DNA and cause inflammation. Therefore alcohol consumption should be limited [Rumgay et al., 2021].

Lack of phytochemicals in the diet

Phytochemicals are a diverse group of plant chemicals which have multiple functions in preventing and repairing DNA damage and inhibiting cancer development and progression [Lui et al, 2004]. Also, many phytochemicals have anti-inflammatory actions [Miller and Snyder, 2012}. See later section in this book for a more in-depth explanation.

Red and processed meat

The mechanistic link between the consumption of red meat and cancer is still unclear. However, what is clear is that vegans and vegetarians have a lower risk of cancer than meat eaters [Watling et al., 2022]. The red pigment in the blood called haemoglobin can be converted to a class of chemicals called N-nitroso's in the intestines by bacteria. These can damage the cells which line our colon resulting in inflammation and increased proliferation and an increased chance of developing mutations which can lead to cancer. Processed meat which contains nitrites can also be converted to N-nitroso compounds in the intestines. Data produced by the World Health Organisation indicates that eating even moderate amounts of processed meat a day increases your risk of developing colon cancer [www.who.int]. Grilling and barbecuing can also create chemicals in meat which can increase the risk of cancer [Chiavarini et al., 2017].

Virus exposure

Some viruses can cause cancer and account for approximately 12 to 20% of worldwide cancers [Morales-Sánchez and Fuentes-Pananá, 2014]. Epstein-Barr virus, human papillomavirus, hepatitis B virus, human herpes virus-8, human T lymphotropic virus type 1 and hepatitis C viruses are the main viruses that contribute to human cancers. Vaccination, exposure prevention and surveillance are the main ways to avoid these viruses and the risk of cancer.

Trans fat

Trans fats can be found in many industrially produced foods and fast food. Regular higher dietary intakes of trans fats, in particular, elaidic acid are associated with elevated breast cancer risk [Matta et al., 2021], although this is emerging evidence. It is not clear as yet whether trans fats are directly carcinogenic or whether their effects are indirectly affecting cellular metabolism in adverse ways.

Additional factors which affect the occurrence and progression of cancer

In addition to these above factors, there are also other factors which can affect the occurrence and progression of cancer. Many of these factors such as hormone influence, growth factors, immunity, inflammation, physical exercise, nutrition and stress are interlinked and may have summative effects.

Hormones and cancer

Hormones are cellular messengers that tell your cells what to do. They are produced and secreted by specialized glands and travel throughout the body within the blood. Some hormones bind to receptors present on the surface of cells or within the cell and influence their metabolism and growth. Increased hormonal stimulation causes cells to proliferate more often and increases the chance of mutations occurring. Therefore excessive hormones such as oestrogen are regarded as carcinogens (cancer-causing). Hormones are implicated in the formation of many cancers including the following:

- Breast
- Prostate
- Uterine
- Ovarian
- Testicular
- Thyroid
- Bone cancers

In particular, for the hormone oestrogen increased exposure in females increases the risk of breast cancer although the extent of this risk is still being assessed. Early onset of menstruation, late first pregnancy, being overweight, late menopause and the use of oral contraceptives can increase the exposure of breast tissue to oestrogen [Santen et al., 2022; Wiggs et al, 2021]. Similarly, increased exposure to the male sex hormone testosterone has been implicated in the development of prostate cancer [Watts et al., 2022]. It should be noted that animal products contain very similar hormones and that individuals who consume animal products have higher circulating levels of these hormones [Malekineiad and Rezabakhsh, 2015] which can in theory result in higher risks of cancer. Oestrogen acts by binding to oestrogen receptors within cells which when activated can turn on genes involved in cell growth (see the figure overleaf).

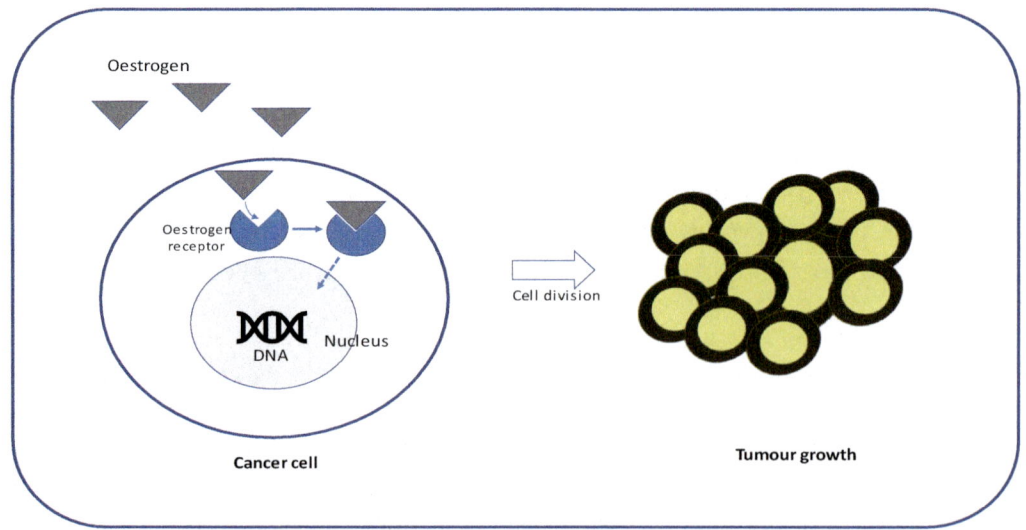

Cell division of cancer cells can be enhanced by oestrogen

Stress and cancer

Studies suggest that there may be a relationship between stress and the development of cancers [www.cancer.gov]. However, research in this area is not clear-cut. What is clear is that there is a consensus among scientists that chronic stress can create a physiological environment conducive to the increased proliferation, migration, invasion, drug resistance, and recurrence of existing cancer cells [Wendel et al., 2021]. The major stress signalling molecules include the hormones cortisol and catecholamines which are released into our bloodstream and travel around our body informing our cells how to act. A summary of the main mechanisms influenced by these signalling molecules include:

- effect on cancer spread via the lymphatic system
- cell growth
- DNA repair
- resistance to apoptosis (cell death)
- immunity
- effect on cell migration via the extracellular matrix
- cancer recurrence
- angiogenesis inhibition (formation of blood vessels in a tumour)
- inhibit chemotherapy-induced cancer cell apoptosis and promote cancer cell survival

Cortisol is a hormone that acts to regulate your body's response to stress and can also suppress inflammation and control metabolism in muscle, fat, liver and bone cells. In particular, cortisol can regulate blood pressure, blood sugar levels and your sleep cycle. Nearly all the cells in your body have receptors for cortisol. There are optimum levels of cortisol needed to function but having chronically high cortisol can have adverse effects on your health as well as influencing the progression and reoccurrence of cancer [Wendel et al., 2021].

Catecholamines are released into the body in response to physical or emotional stress. The main types of catecholamines are dopamine, norepinephrine, and epinephrine. Epinephrine is also known as adrenaline. Dopamine is a neurotransmitter that sends signals throughout the nervous system. It helps regulate movement, emotions, memory and the brain's reward system. Norepinephrine and epinephrine are hormones synthesized by the adrenal glands, located above your kidneys. When they circulate through the body at higher levels, this can have effects including increased heart rate, blood pressure, breathing rate, muscle strength and mental alertness – known as the "flight or fight syndrome" which is useful in a dangerous situation. However, having chronic high levels of catecholamines is detrimental to health for example if you are anxious about your health. Lowering stress levels can be achieved by getting quality sleep, exercising regularly, limiting stressful thinking patterns, practising breathing exercises, taking part in hobbies and enjoyable activities and maintaining healthy relationships.

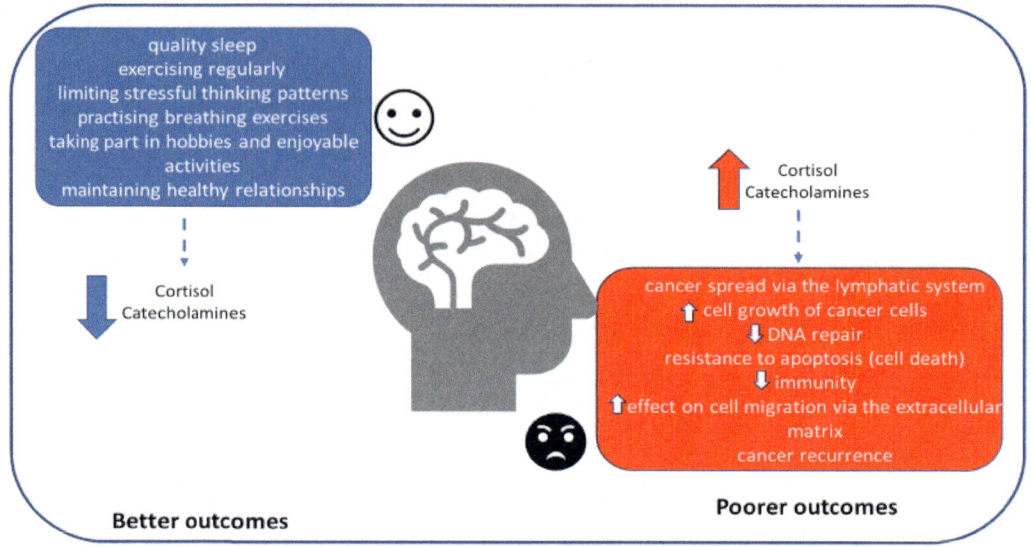

Stress can result in poorer outcomes for cancer

The role of growth factors in cancer

Growth factors are messengers released by cells which travel within our blood. Growth factors can bind to receptors on or within cells. When a growth factor binds to a receptor on or within a cell the receptor is activated and can tell our DNA to instruct the cell to divide. There are different types of growth factors and receptors. One of the most important in terms of increasing the risk of cancer is insulin-like growth factor (IGF). Insulin-like growth factors (IGF) have an important role in the growth and function of many cells in the body. One of them IGF-1 is essential for human development and is made primarily by the liver, but also by many other tissues. At birth, IGF-1 starts at a low level but rises as growth/development begins, rising to a peak in puberty. Levels of IGF-1 vary depending on age, gender, genetics, nutrition, physical activity, and stress. IGF-1 has direct and indirect effects on cells. The most important indirect effect of IGF-1 is on the regulation of other growth hormones which controls cell growth and metabolism. Direct effects occur when IGF-1 binds to its receptor on the surface of cells and activates pathways involved in metabolism, cell death, cell adhesion and angiogenesis (the formation of new blood vessels). We are still learning about the role of IGF-1 in the health of humans and in cancer. IGF-1 can have both positive and negative effects depending on levels in the body. Positive effects include the promotion of growth in children and tissue repair and negative effects include the potential for reducing glucose tolerance and possible links with diabetes, heart disease and some cancers. Some studies have found an especially strong association between circulating IGF-1 concentrations and the risk of breast cancer in premenopausal but not postmenopausal women [Shi et al., 2004]. Note that IGF-1 levels are reported to be elevated in people who are overweight. It's still not entirely clear how IGF-1 may contribute to cancer. Some believe that IGF-1 might cause increased cell transformation, cell migration, metastasis and growth of tumours [Kaaks, 2004]. It seems that IGF-1 doesn't cause cancer but may allow it to progress and spread more quickly.

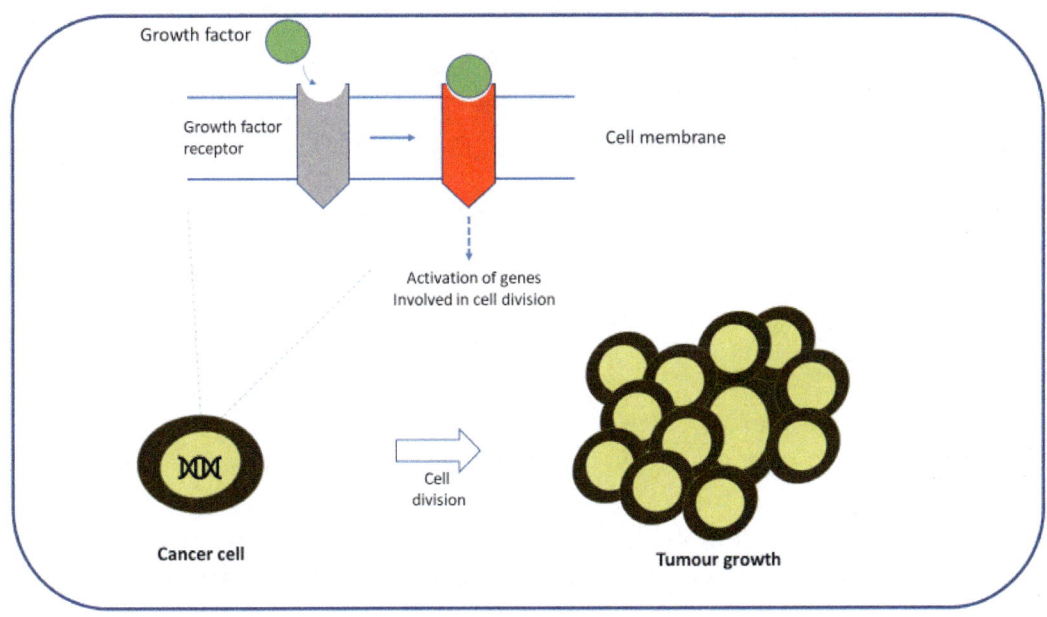

Growth factors within the body can enhance the growth of cancer cells

Inflammation and cancer

Inflammation is present in our bodies all the time caused by both external and internal agents. Generally inflammation occurs when cells are damaged which activates the immune system. Scientists have discovered that inflammation is an important factor in cancer. This could be caused by cigarette smoke, air pollution, food products, UV light, alcohol, or viruses. Long-term inflammation can result in an increased risk of cancer. Some researchers have found that mutations alone are not necessary to initiate cancer but that inflammation is an additional necessary triggering factor [Greten and Grivennikov, 2019]. Being overweight is a significant factor in cancer risk. Being overweight is the third highest cause of cancer in the UK and many other Western countries. The mechanisms are likely multiple and are still being discovered but one factor may be that visceral adipose tissue may be starved of oxygen which causes inflammation. Inflammation can be countered in many ways such as through physical activity and nutritious food containing anti-inflammatory chemicals.

The immune system and cancer

The immune system is a very powerful system to protect us from pathogens (bacteria, fungi, and viruses) and cancer. The way it works is by recognising normal and abnormal cells. Your body has natural physical barriers and defences to prevent pathogens from entering the body but in the case of cancer, these are not applicable as cancer cells develop from within our bodies. The immune system performs its actions through the action of immune cells. This extremely coordinated defence system has two working faces called *innate* and *acquired* immunity.

Innate immunity is the body's first line of defence. The main cells of the innate immune system involved in anti-cancer activity include:

Neutrophils: These short-lived cells are the first line of defence against infection or abnormal cells. They can engulf whole or parts of cancer cells which is particularly effective if the cancer cell is coated with anticancer antibodies produced by B-cells. Additionally, neutrophils release cell-killing granules which can kill cancer cells. They may be affected if your immune system is weakened by certain cancer therapies.

Natural killer cells: These rapid-response cells aggressively attack cancerous and pre-cancerous cells by recognising abnormal cells and releasing cell-killing granules to destroy abnormal cells.

Macrophages: Can engulf whole or parts of abnormal cells and present them to T-cells to activate the acquired immune system.

Dendritic cells: These are the body's surveillance cells, they scout your tissues finding abnormal cells and reporting to T-cells to deliver a more targeted response. Dendritic cells and macrophages are important as they serve as a link between the innate immune system and the acquired immune system by a process called antigen presentation. In this process, abnormal cells are broken into pieces and displayed on the cell surface of dendritic cells and macrophages which present these pieces to T-cells which become activated to provide a targeted immune response.

Acquired immunity - also called adaptive immunity is more sophisticated and takes longer to develop a plan of attack. The cells of the adaptive immune system are:

B-cells: They develop and mature in the bone marrow and make Y-shaped proteins called antibodies that can bind to the surface of cancer cells making them more visible to the other cells of the immune system. Generally B-cells need T- helper cells to activate them.

T-cells: They also form in bone marrow, but mature in the thymus. There are two main types of T-cells: helper T-cells that stimulate B-cells to make antibodies, and killer T-cells that attack cancer cells directly. These different immune cells release signalling molecules called cytokines which allow the cells to talk to each other and coordinate the immune response.

Note that both cancer and cancer treatments may result in the release of pro-inflammatory cytokines which can contribute to adverse side effects.

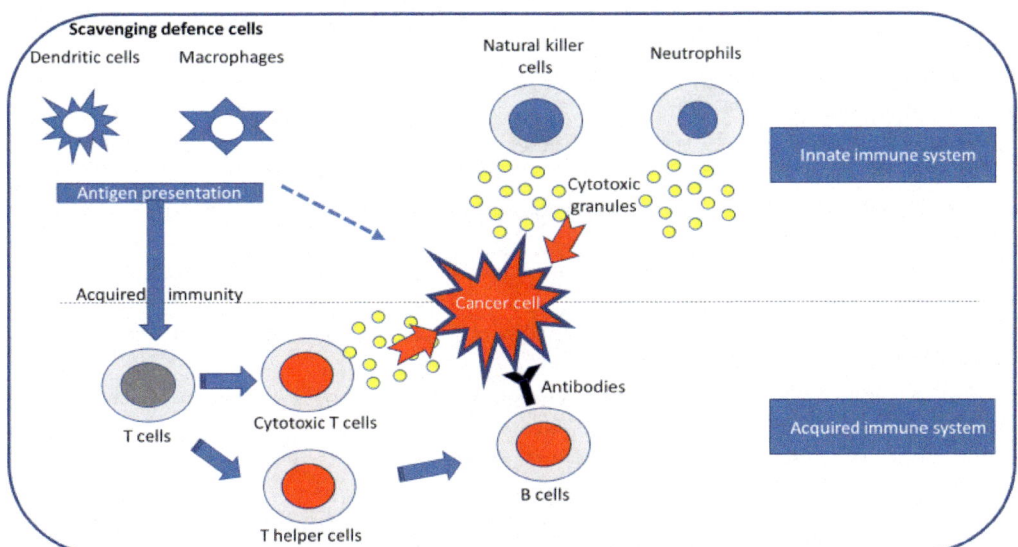

Diagrammatic representation of the main cells and systems of the immune system which are involved in anti-tumourigenic activity.

The immune system can be divided into innate and acquired processes. The innate system is the first line of defence and includes neutrophils, natural killer cells, dendritic cells and macrophages. Dendritic cells and macrophages are scavenger cells which trawl your tissues for abnormal cells. They can engulf abnormal cells or pieces of abnormal cells and present pieces to T- cells in a process called antigen presentation. Neutrophils are also able to engulf abnormal cells and can release cytotoxic granules to kill abnormal cells. Natural killer cells can recognise abnormal cells and aggressively kill them by releasing cytotoxic granules. The acquired or adaptive immune system requires activation via the presentation of antigens from abnormal cells by dendritic cells or macrophages. Once T-cells are activated they can stimulate B-cells to produce anti-cancer antibodies which stick to the surface of cancer cells making it easier for other cells to destroy them. Additionally, T- cells can become cytotoxic T-cells which can hone in on cancer cells and destroy them by releasing cytotoxic granules.

References

Chiavarini M, Bertarelli G, Minelli L, Fabiani R. Dietary Intake of Meat Cooking-Related Mutagens (HCAs) and Risk of Colorectal Adenoma and Cancer: A Systematic Review and Meta-Analysis. Nutrients. 2017 May 18;9(5):514. doi: 10.3390/nu9050514.

Greten FR, Grivennikov SI. Inflammation and Cancer: Triggers, Mechanisms, and Consequences. Immunity. 2019 Jul 16;51(1):27-41. doi: 10.1016/j.immuni.2019.06.025.

Huang Y, Zhu M, Ji M, Fan J, Xie J, Wei X, Jiang X, Xu J, Chen L, Yin R, Wang Y, Dai J, Jin G, Xu L, Hu Z, Ma H, Shen H. Air Pollution, Genetic Factors, and the Risk of Lung Cancer: A Prospective Study in the UK Biobank. Am J Respir Crit Care Med. 2021 Oct 1;204(7):817-825. doi: 10.1164/rccm.202011-4063OC.

Jacob L, Freyn M, Kalder M, Dinas K, Kostev K. Impact of tobacco smoking on the risk of developing 25 different cancers in the UK: a retrospective study of 422,010 patients followed for up to 30 years. Oncotarget. 2018 Apr 3;9(25):17420-17429. doi: 10.18632/oncotarget.24724.

Kaaks R. Nutrition, insulin, IGF-1 metabolism and cancer risk: a summary of epidemiological evidence. Novartis Found Symp. 2004;262:247-60; discussion 260-68.

Malekinejad H, Rezabakhsh A. Hormones in Dairy Foods and Their Impact on Public Health - A Narrative Review Article. Iran J Public Health. 2015 Jun;44(6):742-58

Matta M, Huybrechts I, Biessy C, Casagrande C, Yammine S, Fournier A, Olsen KS, Lukic M, Gram IT, Ardanaz E, Sánchez MJ, Dossus L, Fortner RT, Srour B, Jannasch F, Schulze MB, Amiano P, Agudo A, Colorado-Yohar S, Quirós JR, Tumino R, Panico S, Masala G, Pala V, Sacerdote C, Tjønneland A, Olsen A, Dahm CC, Rosendahl AH, Borgquist S, Wennberg M, Heath AK, Aune D, Schmidt J, Weiderpass E, Chajes V, Gunter MJ, Murphy N. Dietary intake of trans fatty acids and breast cancer risk in 9 European countries. BMC Med. 2021 Mar 30;19(1):81. doi: 10.1186/s12916-021-01952-3.

Miller PE, Snyder DC. Phytochemicals and cancer risk: a review of the epidemiological evidence. Nutr Clin Pract. 2012 Oct;27(5):599-612. doi: 10.1177/0884533612456043.

Morales-Sánchez A, Fuentes-Pananá EM. Human viruses and cancer. Viruses. 2014 Oct 23;6(10):4047-79. doi: 10.3390/v6104047.

Narayanan DL, Saladi RN, Fox JL. Ultraviolet radiation and skin cancer. Int J Dermatol. 2010 Sep;49(9):978-86. doi: 10.1111/j.1365-4632.2010.04474.x.

Pomerantz MM, Freedman ML. The genetics of cancer risk. Cancer J. 2011 Nov-Dec;17(6):416-22. doi: 10.1097/PPO.0b013e31823e5387.

Renehan AG, Soerjomataram I. Obesity as an Avoidable Cause of Cancer (Attributable Risks). Recent Results Cancer Res. 2016;208:243-256. doi: 10.1007/978-3-319-42542-9_13.

Rumgay H, Murphy N, Ferrari P, Soerjomataram I. Alcohol and Cancer: Epidemiology and Biological Mechanisms. Nutrients. 2021 Sep 11;13(9):3173. doi: 10.3390/nu13093173.

Shi R, Yu H, McLarty J, Glass J. IGF-I and breast cancer: a meta-analysis. Int J Cancer. 2004 Sep 1;111(3):418-23. doi: 10.1002/ijc.20233.

Watts EL, Perez-Cornago A, Fensom GK, Smith-Byrne K, Noor U, Andrews CD, Gunter MJ, Holmes MV, Martin RM, Tsilidis KK, Albanes D, Barricarte A, Bueno-de-Mesquita B, Chen C, Cohn BA, Dimou NL, Ferrucci L, Flicker L, Freedman ND, Giles GG, Giovannucci EL, Goodman GE, Haiman CA, Hankey GJ, Huang J, Huang WY, Hurwitz LM, Kaaks R, Knekt P, Kubo T, Langseth H, Laughlin G, Le Marchand L, Luostarinen T, MacInnis RJ, Mäenpää HO, Männistö S, Metter EJ, Mikami K, Mucci LA, Olsen AW, Ozasa K, Palli D, Penney KL, Platz EA, Rissanen H, Sawada N, Schenk JM, Stattin P, Tamakoshi A, Thysell E, Tsai CJ, Tsugane

S, Vatten L, Weiderpass E, Weinstein SJ, Wilkens LR, Yeap BB; PRACTICAL Consortium; CRUK; BPC3; CAPS; PEGASUS; Allen NE, Key TJ, Travis RC. Circulating free testosterone and risk of aggressive prostate cancer: Prospective and Mendelian randomisation analyses in international consortia. Int J Cancer. 2022 Oct 1;151(7):1033-1046. doi: 10.1002/ijc.34116.

Watling CZ, Schmidt JA, Dunneram Y, Tong TYN, Kelly RK, Knuppel A, Travis RC, Key TJ, Perez-Cornago A. Risk of cancer in regular and low meat-eaters, fish-eaters, and vegetarians: a prospective analysis of UK Biobank participants. BMC Med. 2022 Feb 24;20(1):73. doi: 10.1186/s12916-022-02256-w.

Wendel J, Verma A, Dhevan V, Chauhan SC, Tripathi MK. Stress and Molecular Drivers for Cancer Progression: A Longstanding Hypothesis. Biomed J Sci Tech Res. 2021 Jul;37(1):29134-29138. doi: 10.26717/bjstr.2021.37.005953.

Wiggs AG, Chandler JK, Aktas A, Sumner SJ, Stewart DA. The Effects of Diet and Exercise on Endogenous Estrogens and Subsequent Breast Cancer Risk in Postmenopausal Women. Front Endocrinol (Lausanne). 2021 Sep 20;12:732255. doi: 10.3389/fendo.2021

https://www.cancerresearchuk.org/health-professional/cancer-statistics-for-the-uk Accessed March 2023.

https://www.cancer.gov/about-cancer/causes-prevention/risk/obesity/physical-activity-fact-sheet Accessed March 2023.

https://www.cancer.gov/about-cancer/coping/feelings/stress-fact-sheet Accessed March 2023.

https://www.who.int/news-room/questions-and-answers/item/cancer-carcinogenicity-of-the-consumption-of-red-meat-and-processed-meat. Accessed March 2023.

EPIGENETICS

How physical activity and what we eat affects our genetic blueprint, our health and functioning at a genetic level

Prof Chris Palmer

Your genetic blueprint is encoded into your DNA as a linear sequence of chemical bases - guanine, adenine, thymine, and cytosine (GATC) and arranged into 23 pairs of chromosomes. This blueprint is inherited from your parents and forms the basis for building a living organism - you! Your DNA contains sequences termed "genes". Genes are the sections of DNA within your chromosomes that code for the instructions to make a protein, which are formed from a linear sequence of amino acids. Proteins are important as they form structural components in the cell and more importantly enzymes. Enzymes are proteins that catalyse or assist the thousands of metabolic reactions within a cell. Therefore, to direct the function of an individual cell, enzymes are critical in governing this process. Genes are controlled by "promoters" which can be found at the beginning of a gene sequence that act as switches to control the expression of individual genes to synthesize the protein which is encoded by that gene. Different cells in your body will synthesize different proteins for them to fulfil the specific function they have been assigned to in your body. Epigenetics is the control of the expression of a gene to make a protein by mechanisms that are not directly related to the protein-encoding DNA sequence. Your DNA bases termed - G, A, T, C can be modified by chemicals that cause your DNA to change in shape either compacting it, thereby preventing the docking of control factors to the promoter, or opening it, allowing control factors to bind and usually upregulating cellular processes [Al Aboud et al., 2020]. These modifications of your DNA which are termed "the epigenome" are dependent on lifestyle and environmental factors. Our environment, life experiences, and habits mould what and who we are by the nature of their impact on our epigenome and health; as an example, identical twins share the same genome and are phenotypically similar, but they are unique individuals with definable differences. These differences are a result of distinct gene expression influenced by epigenetic factors. Nutrition and physical activity are key environmental epigenetic factors that affect us from gestation to death impacting our health by influencing our DNA through chemical modification. Therefore, food can have dual effects with both positive and negative modifications on our epigenome. These modifications can affect our health and functioning [Dai et al., 2020]. Certainly, it is known that a "Western" diet has a negative impact on our epigenome while a Mediterranean diet has a positive effect on our epigenome in terms of our overall health and that these genome modifications can be inherited by our offspring [Caradonna et al., 2020; Divella et al., 2020]. Therefore it is advised that people take charge of their DNA as nutrition or exercise can have profound effects on the epigenome [Ling and Ronn, 2019; Zam and Khadour, 2017]. For example, in one study after three months following a switch to a plant-based diet over 450 cancer genes were down-regulated and 48 cancer-inhibiting genes were up-regulated regarding prostate cancer [Ornish et al., 2008]

References

Al Aboud NM, Tupper C, Jialal I. Genetics, Epigenetic Mechanism. 2022 Aug 8. In: StatPearls [Internet]. Treasure Island (FL): StatPearls Publishing.

Caradonna F, Consiglio O, Luparello C, Gentile C. Science and Healthy Meals in the World: Nutritional Epigenomics and Nutrigenetics of the Mediterranean Diet. Nutrients. 2020 Jun 11;12(6):1748. doi: 10.3390/nu12061748. PMID: 32545252; PMCID: PMC7353392.

Dai Z, Ramesh V, Locasale JW. The evolving metabolic landscape of chromatin biology and epigenetics. Nat Rev Genet. 2020 Dec;21(12):737-753. doi: 10.1038/s41576-020-0270-8.

Divella R, Daniele A, Savino E, Paradiso A. Anticancer Effects of Nutraceuticals in the Mediterranean Diet: An Epigenetic Diet Model. Cancer Genomics Proteomics. 2020 Jul-Aug;17(4):335-350. doi: 10.21873/cgp.20193.

Ling C, Rönn T. Epigenetics in Human Obesity and Type 2 Diabetes. Cell Metab. 2019 May 7;29(5):1028-1044. doi: 10.1016/j.cmet.2019.03.009.

Ornish D, Magbanua MJ, Weidner G, Weinberg V, Kemp C, Green C, Mattie MD, Marlin R, Simko J, Shinohara K, Haqq CM, Carroll PR. Changes in prostate gene expression in men undergoing an intensive nutrition and lifestyle intervention. Proc Natl Acad Sci U S A. 2008 Jun 17;105(24):8369-74. doi: 10.1073/pnas.0803080105.

Zam W, Khadour A. Impact of Phytochemicals and Dietary Patterns on Epigenome and Cancer. Nutr Cancer. 2017 Feb-Mar;69(2):184-200. doi: 10.1080/01635581.2017.1263746.

PHYSICAL ACTIVITY AND CANCER

Dr Justin Webb

Lifestyle behaviours, such as smoking, alcohol use, an unhealthy diet, and physical inactivity are major risk factors in the development of cancer, as they are for many other diseases [Davies et al., 2011]. Leading a physically active lifestyle, as an independent risk factor, reduces people's risk of developing some cancers [World Cancer Research Fund [WCRF] & American Institute for Cancer Research [AICR], 2018]. Being physically active has also been shown to have many benefits for cancer survivors [Stout et al., 2017].

Physical activity is defined as "any bodily movement produced by skeletal muscles that requires energy expenditure" [WHO, 2010]. Physical activity includes activities of daily living, such as housework and domestic chores, gardening or DIY; active recreation such as walking and cycling; and more structured exercise classes and sports [WHO, 2010]. Dancing is a type of physical activity. The guidelines for physical activity for adults aged 16 to 64 years in the UK are as follows [Davies et al., 2011]:

- To perform a minimum of 150 minutes of moderate-intensity activity over the course of one week, in bouts of 10 minutes or more; or to perform a minimum of 75 minutes or more of vigorous activity over the course of one week or a combination of the two
- To perform physical activity to improve muscle strength on at least two occasions each week
- To keep sedentary time to a minimum

For adults aged 65 years and over, the guidelines also incorporate activities to improve balance and coordination on at least two days a week [Davies et al., 2011].

Moderate-intensity physical activities are those which are between three and six Metabolic Equivalents of Task or METs [WHO, 2011]. One MET refers to the amount of energy expended at rest, so an activity with a MET value of five, such as brisk walking, expends five times the energy (or the number of calories) than at rest. Activities of daily living, for example, hoovering, are rated as three METS, golf four METs, and cycling six METS (Davies, 2004). Physical activities over six METs are classified as vigorous intensity and include activities such as swimming (eight METS) and brisk running (13 METS) [DOH, 2004]. Dancing is classified as between 4 and 10 METS depending on the level of intensity and can therefore be either a moderate or vigorous activity.

Physical activity and cancer prevention

Meeting the recommendations for physical activity can help to prevent and manage many chronic conditions including coronary heart disease, stroke, type 2 diabetes, obesity, mental health problems, and musculoskeletal conditions, as well as reducing the risk of some cancers [Davies, 2011]. Cancer does not occur in isolation; it is reported that 70% of cancer survivors are living with at least one other long-term condition, 47% with two other long-term conditions and 29% with three or more [Macmillan Cancer Support, 2015]. The most common long-term conditions in cancer survivors are estimated to be high blood pressure, obesity, mental health problems, and heart disease [Macmillan Cancer Support, 2015], all of which can be helped by performing physical activity to recommended levels [Davies, 2011].

There is convincing evidence that physical activity protects against colorectal cancer, post-menopausal breast cancer and endometrial cancer [WCRF & AICR, 2018]. There is suggestive evidence to support the role of physical activity in the primary prevention of pre-menopausal breast cancer and cancers of the lung, oesophagus and liver. A dose-response relationship has been reported with those more active having a lower risk of cancer [Li et al., 2016; Moore et al., 2016; Thune & Furberg, 2001; Wannamethee et al., 2001]. As well as protecting against some cancers, physical activity has many benefits for cancer survivors. Studies investigating the benefits of physical activity for cancer survivors have been accumulating since the mid-1980s. Historically, cancer survivors have been told to rest and avoid physical activity, however, the growing body of research challenges this advice [Schmitz et al., 2010]. Physical activity can help cancer survivors tolerate difficult treatments such as surgery and chemotherapy, improve clinical and functional outcomes, and in some cancers improve survival outcomes [Stout et al, 2017].

Physical activity and preparing for cancer treatment

Most people with cancer experience a decline in their physical function, both during and after cancer treatment; this may compound the psychological and emotional issues faced. It has been suggested that those who are physically fit are less likely to experience surgical complications, have higher rates of cardiorespiratory fitness, a quicker return to continence (where this is a consequence of treatment), improved quality of life, and shorter hospital stays [Singh et al., 2013]. Therefore, physical activity is recommended before treatment, particularly in people who are due to undergo surgery, but also more broadly for the wider health benefits, where it is safe, starting slowly and building gradually.

Physical activity during and after cancer treatment

Cancer survivors manage their health daily creating expertise by experience. Physically active cancer survivors report a sense of taking back control of their health and lives [Maley et al., 2013; TNS-BRMB, Webb, 2016]. Being as active as possible during treatment has many benefits. Being active can help to maintain physical function, helping to maintain aerobic fitness and upper and lower body strength. Some may put on body weight and body fat during treatment and being active can help with this too [Speck et al., 2010]. Perceptions of one's own body have been shown to be more positive in those taking part in regular exercise, improving self-esteem; in addition, feelings of sexuality are higher in those who are active compared to those who are not [Mishra et al., 2012].

Being active during and after treatment has been shown to improve emotional well-being and social functioning, whilst also reducing anxiety, depression, and pain [Fong et al., 2012; Mishra et al., 2012]. Confusion, sometimes called 'brain fog' may be experienced by people going through cancer treatment; being active may help with this as cognitive function is suggested to be higher in those who are active compared to those who are not [Cormie et al., 2017]. The current evidence also highlights the role of physical activity in improving bladder and bowel function in those cancer survivors for whom this is an issue [Cormie et al., 2017].

The evidence investigating physical activity in cancer survivors following completion of active treatment is under-represented for the less common cancers, with an over-representation of breast cancer survivors. The balance of the evidence suggests that many of the benefits seen from being active during treatment are experienced by those who have completed their treatment. Physical activity after the completion of treatment improves physical fitness, helps maintain healthy body composition, increases positive views of body image, improves physical and sexual functioning, and helps maintain bone and heart health. Further, physical activity can improve mental well-being, combat depression and anxiety, and increase self-esteem and social functioning [Speck et al., 2010].

The most reported consequence of cancer and its treatments is fatigue. It might seem counterintuitive to be active if fatigued, but the evidence suggests that this too improves with physical activity both during and after cancer treatment, although maybe not for those with a haematological malignancy such as leukaemia, or lymphoma [Bergenthal et al., 2014; Cramp & Daniel, 2008; Fong et al., 2012]. Having a good quality of life is reported by cancer survivors to be as important as cancer outcomes [Lee et al., 2014]; more active cancer survivors report higher scores on health-related quality-of-life measures than those who are less active.

Physical activity and cancer mortality and recurrence

The first epidemiological study investigating the link between physical activity and cancer outcomes was published in 2005 by Holmes et al., [2005]. Holmes and colleagues assessed the cancer outcomes for 2,987 women diagnosed with breast cancer over eight years. The results showed a 35% reduction in death from all causes and a 40% reduction in death from breast cancer as well as a 26% reduction in breast cancer recurrence, for those most active compared to the least physically active. More recent evidence supports the protective effect of physical activity [Cormie et al., 2017; Li et al., 2016] in both preventing cancer in the first place, but also preventing death from cancer and cancer reoccurrence.

Those who are inactive have the most to gain. A rapid decline in the chances of death from cancer is seen in those going from being completely inactive to doing some activity, with a 2% reduction in risk for every one MET-hour-per-week increase in physical activity, that is going from being sedentary to a regular brisk walk.

Physical activity and palliation

The benefits of being physically active are not just limited to those cancer survivors with a good prognosis. A review of a small but growing body of evidence observes that physical activity improves cardiovascular fitness, physical function, fatigue, and quality of life in cancer survivors with advanced disease [Dittus et al., 2017].

Is it safe to be active?

In 2010, the American College of Sports Medicine brought together multidisciplinary experts to review the evidence on physical activity for cancer survivors. This group of experts concluded that physical activity is safe for cancer survivors both during and after cancer treatments, including intensive life-threatening treatments such as bone marrow transplants [Schmitz et al., 2010]. However, some cancer survivors may need to obtain permission from their cancer care team before becoming physically active in case special precautions are necessary [Schmitz et al., 2010], being:

- Those less than eight weeks post-surgery
- Those experiencing extreme fatigue, anaemia or severe balance and coordination problems
- Those with cancer in their bones or bone thinning
- Those with a heart or lung condition
- Those with pain in their chest at rest, during daily activities or when becoming active
- Those with persistent pain in their muscles, bones or joint pain
- Those with swelling or inflammation in the abdomen, groin, or lower extremity

Also, it is advised that cancer survivors with arm lymphedema wear well-fitting compression garments, colon cancer survivors should avoid exercises that increase abdominal pressure, and those with a stoma should avoid participation in contact sports and weight training [Schmitz et al., 2010].

Physical activity is likely to decrease following a diagnosis of cancer and may not increase again to pre-diagnosis levels. People living with and beyond cancer should try to be as active as their abilities allow and aim to reduce sedentary time.

In summary

Increasing physical activity before the start of treatment may help cancer survivors tolerate difficult treatments such as surgery and chemotherapy, and slow the decline in physical function [Singh et al., 2013]. Physical activity can improve functional recovery post-treatment, reduce complications following surgery, and reduce the length of hospital stay [Singh et al., 2013].

Physical activity can improve many common side-effects of cancer treatment, both during and following treatment, including fatigue, psychological distress, and an adverse impact on body composition, as well as improving physical function and quality of life [Fong et al., 2012; Schmitz et al., 2010; Speck et al., 2010]. Physically active cancer survivors report a sense of regaining control of, and some normalcy in, their lives following a cancer diagnosis [Larsson et al., 2008; Maley et al., 2013; TNS-BRMB, Webb, J, 2016]. Increased physical activity is associated with improved survival and reduced disease recurrence with a dose-response relationship reported [Cormie et al., 2017; Li et al., 2016].

Being physically active is safe, however, increasing activity levels should be discussed with healthcare professionals in case special precautions are needed [Irwin, 2012; Schmitz et al., 2010; Stout et al., 2017]. Cancer survivors should avoid inactivity and return to normal daily activities, as soon as possible after surgery and during cancer treatments adhering to the standard age-appropriate physical activity guidelines [Schmitz et al., 2010].

References

Bergenthal, N., Will, A., Streckmann, F., Wolkewitz, K.-D., Monsef, I., Engert, A., et al. (2014). Aerobic physical exercise for adult patients with haematological malignancies. *Cochrane Database of Systematic Reviews*, 45(2), 355–67. http://doi.org/10.1002/14651858.CD009075.pub2

Cormie, P., Zopf, E. M., Zhang, X., & Schmitz, K. H. (2017). The Impact of Exercise on Cancer Mortality, Recurrence, and Treatment-Related Adverse Effects. *Epidemiologic Reviews*, 39(1), 71–92. http://doi.org/10.1093/epirev/mxx007

Cramp, F., & Daniel, J. (2008). Exercise for the management of cancer-related fatigue in adults. *The Cochrane Database of Systematic Reviews*, (2), CD006145. http://doi.org/10.1002/14651858.CD006145.pub2

Davies, S., Burns, H., Jewell, T., & McBride, M. (2011). Start Active, Stay Active. A report on physical activity for health from the four home countries' Chief Medical Officers. 2011.

Dittus, K. L., Gramling, R. E., & Ades, P. A. (2017). Exercise interventions for individuals with advanced cancer: A systematic review. *Preventive Medicine*, 104(C), 124–132. http://doi.org/10.1016/j.ypmed.2017.07.015

Department of Health. (2004). *At least five a week: evidence on the impact of physical activity and its relationship to health. A report from the Chief Medical Officer*. London: Crown copyright.

Fong, D. Y. T., Ho, J. W. C., Hui, B. P. H., Lee, A. M., Macfarlane, D. J., Leung, S. S. K., et al. (2012). Physical activity for cancer survivors: meta-analysis of randomised controlled trials. *Bmj*, 344(jan30 5), e70–e70. http://doi.org/10.1136/bmj.e70

Holmes, M. D., Chen, W. Y., Feskanich, D., Kroenke, C. H., & Colditz, G. A. (2005). Physical activity and survival after breast cancer diagnosis. *Jama*, 293(20), 2479–2486. http://doi.org/10.1001/jama.293.20.2479

Lee, J. A., Kim, S. Y., Kim, Y., Oh, J., Kim, H. J., Jo, D. Y., et al. (2014). Comparison of Health-related Quality of Life Between Cancer Survivors Treated in Designated Cancer Centers and the General Public in Korea. *Japanese Journal of Clinical Oncology*, 44(2), 141–152. http://doi.org/10.1093/jjco/hyt184

Li, T., Wei, S., Shi, Y., Pang, S., Qin, Q., Yin, J., et al. (2016). The dose–response effect of physical activity on cancer mortality: findings from 71 prospective cohort studies. *British Journal of Sports Medicine*, 50(6), 339–345. http://doi.org/10.1136/bjsports-2015-094927

Macmillan Cancer Support. (2015a). *The burden of cancer and other long-term health conditions*. London: Macmillan Cancer Support.

Maley, M., Warren, B. S., & Devine, C. M. (2013). A second chance: meanings of body weight, diet, and physical activity to women who have experienced cancer. *Journal of Nutrition Education and Behavior*, 45(3), 232–239. http://doi.org/10.1016/j.jneb.2012.10.009

Mishra, S. I., Scherer, R. W., Geigle, P. M., Berlanstein, D. R., Topaloglu, O., Gotay, C. C., & Snyder, C. (2012). Exercise interventions on health-related quality of life for cancer survivors. *Cochrane Database of Systematic Reviews*, *8*(29), 6312–380. http://doi.org/10.1002/14651858.CD007566.pub2

Moore, S. C., Lee, I. M., Weiderpass, E., Campbell, P. T., Sampson, J. N., Kitahara, C. M., et al. (2016). Association of Leisure-Time Physical Activity With Risk of 26 Types of Cancer in 1.44 Million Adults. *JAMA Internal Medicine*, *176*(6), 816–10. http://doi.org/10.1001/jamainternmed.2016.1548

Schmitz, K. H., Courneya, K. S., Matthews, C., Demark-Wahnefried, W., GALVÃO, D. A., Pinto, B. M., et al. (2010). American College of Sports Medicine Roundtable on Exercise Guidelines for Cancer Survivors. *Medicine & Science in Sports & Exercise*, *42*(7), 1409–1426. http://doi.org/10.1249/MSS.0b013e3181e0c112

Singh, F., Newton, R. U., Galváo, D. A., Spry, N., & Baker, M. K. (2013). A systematic review of pre-surgical exercise intervention studies with cancer patients. *Surgical Oncology*, *22*(2), 92–104. http://doi.org/10.1016/j.suronc.2013.01.004

Speck, R. M., Courneya, K. S., Mâsse, L. C., Duval, S., & Schmitz, K. H. (2010). An update of controlled physical activity trials in cancer survivors: a systematic review and meta-analysis. *Journal of Cancer Survivorship*, *4*(2), 87–100. http://doi.org/10.1007/s11764-009-0110-5

Stout, N. L., Baima, J., Swisher, A. K., Winters-Stone, K. M., Welsh, J. (2017). A systematic review of exercise systematic reviews in the cancer literature (2005-2017). *Physical Medicine & Rehabilitation*, *9*(Supplement 2), S347–S384. http://doi.org/10.1016/j.pmrj.2017.07.074

Thune, I., & Furberg, A. S. (2001). Physical activity and cancer risk: dose-response and cancer, all sites and site-specific. *Medicine & Science in Sports & Exercise*, *33*(6 Suppl), S530–50– discussion S609–10.

TNS-BRMB, Webb, J [ed.] (2016) *What motivates people with cancer to get active?* London: Macmillan Cancer Support. Available at https://www.webcitation.org/6taiRkTHG

Wannamethee, S. G., Shaper, A. G., & Walker, M. (2001). Physical activity and risk of cancer in middle-aged men., *85*(9), 1311–1316.

World Health Organization. (2010). *Global recommendations on physical activity for health*. Geneva: World Health Organisation

World Cancer Research Fund and American Institute of Cancer Research. (2018). *Food, nutrition, physical activity and the prevention of cancer: A global perspective*. Washington: World Cancer Research Fund and American Institute of Cancer Research

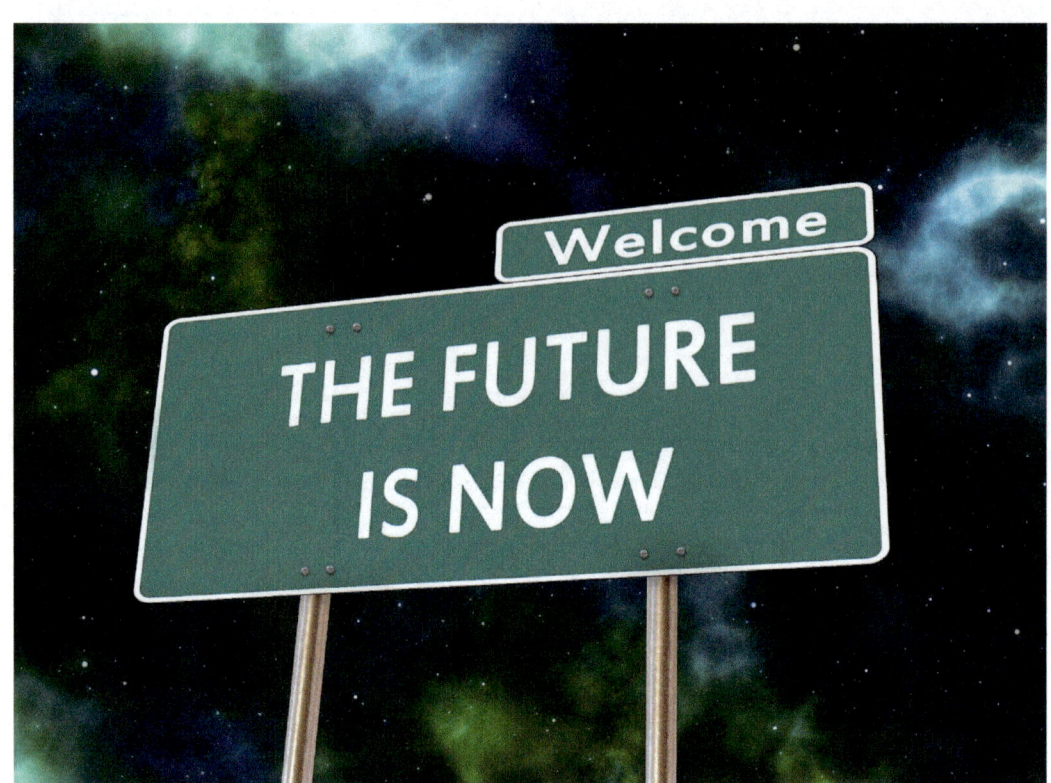

You can't change the past!

MAKING A CHANGE WHEN CHANGE IS HARD

Dr Justin Webb

As identified in the previous chapter, being physically active has multiple benefits for cancer survivors. Physical activity can improve many common side effects of cancer treatments, such as fatigue, psychological distress, and adverse impact on body composition, as well as improving physical function and quality of life [Fong et al., 2012; Schmitz et al., 2010; Speck et al., 2010]. In addition, increased physical activity is associated with improved survival and reduced disease recurrence. Physically active cancer survivors report a sense of regaining control of their lives [Macmillan Cancer Support, 2015; Marley et al., 2013] and some normalcy [Larsson et al., 2008] following a cancer diagnosis. Engaging in physical activity is not only recommended but also safe both during and after cancer treatments [Schmitz et al., 2010]. The American College of Sports Medicine [Schmitz et al., 2010] advises that cancer survivors avoid inactivity and return to typical daily activities as soon as possible after surgery and during and after cancer treatments, working toward the standard age-appropriate physical activity guidelines [Davies et al., 2010] which are to take part in 150 minutes of moderate-intensity activity each week, plus activities to maintain or build strength, balance and coordination. However, many people are not active to a level to benefit their health. Physical inactivity is rising in the UK adult population, particularly in those with a long-term health condition (*New strategy to tackle inactivity*, no date).

What is behaviour?

Behaviour is defined as the way in which a person behaves in response to a particular situation or stimulus. Mental processes, emotions, thoughts, and feelings are not behaviours but they do influence our behaviour. Behaviours can be seen or heard; they are observable actions. We are creatures of habit. Our behaviours might take place without us even realising that we are doing them, for example, automatically taking the lift instead of the stairs at work, jumping in the car to take the short journey to the shops to pick up the essentials, or sitting at a desk all day rarely getting up to stretch our legs. On the other hand, our behavioural decisions may be conscious, driven by impulse, or our past experiences, by social norms, or by our views on the expectations of others. Being physically active is a behaviour. Our levels of physical activity (or lack of it) may be driven by our habits. In many ways we have designed physical activity out of our lives; It has been reported that people in the UK are around 20% less active now than they were in the 1960s (*Health matters: getting every adult active every day*, no date).

Dancing is a great way to keep active. Other ways to become active can include incorporating activity into our daily life, walking more, gardening, as well as more structured exercise and fitness classes. It is important to start slow and build gradually if you have had low levels of activity for some time. Pick an activity that you enjoy and a level that is right for you, building up to the recommended guidelines for physical activity. Changing behaviour is rarely a simple and smooth process. It can take a long time. Try and build on small achievements, acknowledging and learning from the setbacks along the way. Changing behaviour to become physically active is difficult, particularly for people who have had a cancer diagnosis. This chapter provides some strategies to help those ready to make a behavioural change to become more active.

Helping you to get started

It can be useful to write down why you are planning on making a lifestyle change and what you hope to achieve from making this change.

Using the space below or on a sheet of paper, write down what it is that you are thinking of changing.

```
The change that I would like to make is:



```

Now think of your reasons for making this change

1. _____
2. _____
3. _____

How would your life be better if you make the change outlined in the previous section?

If you do not make the change outlined above, what would life be like?

You should now set yourself a goal. Setting realistic goals is a great way to help you change your behaviour. A big goal or aim can be broken down into smaller goals. The best way to set yourself a goal or series of goals is to follow the SMART goal-setting principle.

Goals should be:

Specific: Your goal should be precise and clear. To help with this think about what you are going to do, when and where, how you are going to do it and who are you going to do it with.

Measurable: Making a goal specific will allow you to measure if your goal has been achieved or not.

Achievable: Make sure that the goal that you set yourself is not too easy and not too hard; it should be within your reach.

Relevant: Make sure that the goal is relevant to what it is that you are hoping to achieve as a consequence behaviour.

Timely: Is this goal right for you right now? If it is, then set yourself a time by which you hope to achieve your goal. If it is not the right time, then consider setting a different goal.

What might stop me from achieving my goal?	How can I overcome this barrier?

Have a go at setting your first goal using the SMART principle.

Keeping a diary

Keeping a diary is a great way to track your progress and help you stay motivated. Keeping a diary can also help you re-evaluate your goals over time, was the goal too easy or too hard? Do you need to set yourself a new goal? You may want to keep a weekly diary somewhere visible, maybe stick it on your fridge as a daily reminder.

Reward yourself!

Rewarding yourself when you have achieved a goal can encourage you to keep progressing.

Take some time to think of rewards that would motivate you to achieve your goals.

Managing setbacks

Changing behaviour is hard. Maintaining a behaviour can be even harder; there will be ups and downs along the way. Do not get disheartened by setbacks, they are to be expected and provide an opportunity for learning and goal re-evaluation. If you do suffer a setback in pursuit of your goal, take the time to review your goal and make sure it is still SMART; if your goal needs to be changed, this is the time to do so. Also, take the time to review the list of barriers to achieving your goal and how you might overcome these; ask yourself if you need to make any changes or list any more barriers. Behaviour change is a gradual process. Keep persevering until the change becomes a habit.

Step by step

1. Keep in mind what it is you want to achieve and the benefits of making a change.
2. Set SMART goals and re-evaluate them regularly.
3. Make a firm commitment by sharing your plans with other people.
4. Think about what might get in your way and how you might overcome this.
5. Keep a diary.
6. Reward yourself.
7. Expect setbacks, re-evaluate and try again.

Tips for exercising safely

1. Start slowly with gradual increases.
2. If you are not feeling well, then take a break and do not exercise.
3. If you have bone problems, avoid activities where there is an increased risk of falling and high-impact activities.
4. Wear appropriate clothing for the activity that you are undertaking.
5. Make sure that you are well hydrated.
6. Stop exercising if you experience any sudden symptoms such as feeling sick or dizzy, pain or headache or a racing heart. Get medical advice before starting again.

References

Davies, S., Burns, H., Jewell, T., & McBride, M. (n.d.). Start Active, Stay Active. A report on physical activity for health from the four home countries' Chief Medical Officers. 2011.

Fong, D. Y. T., Ho, J. W. C., Hui, B. P. H., Lee, A. M., Macfarlane, D. J., Leung, S. S. K., et al. (2012). Physical activity for cancer survivors: meta-analysis of randomised controlled trials. *Bmj*, *344*(jan30 5), e70–e70. http://doi.org/10.1136/bmj.e70

Larsson IL, Jönsson C, Olsson AC, Gard G, Johansson K. Women's experience of physical activity following breast cancer treatment. *Scand J Caring Sci*. 2008 Sep;22(3):422–9. doi: 10.1111/j.1471-6712.2007.00546.x.

Li, T., Wei, S., Shi, Y., Pang, S., Qin, Q., Yin, J., et al. (2016). The dose–response effect of physical activity on cancer mortality: findings from 71 prospective cohort studies. *British Journal of Sports Medicine*, *50*(6), 339–345. http://doi.org/10.1136/bjsports-2015-094927

Macmillan Cancer Support. (2015a). *The burden of cancer and other long-term health conditions*. London: Macmillan Cancer Support.

Maley, M., Warren, B. S., & Devine, C. M. (2013). A second chance: meanings of body weight, diet, and physical activity to women who have experienced cancer. *Journal of Nutrition Education and Behavior*, *45*(3), 232–239. http://doi.org/10.1016/j.jneb.2012.10.009

Santen RJ, Stuenkel CA, Yue W. Mechanistic Effects of Estrogens on Breast Cancer. Cancer J. 2022 May-Jun 01;28(3):224-240. doi: 10.1097/PPO.000000000

Schmitz, K. H., Courneya, K. S., Matthews, C., Demark-Wahnefried, W., Galvao, D. A., Pinto, B. M., et al. (2010). American College of Sports Medicine Roundtable on Exercise Guidelines for Cancer Survivors. *Medicine & Science in Sports & Exercise*, *42*(7), 1409–1426. http://doi.org/10.1249/MSS.0b013e3181e0c112

Speck, R. M., Courneya, K. S., Mâsse, L. C., Duval, S., & Schmitz, K. H. (2010). An update of controlled physical activity trials in cancer survivors: a systematic review and meta-analysis. *Journal of Cancer Survivorship*, *4*(2), 87–100. http://doi.org/10.1007/s11764-009-0110-5

Other resources used in the development of this chapter

Michie, S., Rumsey, N., Fussell, A., Hardeman, W., Johnston, M., Newman, S., Yardley, L. (2004). *Improving health: changing behaviour. NHS Health Trainer Handbook*. Department of Health and the British Psychological Society. London.

Macmillan Cancer Support. (2019). *Physical activity and cancer*. Macmillan Cancer Support. London; UK.

Webb J, Fife-Schaw C, Ogden J, Foster J. (2017). The Effect of the Move More Pack on the Physical Activity of Cancer Survivors: Protocol for a Randomized Waiting List Control Trial with Process Evaluation. JMIR Res Protoc. 2017 Nov 9;6(11):e220. doi: 10.2196/resprot.7755.

THE HEALTH BENEFITS OF DANCE

Prof Christopher Palmer and Dr Ebru Aydar

Dancing is a great activity for people of all ages. You do not have to be good or talented at dancing to enjoy the tremendous benefits of dancing which include physical, mental and social benefits, many of which are applicable even when receiving treatment for cancer so long as the mode, duration, intensity, and frequency of the physical activity are appropriate for the stage of disease and nature of treatment [Campbell et al., 2019]. Dancing is uniquely a whole-body physical activity unlike other forms of exercise which target a particular muscle group in an unidirectional manner. Varying tempos of dancing will switch your body in and out of aerobic exercise and different poses and dynamic movements in a three-dimensional space will strengthen your skeletal muscular system in an entirely natural way making it a suitable fitness program for anybody of any age, size, shape or ability. It is not about performance but feeling your joy of movement in your own unique way. Some of the benefits of dance are discussed below:

Improved condition of your heart and lungs

It is well-established that physical activity can improve the cardiovascular system but what about dance? Dancing increases your heart rate as it pumps blood to your muscles. This increase in heart rate strengthens your heart and keeps muscles conditioned. Keeping your heart healthy through dance can help to reduce stress, high blood pressure and the risk of heart disease. In terms of cardiovascular disease in a large cohort of subjects moderate dance intensity was shown to significantly reduce cardiovascular disease. These benefits were similar but greater than compared to walking as an exercise [Merom et al., 2016]. The exact mechanisms were not investigated, however, previously it has been shown that the pulse rate of the dancer can range from 60% to 95% of the maximum heart rate [Blanksby and Reidy, 1988; Cohen et al., 1982]. Fitness guidelines suggest that people who wish to improve their cardiovascular fitness should exercise between either:

- 64 and 94 % of their HRmax, a measure of a person's maximum heart rate
- 40 to 85 % of VO2 max, a measure of the maximum volume of oxygen a person can use

Practically, dancing can be a great alternative to get a cardiovascular workout for those who are not keen on going to a gym. Additionally, dance moves can be performed in a wheelchair for those with less lower-body mobility. It should also be noted that dancing is a social activity and this may have benefits in stress reduction which in the long term can result in cardiovascular benefits.

Subjectively, dancing is more fun as a group activity than joining a gym class so this can motivate you to attend regular sessions and it is possible to get cardiovascular benefits without feeling you are over-exerting yourself compared to other traditional cardiovascular workouts. The best workouts are those which incorporate both aerobic and anaerobic exercise. Dance is a great way to get both types during a class. By engaging the motions of changing direction, jumping, and short sequences across the room, you can get a quality aerobic workout at the same time. Working your muscles through balancing, suspensions can achieve an anaerobic workout at the same time.

Blood pressure (hypertension)

Blood pressure is a measure of the force that the heart uses to pump blood around your body. Blood pressure is important as high blood pressure can lead to long-term health problems such as kidney disease and heart disease. High blood pressure is often related to unhealthy lifestyle habits, such as smoking, drinking too much alcohol, being overweight and not exercising enough. Although hypertension is commonly treated with drugs, for a significant proportion of people these drugs are ineffective. In general, it is better to treat the root causes of a disease rather than its effects. Studies have indicated that dance can significantly reduce hypertension in as little as 12 weeks [Maruf et al., 2016].

Weight management

There are many diseases in which being overweight is a contributory factor including diabetes, cancer, heart disease, metabolic syndrome and susceptibility to infections. Being overweight is an important risk factor for cancer occurrence and therefore as a priority, it is important when thinking about reducing the risk of these diseases to concentrate on sustainably losing weight. In terms of cancer prevention, if you are overweight rather than searching for some miracle diet or consuming often published "superfoods" it is better to focus on sustainable weight loss. Additionally, being overweight is a contributory factor in cancer reoccurrence [Demark-Wahnefried et al., 2012]. Weight loss can be achieved by a combination of dietary changes and physical exercise. Dance is a great form of physical exercise; obviously more vigorous dance forms will burn more calories. Shown below are examples of calories utilised for a 60 mins dance class for someone who weighs 75 kg. If you weigh more you will burn more, if you weigh less you will burn less:

- Ballet   358 calories
- Ballroom   236 calories
- Hip hop   414 calories
- Salsa   286 calories
- Swing   414 calories
- Tap   328 calories
- Flamenco   300 calories

To achieve significant weight loss (at least 5% of body weight) it is recommended to undertake at least 300 minutes of moderate-intensity exercise per week so including a few dance classes in your fitness regime along with other forms of exercise can achieve this aim. Think of ways you can incorporate exercise into your daily routine. For example walking or biking to work, getting off the bus a few stops early, and taking the stairs instead of the elevator can also add to your weekly activity.

Stronger bones and reduced risk of osteoporosis

Insufficient exercise can result in a reduction in bone density and strength. Eventually, low bone density can lead to osteoporosis where your bones become brittle and more likely to fracture. Peak bone density is achieved between the ages of 15-20 years of age and declines as we age. In particular, lower oestrogen levels associated with menopause can result in further declines in bone density. Bones are in a state of flux, continually breaking down and reforming so as you get older it is important to maintain bone density to delay degeneration. As well as eating foods rich in calcium and vitamin D, getting weight-bearing exercise is very important for maintaining strong bones. Weight-bearing activity means an activity that puts tension and pressure on your bones so swimming and cycling would not achieve that effect. Dance is a great type of weight-bearing activity which works in a multi-directional manner with bones, muscles and tendons being strengthened in different directions. A study looking at bone density in ballet dancers and non-dancers found higher bone density, particularly in the legs and pelvis of dancers [van Marken Lichtenbelt et al., 1995].

Balance and dancing

Daily activities like walking, cycling or swimming involve limited mono-directional movement, often fixing your body in a particular pose. Dance on the other hand involves 3-dimensional movement as well as the possibility of turns, jumps, and hops. Your pelvis and postural muscles will be constantly adjusting themselves to control your movement, often without you being aware of it. Your core will receive a workout moving your body and improving your balance and coordination. Falling over and breaking bones is a major cause of physical impairment and hospitalization in older people therefore dance can be a way to prevent this.

Increased confidence, self-esteem and mental benefits

A serious illness can affect our confidence resulting in negative thoughts and possibly depression. Dancing is a great way to improve our mental confidence by improving the following factors:

- cognition
- mental functioning
- mobility and flexibility
- memory and attention

Dancing is not just a physical activity but also a mental workout. If you are new to dance then you may be amazed at the ability of your classmates to remember complex sequences. Do not worry as this ability will quickly improve if you are new to dance. Learning a dance combination is akin to a mental push-up as you challenge your brain to remember and reproduce steps and improve the plasticity of your brain. As a bonus dancing helps prevent age-related mental impairments like poor memory and attention [Zhu et al., 2020].

Dance is a sociable activity. During dance classes, we engage with other people making verbal and non-verbal connections. Often in times of ill health, we rely on our family to support us. However, sometimes we are unable to express our emotions to those close to us or possibly they do not know how to talk to us about our situation, or are afraid of upsetting us. But dance presents a space where new friends and connections can be made with people with a shared love of dance. These connections, even if it is just sharing the same space, and moving to the same music, are still valuable and important to our mental well-being. As a result, dancing can be a way to combat isolation, stress and loneliness.

Effect of dance on neurotransmitters

Physical activity in general has been associated with a sense of feeling good which may be linked with physiological and psychological effects. People who participate in dance have reported feelings of happiness, elation, energy, and euphoria as well as relaxation and calm [https://taniasoubry.com/the-potential-power-of-the-clubbing-and-dance-culture-event/]. Furthermore, quantitative studies found positive effects of recreational dance interventions on physical and psychosocial health and well-being in children and adolescents (Burkhardt & Brennan 2012) as well as in the older population (Connolly & Redding 2010). This is in part due to the neurotransmitters released in the brain when people dance such as dopamine, oxytocin, serotonin, and endorphins. Other neurotransmitters which may be affected by dance include cortisol and norepinephrine. Cortisol has a major role in reducing stress and anxiety while norepinephrine plays a central role in mediating and modulating behaviours that are disrupted in depression.

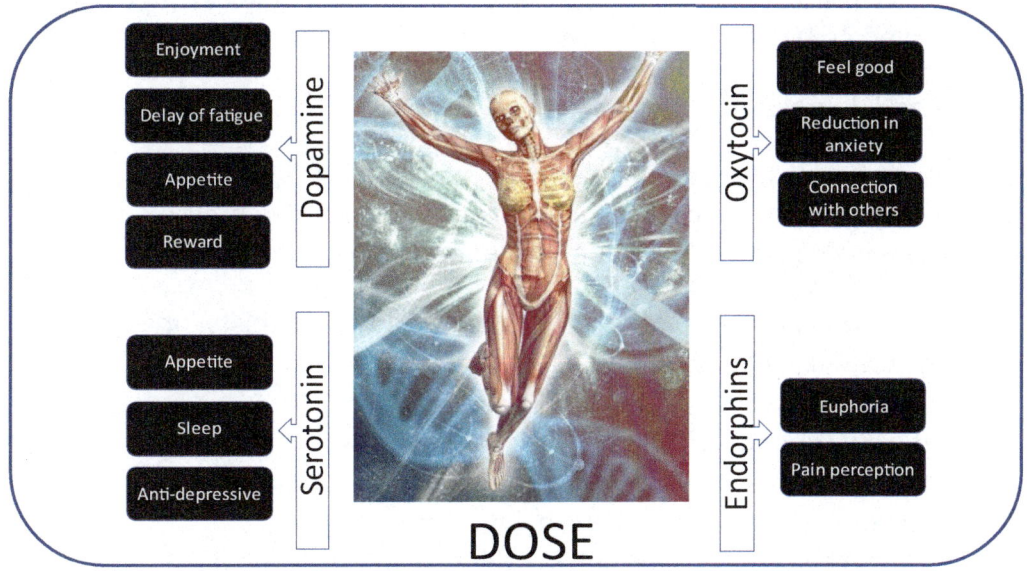

The effects of dancing on neurotransmitters within the body

Improved emotional expression

Keeping feelings and emotions inside us can be damaging to our minds leading to depression and poorer health outcomes. Dancing can result in improved emotional expression. Happy music can allow us to dance in a happy way, and sad music can help us to dance in a sad way, both are good. As we exercise our emotional "muscles" we can release negative feelings which we may not realise we are suppressing. It is good in some ways to be mentally tough but better to be mentally pliable, acknowledging when things get rough and letting go of emotions. Acceptance of ill health can be a route to recovery, denial can result in a block of emotions and a build-up of negative thoughts causing stress which we can hold within ourselves and which can have a detrimental effect on our physical health. Ultimately, dance can be effective as a moving meditation when we stop thinking but allow a sub-conscious synergy in the joy of movement to shape our mental, emotional and spiritual worlds. It is good to talk to people when life gets tough but dance is a form of non-verbal communication where we can work through our emotions in our own unique way. Therefore dance is useful when we feel isolated or unable to communicate verbally. Mental benefits of dance can be seen at any age, for example dance can help adolescents cope with emotional distress showing less nervousness, anxiety for those regularly attending dance classes [Tao et al., 2022]. Regardless of dance style, people of all ages and cultural groups report a greater sense of happiness, social connectedness and life satisfaction through dance participation [Sheppard et al., 2020].

Dancing and depression

Participating in activities you once enjoyed may be hard if you are depressed. However, engaging in dancing could boost your mood and improve your symptoms in some cases. The symptoms of depression may include:

- low mood in the form of sadness, hopelessness, irritability, or anger
- fatigue and low motivation
- unexplained aches and pains
- difficulty experiencing joy
- trouble focusing
- changes in sleeping and eating habits
- feeling restless or moving and speaking slower than usual
- thoughts of self-harm and death

If you are depressed you may not feel motivated but some dancing activities may make you feel better. Studies indicate that regular dance sessions can aid with boosting mood. Yoga also scored high in reducing symptoms of depression [Seshadri, 2020]. In a meta-analysis of 28 studies on adult depression symptoms, stress and anxiety were reduced following 2.5 hours of dance per week (Salihu et al, 2021). Dance can affect your mental health by enhancing neurotransmitter activity and the release of endorphins (a feel-good hormone). Dancing can aid with intrusive thoughts by bringing you into the present, temporarily freeing your mind from negative thoughts. One way to view it is that dancing can be a moving meditation breaking a cycle of racing unwanted thoughts. One study revealed that dancing more than once a week was associated with an increase in mindfulness, reduced distress and improved quality of life (Laird et al, 2021). Traumatic experiences can result in depression since trauma can be stored in the body. Dancing can help people through somatic interventions by "moving" through difficult memories to aid mental healing (https://psychosocialsomatic.com/dance-therapy/).

Dementia

Dancing is a challenging cognitive activity activating pathways including coordination, memory, cognition and attention. The brain is stimulated when we recall dance movements activating regions of the brain that contribute to learning and performance. A study of 469 people over age 75 indicated that "participation in leisure activities is associated with a reduced risk of dementia." The study called for further evaluation but stated that "dancing was the only physical activity associated with a lower risk of dementia" [Verghese et al, 2003].

Improved lymph circulation

Lymph nodes form a network of interconnecting channels which collect fluids from our cells and return this fluid to the blood circulation. Lymph nodes also act as a screen to catch and scan for abnormal cells and consequently neutralize them. The lymph fluid circulates our bodies through the action of bodily movement in effect squeezing the fluid from cells through the lymph nodes and eventually to the main circulation. For this to efficiently occur movement/activity is required for optimal action and dance can very effectively achieve this.

Improved immune system

A lifestyle that is considered active reduces the risk of cancer developing [McTiernan et al., 2019], with very active lifestyles reporting lower risk for oesophageal adenocarcinoma, liver, lung, kidney, gastric cardia, endometrial, myeloid leukaemia, myeloma, colon, head and neck, rectal, bladder, and breast cancers with reductions in risk ranging from 10 to 42% [Moore et al, 2016]. One of those factors which has significant implications on cancer is the effect of physical activity on the immune system. The immune system plays a fundamental role in the elimination of malignant cells, although it should be noted that some aspects of immune function can contribute to tumour progression [Gonzalez et al, 2018]. A lower incidence of cancer is observed in people with higher natural killer cell cytotoxicity in the blood [Moon et al, 2019]. Note that cancer therapy – primarily chemotherapy and radiotherapy, can detrimentally affect the immune system. Thus it is important to maintain the functioning of the immune system through physical exercise and nutrition during treatment to avoid bacterial and viral infections. The immune system can be influenced both positively and negatively by physical activity such as dance determined primarily by the intensity and duration of exercise. Both the innate and adaptive responses of the immune system can be affected by physical activity. The innate immune system is the first defence against pathogens and abnormal cells. Fast-responding neutrophil cells can recognise pathogens and remove them by engulfing them, destruction by reactive oxygen species (ROS), antimicrobial peptides (AMPs) and inflammatory cytokines (immune signalling protein molecules). Dance of moderate intensity is beneficial via a reduction of pro-inflammatory molecules and elevating anti-inflammatory proteins. Additionally, neutrophil numbers and functioning are improved [Borges et al., 2019]. However acute high-intensity dance affects neutrophils by increased production of pro-inflammatory molecules [Borges, 2018] which would indicate susceptibility to infection. Further investigation suggested that high-intensity dance could induce a transient level of immunosuppression, making the dancer more susceptible to infection. Natural killer cells are an effective type of cell which can target abnormal cells. The recruitment of NK cells occurs through cellular stress promoted by exercise [Evans, 2017]. However, physical activity lasting more than three hours causes the concentration of NK cells to return to the pre-exercise state or even lower than this [da Silveira et al., 2021]. High amounts of IgA found at mucosal membranes correlate with lower susceptibility to upper respiratory tract infection, URTI [Hanson, 1983]. Moderate physical activity can improve mucosal IgA levels while intense exercise can temporarily impair IgA levels [Peters, 1997; Gleeson et al., 1999] and compromise anti-viral defences [Levando et al., 1988; Gleeson and Pyne., 2000]. Finally, cortisol is a stress hormone that can exert immunosuppressive activities; direct social interaction and a conducive environment for aerobic dance, have both been demonstrated to reduce cortisol levels in saliva, hence alleviating stress and restoring immune competence [Ramania et al., 2020]. Since excessive physical activity may temporarily suppress the innate immune system it is sensible when undergoing cancer treatment not to undertake excessive exercise which may leave the person susceptible to opportunistic bacterial and virus infections.

Better sleep

Sleep is very important for our physical and mental well-being. Dance can improve sleep by improving your sleep quality by increasing your deep sleep which is crucial for your body to relax, regenerate cells, heal and improve your memory. Improved sleep can decrease stress and anxiety and reduce blood pressure. One study indicated that dance therapy can be a useful complementary therapy protocol, contributing to controlling blood pressure and enhancing sleep quality and, in general, the quality of life in pre-hypertensive and hypertensive middle-aged women [Maruf et al., 2016].

Muscle strength and endurance

Dancing involves strength, stamina and endurance. Partaking in regular dance classes will build muscular strength in particular in your legs and torso. By creating opportunities for tension within your musculoskeletal system you strengthen this system in a multi-directional manner leading to a stronger body. Few types of exercise or activity can mimic this without the need to build bulky muscles, whereas dance also lengthens the muscles in the body. There are many different muscles in our body and dancing can activate the major and minor muscles in the body that other forms of activity may neglect. Studies indicate that attending 3 dance classes a week will result in stronger legs and enhanced endurance in 12 weeks [Pilch et al, 2017].

Mobility and flexibility

Dancing can strengthen joints, maintain flexibility and help people with mobility issues such as people with Parkinson's disease. Recent research revealed regular dance classes improved the functional ability of people with Parkinson's and slowed the progression of the disease [Beers and De Souza, 2021].

Anti-cancer benefits of physical activity

Physical activity can have anti-cancer benefits. However, the exact mechanisms are still being investigated. Regular aerobic exercise increases transit time, reducing mucosal exposure to potentially carcinogenic substances which potentially reduces the risk of colon cancer [Oruç and Kaplan, 2019]. It is speculated that physical activity reduces exposure to oestrogen, possibly due to delayed menarche and reduced ovulatory cycles resulting in a reduced incidence of breast cancer [Kossman et al., 2011]. Exercise can induce higher levels of globulin being produced in the blood which can bind and reduce exposure to testosterone which is linked to an increased risk of prostate cancer [Brown et al, 2012]. Other mechanisms include reducing oxidative stress and inflammation, limiting adipose tissue accumulation, improving immune surveillance, and modulating the insulin-like growth factor axis [Gill et al, 2010].

Beneficial effects of music

Music is often an integral part of dance. Music can result in the following effects:

- Boost self-esteem
- Induces relaxation

- Evokes emotion
- Reduces anxiety and stress
- Improves sleep
- Improved healing
- Better pain management
- Fatigue reduction
- Improved Immune system

When we hear music that stimulates us our body releases dopamine which is a neurotransmitter that is released during enjoyable activities such as sex or eating. Dopamine gives us a feeling of well-being and reward and is associated with motivation and attention which can boost self-esteem. Music evokes emotions which involves a part of the brain called the pre-frontal cortex which is involved in memory. Thus music can tap into memories, evoking emotions. Music can also reduce agitation by stimulating oxytocin release which provides a positive feeling and increased social connection and bonding. Cortisol is the body's chief stress hormone. While cortisol levels may increase temporarily, the long-term elevation of cortisol levels is detrimental to our health. Listening to music can help reduce cortisol levels and in turn have a relaxing effect so we feel less stressed, with proven reductions in blood pressure and improved heart rhythms [Thorna et al, 2013]. Music can be beneficial to our sleep by increasing oxytocin and decreasing cortisol and as such we are more likely to get better quality sleep [Trahan et al, 2018]. One study found that music can stimulate the pituitary gland, releasing growth hormones that are associated with improved healing rates [Thorna et al, 2013]. Other effects of music include small intestine regulation, pain reduction, thyroid regulation, adrenaline release, immune regulation and adrenal gland regulation [Myskja and Lindbaek, 2000].

In summary dance can have multiple health benefits both physical and mental. Individuals diagnosed with cancer frequently have other health conditions such as cardiovascular problems, high blood pressure, diabetes, obesity, dementia and metabolic syndrome as such dance can have beneficial impacts for a person's overall well-being which can feed back to better outcomes after cancer treatment.

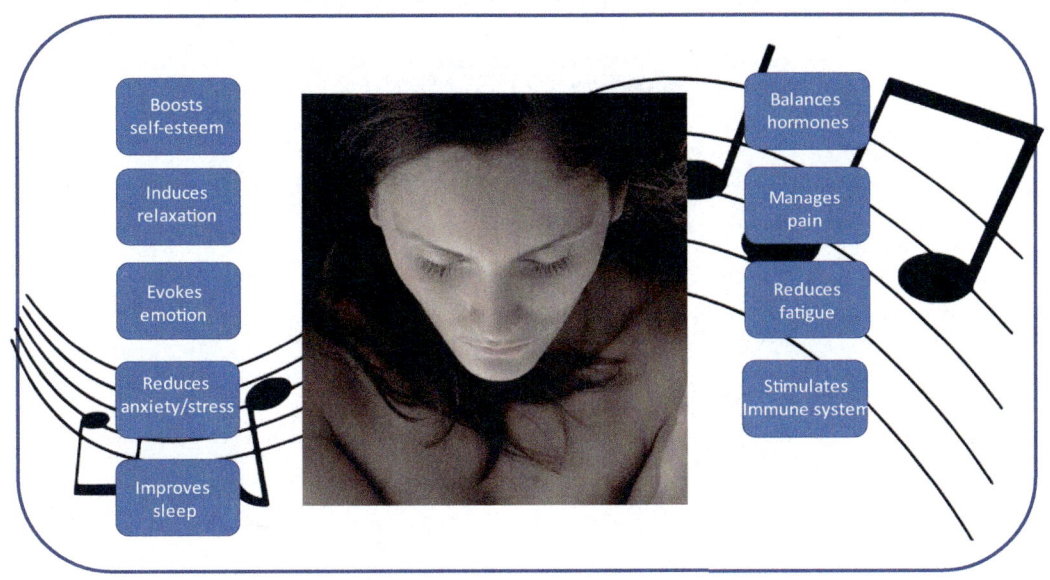

Beneficial effects of music

References

Bearss KA, DeSouza JFX. Parkinson's Disease Motor Symptom Progression Slowed with Multisensory Dance Learning over 3-Years: A Preliminary Longitudinal Investigation. Brain Sci. 2021 Jul 7;11(7):895. doi: 10.3390/brainsci11070895.

Blanksby BA, Reidy PW. Heart rate and estimated energy expenditure during ballroom dancing. Br J Sports Med. 1988 Jun;22(2):57-60. doi: 10.1136/bjsm.22.2.57.

Borges L, Dermargos A, Gray S, Barros Silva MB, Santos V, Pithon-Curi TC, et al. Neutrophil Migration and Adhesion Molecule Expression after Acute High-Intensity Street Dance Exercise. J Immunol Res. 2018;2018:1684013.

Borges L, Gorjão R, Gray SR, Martins TR, Santos VC, Momesso CM, et al. Lymphocyte activation after a high-intensity street dance class. PLoS One. 2020;15(9):e0239516.

Borges L, Passos MEP, Silva MBB, Santos VC, Momesso CM, Pithon-Curi TC, et al. Dance Training Improves Cytokine Secretion and Viability of Neutrophils in Diabetic Patients. Mediators Inflamm. 2019;2019:2924818.

Brown JC, Winters-Stone K, Lee A, Schmitz KH. Cancer, physical activity, and exercise. Compr Physiol. 2012 Oct;2(4):2775-809. doi: 10.1002/cphy.c120005.

Jan Burkhardt & Cathy Brennan (2012) The effects of recreational dance interventions on the health and well-being of children and young people: A systematic review, Arts & Health, 4:2, 148-161, DOI: 10.1080/17533015.2012.665810

Campbell KL, Winters-Stone KM, Wiskemann J, May AM, Schwartz AL, Courneya KS, Zucker DS, Matthews CE, Ligibel JA, Gerber LH, Morris GS, Patel AV, Hue TF, Perna FM, Schmitz KH. Exercise Guidelines for Cancer Survivors: Consensus Statement from International Multidisciplinary Roundtable. Med Sci Sports Exerc. 2019 Nov;51(11):2375-2390. doi: 10.1249/MSS.0000000000002116.

Cohen JL, Segal KR, Witriol I, McArdle WD. Cardiorespiratory responses to ballet exercise and the VO2max of elite ballet dancers. Med Sci Sports Exerc. 1982;14(3):212-7.

Connolly, M., & Redding, E. (2010). *Dancing towards well-being in the third age: Literature review on the impact of dance on health and well-being among older people*. London: Trinity Laban Conservatoire for Music and Dance.

da Silveira MP, da Silva Fagundes KK, Bizuti MR, Starck É, Rossi RC, de Resende E Silva DT. Physical exercise as a tool to help the immune system against COVID-19: an integrative review of the current literature. Clin Exp Med. 2021 Feb;21(1):15-28. doi: 10.1007/s10238-020-00650-3. Epub 2020 Jul 29.

Demark-Wahnefried W, Platz EA, Ligibel JA, Blair CK, Courneya KS, Meyerhardt JA, Ganz PA, Rock CL, Schmitz KH, Wadden T, Philip EJ, Wolfe B, Gapstur SM, Ballard-Barbash R, McTiernan A, Minasian L, Nebeling L, Goodwin PJ. The role of obesity in cancer survival and recurrence. Cancer Epidemiol Biomarkers Prev. 2012 Aug;21(8):1244-59. doi: 10.1158/1055-9965.EPI-12-0485. Epub 2012 Jun 13.

Evans W. NK cell recruitment and exercise: Potential immunotherapeutic role of shear stress and endothelial health. Med Hypotheses. 2017 Nov;109:170-173. doi: 10.1016/j.mehy.2017.10.015. Epub 2017 Oct 17.

Gill JK, Wilkens LR, Pollak MN, Stanczyk FZ, Kolonel LN. Androgens, growth factors, and risk of prostate cancer: the Multiethnic Cohort. Prostate. 2010 Jun 1;70(8):906-15. doi: 10.1002/pros.21125.

Gonzalez H, Hagerling C, Werb Z. Roles of the immune system in cancer: from tumor initiation to metastatic progression. Genes Dev. 2018 Oct 1;32(19-20):1267-1284. doi: 10.1101/gad.314617.118.

Gleeson M, Hall ST, McDonald WA, Flanagan AJ, Clancy RL. Salivary IgA subclasses and infection risk in elite swimmers. Immunol Cell Biol. 1999 Aug;77(4):351–5.

Gleeson M, Pyne DB. Special feature for the Olympics: effects of exercise on the immune system: exercise effects on mucosal immunity. Immunol Cell Biol. 2000 Oct;78(5):536–44.

Hanson, L.A., Bjorkander, J. and Oxelius VA. Selective IgA deficiency. In: Primary and secondary immunodefieciency disorders. Churchill Livingstone, Edinburgh.; 1983. p. 62–84.

Kossman DA, Williams NI, Domchek SM, Kurzer MS, Stopfer JE, Schmitz KH. Exercise lowers estrogen and progesterone levels in premenopausal women at high risk of breast cancer. J Appl Physiol (1985). 2011 Dec;111(6):1687-93. doi: 10.1152/japplphysiol.00319.2011.

Levando, V.A., Sazdal'nitskii, R.S., Perstin, B.B., Zykov MP. Study of secretory and antiviral immunity in sportsmen. Sport Train Med Rehab. 1988;1:49–52.

Maruf FA, Akinpelu AO, Salako BL, Akinyemi JO. Effects of aerobic dance training on blood pressure in individuals with uncontrolled hypertension on two antihypertensive drugs: a randomized clinical trial. J Am Soc Hypertens. 2016 Apr;10(4):336-45. doi: 10.1016/j.jash.2016.02.002.

McTiernan A, Friedenreich CM, Katzmarzyk PT, Powell KE, Macko R, Buchner D, Pescatello LS, Bloodgood B, Tennant B, Vaux-Bjerke A, George SM, Troiano RP, Piercy KL; 2018 PHYSICAL ACTIVITY GUIDELINES ADVISORY COMMITTEE*. Physical Activity in Cancer Prevention and Survival: A Systematic Review. Med Sci Sports Exerc. 2019 Jun;51(6):1252-1261. doi: 10.1249/MSS.0000000000001937.

Merom D, Grunseit A, Eramudugolla R, Jefferis B, Mcneill J, Anstey KJ. Cognitive Benefits of Social Dancing and Walking in Old Age: The Dancing Mind Randomized Controlled Trial. Front Aging Neurosci. 2016 Feb 22;8:26. doi: 10.3389/fnagi.2016.00026.

Moon WY, Powis SJ. Does Natural Killer Cell Deficiency (NKD) Increase the Risk of Cancer? NKD May Increase the Risk of Some Virus Induced Cancer. Front Immunol. 2019 Jul 19;10:1703. doi: 10.3389/fimmu.2019.01703.

Moore SC, Lee IM, Weiderpass E, Campbell PT, Sampson JN, Kitahara CM, Keadle SK, Arem H, Berrington de Gonzalez A, Hartge P, Adami HO, Blair CK, Borch KB, Boyd E, Check DP, Fournier A, Freedman ND, Gunter M, Johannson M, Khaw KT, Linet MS, Orsini N, Park Y, Riboli E, Robien K, Schairer C, Sesso H, Spriggs M, Van Dusen R, Wolk A, Matthews CE, Patel AV. Association of Leisure-Time Physical Activity With Risk of 26 Types of Cancer in 1.44 Million Adults. JAMA Intern Med. 2016 Jun 1;176(6):816-25. doi: 10.1001/jamainternmed.2016.1548.

Myskja A, Lindbaek M. Hvordan virker musikk på menneskekroppen? [How does music affect the human body?]. Tidsskr Nor Laegeforen. 2000 Apr 10;120(10):1182-5. Norwegian.

Oruç Z, Kaplan MA. Effect of exercise on colorectal cancer prevention and treatment. World J Gastrointest Oncol. 2019 May 15;11(5):348-366. doi: 10.4251/wjgo.v11.i5.348.

Peters EM. Exercise, immunology and upper respiratory tract infections. Int J Sports Med. 1997 Mar;18 Suppl 1:S69-77.

Pilch W, Tota Ł, Sadowska-Krępa E, Piotrowska A, Kępińska M, Pałka T, Maszczyk A. The Effect of a 12-Week Health Training Program on Selected Anthropometric and Biochemical Variables in Middle-Aged Women. Biomed Res Int. 2017;2017:9569513. doi: 10.1155/2017/9569513.

Ramania, N.S., Iwo, M.I., Apriantono, T. and Winata B. The effect of social interaction and environment during aerobic dance on salivary cortisol. Physiother Q. 2020;28:14–20.

Salihu D, Kwan RYC, Wong EML. The effect of dancing interventions on depression symptoms, anxiety, and stress in adults without musculoskeletal disorders: An integrative review and meta-analysis. Complement Ther Clin Pract. 2021 Nov;45:101467. doi: 10.1016/j.ctcp.2021.101467.

Sheppard A, Broughton MC. Promoting wellbeing and health through active participation in music and dance: a systematic review. Int J Qual Stud Health Well-being. 2020 Dec;15(1):1732526. doi: 10.1080/17482631.2020.1732526.

Seshadri A, Adaji A, Orth SS, Singh B, Clark MM, Frye MA, Fuller-Tyszkiewicz M, McGillivray J. Exercise, Yoga, and Tai Chi for Treatment of Major Depressive Disorder in Outpatient Settings: A Systematic Review and Meta-Analysis. Prim Care Companion CNS Disord. 2020 Dec 31;23(1):20r02722. doi: 10.4088/PCC.20r02722.

Tao D, Gao Y, Cole A, Baker JS, Gu Y, Supriya R, Tong TK, Hu Q, Awan-Scully R. The Physiological and Psychological Benefits of Dance and its Effects on Children and Adolescents: A Systematic Review. Front Physiol. 2022 Jun 13;13:925958. doi: 10.3389/fphys.2022.925958.

Thoma MV, La Marca R, Brönnimann R, Finkel L, Ehlert U, Nater UM. The effect of music on the human stress response. PLoS One. 2013 Aug 5;8(8):e70156. doi: 10.1371/journal.pone.0070156.

Trahan T, Durrant SJ, Müllensiefen D, Williamson VJ. The music that helps people sleep and the reasons they believe it works: A mixed methods analysis of online survey reports. PLoS One. 2018 Nov 14;13(11):e0206531. doi: 10.1371/journal.pone.0206531.

van Marken Lichtenbelt WD, Fogelholm M, Ottenheijm R, Westerterp KR. Physical activity, body composition and bone density in ballet dancers. Br J Nutr. 1995 Oct;74(4):439-51. doi: 10.1079/bjn19950150. PMID: 7577885.

Verghese J, Lipton RB, Katz MJ, Hall CB, Derby CA, Kuslansky G, Ambrose AF, Sliwinski M, Buschke H. Leisure activities and the risk of dementia in the elderly. N Engl J Med. 2003 Jun 19;348(25):2508-16. doi: 10.1056/NEJMoa022252.

Zhu Y, Zhong Q, Ji J, Ma J, Wu H, Gao Y, Ali N, Wang T. Effects of Aerobic Dance on Cognition in Older Adults with Mild Cognitive Impairment: A Systematic Review and Meta-Analysis. J Alzheimers Dis. 2020;74(2):679-690. doi: 10.3233/JAD-190681.

https://psychosocialsomatic.com/dance-therapy/ 2022 Accessed March 2023.

https://taniasoubry.com/the-potential-power-of-the-clubbing-and-dance-culture-event/ 2013 Accessed March 2023.

The power of transformation

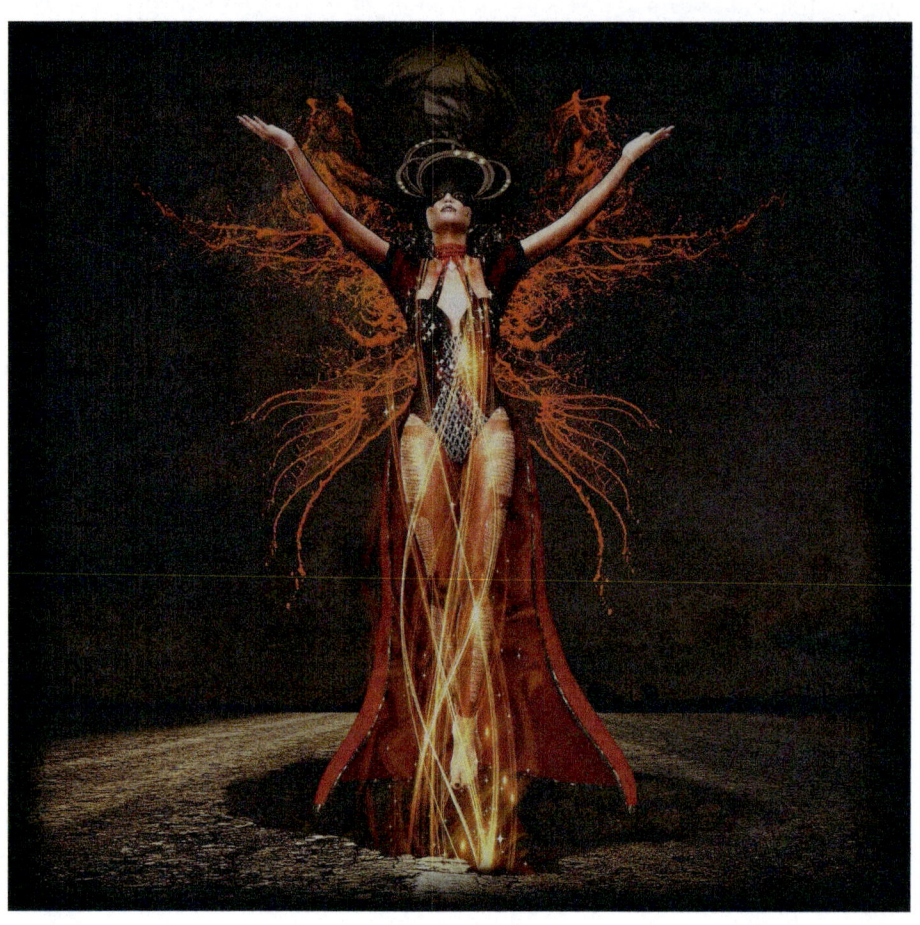

TIPS FOR TAKING UP DANCING

Fenella J Barker

To dance is a human instinct and there are so many reasons why people dance. I'm going to discuss here tips for taking up dance in regards to studying dance and/or participating in group dance activities at a recreational rather than professional level (not that either are mutually exclusive). During my career, I have worked as a professional dancer in a variety of dance styles and also taught all ages and abilities, predominantly in adult education, but also in small dance studios, vocational dance schools, state schools, schools for children with special educational needs and in further and higher education. My youngest student was about 3 years old and my oldest is 90.

So, why dance?

It might be because you love the music or the culture associated with a particular style of dance, you might be looking to make friends, it might be for medical reasons (fitness, mental health, physical recuperation), you might want to perform or you might want to dance on your own, you might just be curious or maybe it's all or none of these. Above all, dancing should be fun, often challenging too but if you're not enjoying your dance classes then maybe it's time to look for a different dance style, a different class level or a different teacher. Whether it's for work or pleasure, I dance for fun, friendship, fitness, the music and, for me, sometimes it's for nostalgia too.

So, what should you initially consider when you're thinking about joining a dance class?

1. Maybe the first thing to decide is what your current level of fitness is, but obviously this shouldn't preclude any styles as the teacher should be able to adapt to your level of fitness. However, some styles are more energetic than others.
2. Do you want to dance on your own, in a group, or with a partner?
3. Do you want to be inspired by music, physicality, culture, or your mind (i.e. more meditative dance styles)? It might be all of these - if so, which ones are more predominant?
4. Is there a particular music style that you love to listen to and would get inspired by? What styles of dance are taught to this music?
5. Are there any cultures you are interested in knowing more about? What are the traditional dance styles associated with these cultures?

6. If you are not sure what style of dance to try, look for open days and taster workshops, where you can either watch or join in with a variety of beginner-level classes. The adult education college I work for has an annual day of dance where they offer free 20-minute taster workshops in an enormous range of dance styles. There may be a style you've never heard of or have dismissed for various reasons and in a taster class you may find you fall in love with it. I had a student who walked into one of my beginner flamenco classes by accident, looking for a salsa class. She decided to stay and try the class and she's never left.

Once you have decided what style or styles of dance, you need to then consider the following:

1. Decide on your level, which would be beginner or introduction if you're new to dance or if it's a style that's new to you.
2. How do you want to study? Do you want to study in a class in a dance studio or classroom? Do you want to study online? Since Covid-19 there has been a rise in dance classes offered live online as well as in studios or classrooms. There are also classes offered on video but I would not recommend this as your main source of dance training unless you are very experienced, know your own strengths and weaknesses and can self-correct. However, videos of classes or short video tutorials of elements of classes can be very beneficial if they are used to supplement studio or online lessons.
3. Do you want to study with other students or in private lessons?
4. If you want to study with other students, do you want to be in a big or a small class and do you mind what age the other students are?
5. Do you want a slower-paced, more relaxed class or do you want a class where you are encouraged to achieve at a faster pace?
6. How much can you afford to pay for your classes?

Now you've considered all of the above, it's time to think about possibly the most important aspect of learning to dance – your teacher:

1. The first thing you should consider is whether your teacher is qualified to teach you and whether they're insured. There are several dance teaching associations (eg RAD, IDTA, SDS, BBO, and ISTD to name but a few) that have lists of qualified and insured teachers. There are also dance advocate organisations such as People Dancing (Foundation for Community Dance), One Dance (formerly Dance UK) and the Council for

Dance and Musical Theatre (CDMT, formerly CDET Council for Dance Education & Training) that can recommend qualified and insured teachers.
2. Don't be worried about approaching a prospective teacher to ask to talk to them or to e-mail them with some questions. They will be happy to help.
3. It is also advisable to ask for a trial class (most teachers offer this, many for free) and to talk to some of the students in the class, either before or after the class, to see how they feel about the teacher and the class in general. You should look in your trial class for a happy, friendly, non-judgemental feel to the class, a teacher who pays attention to the students and their needs and offers appropriate feedback.
4. If you are interested in performing, ask the teacher what the performance opportunities are for students.
5. If you are interested in taking exams, ask the teacher if they offer syllabus classes, in which dance styles and with which organisations.

Other things to consider are:

1. How close to your home or work the dance studio is and if it is near public transport and/or has parking available.
2. Does the studio have adequate dance flooring, fitness equipment, mirrors and/or barres (depending on what style of dance you are studying)?
3. What size is the studio?
4. Does it have adequate lighting and is it well-ventilated?
5. Is the sound equipment (either for pre-recorded music or live musicians) adequate?
6. Are there showers / toilets / changing rooms?
7. Is there access to drinking water?
8. Is there somewhere to relax and socialise before /after the class?

If you have any health issues (e.g. are undergoing cancer treatment) or special needs:

1. Please ask to speak to your teacher privately before or after the class or by telephone.
2. It is really important that you let your teacher know immediately if you have health issues, are undergoing treatment, have an injury or have any other special needs (including things like depression or bereavement). You might want to keep things to yourself but it is essential that your

teacher knows of anything that will affect you physically and it will also help your teacher to give you the best possible experience if you let them know of any mental or emotional problems you may be having.
3. It is also important that your teacher knows if you are dyslexic, on the autistic spectrum or have any other special educational needs and which learning styles suit you best. This will help your teacher to help you to learn in the way that works best for you – we all learn differently so your teacher should by default include a range of learning and teaching methods in their classes but it is always useful for them to know if there is something specific that helps you to learn.

If you are undergoing intermittent treatment (e.g. for cancer or any other condition) or have a condition that causes fatigue so that you are not always able to attend class:

1. Check if your teacher offers a live online feed from your class so that you can still do or even watch the class at home.
2. Check if your teacher offers videos of the class so that you can continue to study in your own time as and when you are well enough.
3. Check if your teacher offers short video tutorials of the work studied each week so that you can just quickly dip into what was covered. This will help you to still feel connected to the class during times when you can't attend or can't use the online or full-class video options. The more connected to your class that you continue to feel, the easier it will be to return after a period of absence.
4. Listen to your body and rest when you need to.

Most importantly, dancing (and especially dancing through cancer) is about enjoyment, escapism, strengthening mind and body and friendship. It might take a few weeks or even a month or so to feel really comfortable in your new dance class. However, if, after a couple of months or a term, you don't feel you are enjoying the experience, just go and find a different dance style, a different class level or a different teacher or maybe all three! Happy dancing!

MENTAL HEALTH AND CANCER

Professor Chris Palmer and Dr Ebru Aydar

Receiving a cancer diagnosis can evoke a host of different emotions which may be difficult to cope with making you feel overwhelmed. Partners, friends and family may have similar feelings. Some common feelings include:

- Shock
- Anxiety
- Depression
- Frightened
- Sad
- Guilty
- Isolated

When you are first diagnosed it may be hard to believe and you may feel shocked and numb. Not only that but you may have a lot of questions and new information to understand which cycle round in your mind. At first, you may find it hard to talk about or you may find it difficult to think or talk about anything else. Everybody is different and these reactions are normal, be reassured that these feelings will get easier over time. Anxiety about future or current treatments is common, it is not something you can control but you can cope with it by focusing on things you can control by continuing to undertake things you enjoy or finding new things to enjoy. Feeling uncertain about your future is a normal reaction which may make you feel sad. However, for most people, these periods of sadness improve. Anger, resentment, guilt and blame are also common feelings especially when you feel frightened, stressed or unwell. Try and recognise these feelings and realise they are not you or part of you but a temporary feeling that will pass. It is possible that you feel alone or isolated and that you do not have support. Talk about your feelings -reach out to family and friends and particularly other cancer survivors. Note that people with cancer have a heightened risk of developing mental health problems such as depression and anxiety [Niedzwiedz et al, 2019]. Research indicates that many cancer patients with clinical depression do not receive adequate mental support [Wang et al, 2020]. Additionally, depression can worsen cancer-related outcomes as people may miss treatment appointments, be less likely to exercise and may be more susceptible to alcohol abuse. Patients who received treatment for depression and had fewer depression symptoms were found to have longer survival times than those with more depression symptoms [Wang et al, 2020].

Therefore it is important in cancer to not only receive medical treatment for your body but to take proactive care of your mind. Depression is more prevalent in people with cancer compared to the general population [Hartung et al, 2017] and inadequate recognition of depression is related to a reduction in quality of life and survival. Furthermore, some cancers for example, pancreatic and lung cancer can release depression-causing chemicals and some cancer treatments such as corticosteroids and chemotherapy can cause depression.

Depression is not just a feeling of sadness. Depression is when someone experiences at least one of the following symptoms for more than two weeks:

- Feeling sad most of the time
- Loss of pleasure and interest in activities you used to enjoy
- Changes in eating and sleeping habits
- Unexplained tiredness
- Feeling worthless
- Feeling guilt for no reason
- Slow physical and mental response
- Decreased concentration ability
- Thoughts of death or suicide
- Nervousness

If you notice any of these symptoms for more than two weeks which affect your day-to-day activities, talk to your doctor about treatment options such as counselling, medication and therapy. In the past, it was thought that depression and anxiety are caused by an imbalance of chemicals (neurotransmitters) in the brain which allow nerve cells to talk to each other. However, later research indicates that it is more complex than that and that several factors including genetic vulnerability, faulty mood regulation, and a stressful life event can contribute to depression with many different neurotransmitters involved acting in synergy. The neurotransmitters dopamine and serotonin are often referred to as "happy hormones" as they are known to promote mental well-being. Dopamine, also known as the "feel-good" hormone, is associated with the brain's reward system and produces pleasant sensations. Serotonin can help increase happiness by alleviating depression and anxiety. Therefore it is important to maintain a lifestyle which naturally increase the levels of these neurotransmitters to ward off the likelihood of depression. This can be achieved through physical activity, nutrition, meditation, music, reducing stress and paying attention to our need for sleep. Some additional ways to improve your psychological well-being daily include the following:

- Find a new outlook or activity
- Make healthy lifestyle choices
- Talk about your feelings, reach out to family and friends, other cancer survivors
- Attend to your needs for nutrition, exercise, rest, sleep
- Try mind-body techniques, such as relaxation therapies, meditation, psychotherapy

In summary, we do not understand everything about what causes anxiety and depression but in many cases, we can take action to help improve our mental health.

References

Hartung TJ, Brähler E, Faller H, Härter M, Hinz A, Johansen C, Keller M, Koch U, Schulz H, Weis J, Mehnert A. The risk of being depressed is significantly higher in cancer patients than in the general population: Prevalence and severity of depressive symptoms across major cancer types. Eur J Cancer. 2017 Feb;72:46-53. doi: 10.1016/j.ejca.2016.11.017.

Niedzwiedz CL, Knifton L, Robb KA, Katikireddi SV, Smith DJ. Depression and anxiety among people living with and beyond cancer: a growing clinical and research priority. BMC Cancer. 2019 Oct 11;19(1):943. doi: 10.1186/s12885-019-6181-4.

Wang YH, Li JQ, Shi JF, Que JY, Liu JJ, Lappin JM, Leung J, Ravindran AV, Chen WQ, Qiao YL, Shi J, Lu L, Bao YP. Depression and anxiety in relation to cancer incidence and mortality: a systematic review and meta-analysis of cohort studies. Mol Psychiatry. 2020 Jul;25(7):1487-1499. doi: 10.1038/s41380-019-0595-x.

WHAT WAS LOST?

How Dance/Movement Therapy Can Support the Retention and Repair of Cognitive Abilities in Cancer Patients

Sarah Menser

As if surviving cancer was not challenging enough, patients are often faced with the residual effects from chemotherapy treatment - the most common being reports of cognitive dysfunction. This dysfunction can force individuals to relearn how to retain information or function in day-to-day life. For survivor Christina, her struggles began after treatment ended and she returned to college. A once successful student who learned with ease, she was faced with lower test scores compared to her classmates (Fernandez, 2018). She reported having to "read and reread the same paragraph, but could not grasp the information," as well as "taking twice the time to learn new concepts" (Fernandez, 2018). Trying everything she could to combat these difficulties, including reciting her notes into a voice recorder and preparing discussion questions in advance so as not to stumble over her words, Christina was forced to learn how her "new" brain functioned (Fernandez, 2018). For survivors, just getting by in daily life can be physically and mentally exhausting. And I am one of them.

I was diagnosed with Stage IV Hodgkin's Lymphoma in the Winter of 2019. I was right in the middle of completing my Masters in Clinical Mental Health Counseling with a Specialization in Dance/Movement Therapy. I watched my cognitive abilities suffer due to my chemotherapy treatments. I watched my physical activity be traded for days on the couch under a blanket. Without exercising my mind and my body, my brain began to suffer. I was always a bright student and brilliant writer. I felt as if I had a strong command of words and could relay my point artistically and poignantly. Attempting to continue to do schoolwork while experiencing cancer-related cognitive impairment (CRIC) was difficult. Reading and comprehending became a challenge. My memory was not as deep as it used to be. Typing became difficult, as I struggled to hit the keys in the correct order. I was no longer the student I used to be. This also took a toll on my practice in being a dance/movement therapist during my internship. I was inclined to sit and act as an observer of my own sessions, allowing the individuals to follow my prompts, but never model them myself. It was apparent to me the cognitive impairments I suffered hindered my daily life.

Cancer-related cognitive impairment (CRCI), or chemo-brain to the lay person, has been defined as the loss of mental acuity associated with cancer and its subsequent treatment (Salerno et al, 2019). Although a broad range, it is reported that an estimated 17-75% of cancer patients experience CRCI in relation to their treatment, affecting their day to day functioning (Campbell, et al., 2017; Myers, 2008; Wefel, et al, 2004). Since CRCI has only been recently addressed on a more consistent basis in literature, it is important to understand the transformations that occur in an individual's quality of life. Patients describe the effects of CRCI as "forgetfulness, absentmindedness, and an inability to focus when performing daily tasks" (Myers, 2008). He (2008) also reports that "patients have expressed concern about CRCI and their subsequent ability to resume previous profession, scholastic, and social activities". It is important to remember there are many different types of chemotherapy and its side effects do not discriminate based on the cancer it is treating. These self-reported side effects and concerns are clearly a detriment to everyday life for a cancer patient, creating challenges that were not previously present in their lifestyle. These changes in "memory, attention, focus, and ability to multitask has now been documented on cognitive tests as well as functional MRIs" (Love et al, 2015). This can be discouraging and frustrating for many and requires an adjustment to their lifestyle. Although chemotherapy has been the typical treatment method for cancer, the exact cause or precise mechanisms that contribute to changes in the brain are unclear (Campbell et al, 2020). It is only recently that this side effect is being recognized in research. With the "potential for significant impact on patients' quality of life," it is shocking that this topic is only now being taken seriously, showing that chemotherapy may damage the hippocampus which leads to cognitive impairments (Myers, 2008). Most notably, the fornix is shown to see significant impact during chemotherapy. The fornix plays an "important role in the encoding, consolidation, and recall of declarative and episodic memory" and is the major output tract of the hippocampus (Burzynska, et al., 2017). The hippocampus can be attributed to assisting in working memory. The fractional anisotropy (FA) values in the fornix have shown decline after chemotherapy and can be linked to the earliest sign of cognitive decline and a predictor of CRCI (Mo, et al., 2017). These are all vital for daily functioning for an individual.

The degeneration of cerebral white matter (WM) is a leading cause in cognitive decline for older adults, similar to what has been seen with chemotherapy patients and the changes in their WM, often affecting processing speed (Burzynska, et al., 2017). Researchers believe that by incorporating physical, cognitive, and social engagements, patients may see an improvement in their cognitive abilities. The one activity that can fully encompass all of the previously mentioned themes is dance. "Improving WM integrity is key in preserving cognitive performance" (Burzynska, et al., 2017). Through this study, 174 participants underwent six months of observation, participating in intervention groups such as dancing, walking, walking + nutrition, and an active control. One of the main purposes of this study was to observe the changes in fractional anisotropy (FA), measuring the levels of fiber integrity in orientation and density in the fornix (Burzynska, et al., 2017). Notably, the dance group worked on social engagement and memorization with learning social dances over the course of one-hour weekly sessions. From this intervention, it was observed that the FA in the fornix increased over the six-month period of engagement in dance, while the other groups witnessed a decline (Burzynska, et al., 2017). The combination of physical and social interventions led to a more positive result, demonstrating dance to be a holistic intervention. The combination of physical and social interventions also can lead to longer-lasting effects (Burzynska, et al., 2017). With this new wealth of information, dance and movement can now be used as an intervention to assist in retention and repair of WM to better handle cognitive functioning. Research by Kattenstroth et al., 2013 also acknowledged the diverse features within treatment interventions involving dance or movement, making it a strong neuroplasticity inducing tool. An overall widespread growth encompassing both attention and cognition is demonstrated after the initiating of dance into the lives of those experiencing cognitive dysfunction. The incorporation of movement for its cognitive, physical, and social benefits for WM health is "key in preserving cognitive performance" (Burzynska, et al., 2017). Studies have also shown that "the aging of the brain is detectable on the scale of 6-months, which highlights the urgency of finding effective interventions to slow down this process" (Burzynska, et al., 2017).

Pace and Villani (2012) studied the effects of chemotherapy on the brain of women with breast cancer. Their study showed that white matter tracts decreased in the frontal, parietal, and occipital lobes of the brain due to the introduction of chemotherapy. The women in the study who had received chemotherapy had a lower score on attention tests, psychomotor speed tests, and memory tests than those who did not. These lower test scores were a direct reflection of the effects that chemotherapy had on the brain, primarily on the demyelination that effects cognitive abilities. Throughout my experience with cancer and chemotherapy, I never had any scans that involved my brain that would assist me in viewing my changes in the fornix or any white matter. I am able to discern from research that these changes are prominent in many cancer patients, but I do not have the ability to use myself as an example in this case. Chemotherapy creates a disturbance in functions that are shown to be durable for some up to ten years (Tannock, et al., 2004). As a natural bridge between the mind-body connection, dance/movement therapy (DMT) is an underexplored supplement to chemotherapy throughout a cancer patient's experience in assisting with the effects of CRCI.

"At its very core, dance/movement therapy emphasizes the holism of mind and body, thereby, providing a new avenue for exploring the complicated inter-relationship of factors involved in coping with cancer" (Cohen & Walco, 1999). The integration of the mind and body can assist in internalizing and understanding of oneself, that can work to explore how the mind is affected during chemotherapy. When moving, the individual can understand more on how functioning occurs within oneself. By introducing movement into the body, the mind will also benefit, creating a cyclical effect to improve one's quality of life. Recently, more studies have been conducted in correlation with exercise to cognitive abilities in cancer patients. While these studies are providing results that support the introduction of physicality during chemotherapy, there are none that focus solely on the effects of DMT.

With a closer relation to the mind-body connection, yoga has also been used to improve both mental and physical health through a therapeutic lens (Mackenzie, et al., 2014). The idea of "mindfulness" is on the forefront of this practice, helping to bridge the gap between standard exercise and the physical activity associated with DMT. Studies show that "within exercise settings, mindfulness builds upon associative attention by refining perceptions of exertion on a moment-by-moment basis via increased sensitivity to a host of cognitive and interoceptive cues, and concurrently limits emotional reactivity to these cues" (Mackenzie, et al., 2014). Turning the focus on an internal lens, "the strong mind-body interaction within contemporary yoga practice adds a unique contemplative dimension to exercise that has been referred to as 'mindfulness in motion'" (Mackenzie, et al., 2014).

While there is a lack of research done to understand how DMT can support the retention and repair of cognitive abilities related to chemotherapy, other studies that encapsulate the benefits of this type of therapy are extensive. It is important to note that the simple introduction of dance alone is not what results in the largest benefit for individuals experiencing CRCI or other forms of cognitive dysfunction. The "broad, multimodal stimulation had greater benefit for WM integrity than aerobic exercise alone" (Burzynska, et al., 2017). Kattenstroth, et al. (2013) states that "dancing is increasingly used as an intervention because it combines many diverse features making it a promising neuroplasticity-inducing tool". For dancing to be a fully beneficial intervention, it must be taken from the lens of DMT to provide the most multidimensional approach. DMT can be structured to provide a lower impact form of physical activity. Working towards the mind-body connection will assist in not only the physical aspect, but also the mental aspect that is so affected by chemotherapy. DMT supports the "emotional, social, cognitive, and physical integration of the individual, for the purpose of improving health and well-being" (Welling, 2019). This multi-tiered approach is what makes it to be a strong tool in retaining and repairing cognitive abilities in cancer patients, for those both actively receiving chemotherapy and in recovery. The benefits are clear from the research published that including exercise in a daily routine while battling cancer is effective in helping cognitive abilities, as much as they are clear from DMT supporting cognitive growth from other populations experiencing dysfunction. With this wealth of information available, DMT should be utilized in the oncology setting to work to improve the cognitive abilities of those affected by chemotherapy.

There is research demonstrating the benefits of DMT for cancer patients, but for other areas than assisting with CRCI. Being known for encompassing "dance, movement, emotional expression, social support, and creative activity in a single intervention approach," DMT has been used as an intervention to address many problems presented associated with receiving chemotherapy (Goodill, 2018). Allowing for patients to explore new ways to express themselves and understand their bodies, "the body level learning that occurs in this embodied, enactive work means that newly learned patterns could be easily generalized into everyday life (Goodill, 2018). Goals of DMT sessions for cancer patients currently include: overall quality of life, stress management, and perceived stress, pain management, reduction of anxiety, and fatigue, increases in sense of vitality, and energy, body awareness, and body image, social support, and the recognition of need for support, self-efficacy, and improved self-care, meaning making, and increases in resilience, and the installation of hope (Goodill, 2018). DMT is also known to support more "diversified and less monotonous approach compared to conventional fitness programmes" (Sturum et al, 2014). Offering these diverse approaches is what helps to make DMT stand out amongst other treatment approaches. DMT has been recognized as a positive outlet that "allows the patients to creatively and kinesthetically process the assaults of cancer and its treatment, and thus establish a stronger sense of self and improved quality of life" (Madden et al, 2010). The connections between the body and mind through creative interventions can assist in improving a patient's overall quality of life, demonstrated in both pediatric and adult patients (Madden, et al., 2010). Suzi Tortora explored the positive effects of DMT for children hospitalized for cancer. With her idea that movement and expression through dance are natural parts of childhood, one can translate this sentiment into adulthood. When they are compromised with a life-threatening disease such as cancer, it becomes more difficult to achieve movement, leaving them feeling a "sense of disempowerment and loss of control of one's body and stress physiology when facing a threatening, traumatic life event" (Tortora, 2019). Being able to move brings ownership and control back over the body. This somatic empowerment can help patients feel as if they can manage their illness. Intervening with a cancer diagnosis from a multi-dimensional kinesthetic approach can be called 'integrative oncology'. DMT, while still new to this field, definitely can be categorized into integrative oncology.

The opportunities for DMT to be used in an oncology setting are vast, as demonstrated here, but are not limited to quality of life, expression, or physical and mental health. There are many rich benefits to movement-based interventions for those undergoing chemotherapy treatments. With DMT stressing the idea of the mind-body connection, it is hoped that research broadens its lens to examine how DMT can support the retention and repair of cognitive abilities that are damaged during chemotherapy. In a DMT session focused around cognitive repair, patients can focus on meditation or other embodiment exercises, becoming mindful of their own bodies and bringing focus internally. They can utilize light stretching, similar to what is seen in yoga, and be modified to be done from a chair if energy levels are too low to be standing. Light movement around a space can be done to get the body active, while interacting and socializing with others around them. A group or an individual can work on memorizing a short movement phrase, building week to week to test their memory and retention. Movement patterns can be performed in a sequence, asking for them to be mirrored back to improve the ability to quickly recall. Not only are all of these activities focusing on getting the body moving, they are also pushing the brain to be just as active.

The research discussed in this literature review has shown altered states of grey and white cerebral matter. This visible change leads me to believe that there is more research that can be done to further understand the physiology and etiology of CRCI. The addition of movement into a patient's day to day life showed the physical changes in the brain, further proving the idea of the mind-body connection. My experience with the mind-body connection had promising results. Not only was I moving with my clients at my internship site instead of being an active observer on the sidelines, I went on short walks during available time. I took the time to move for myself and tap into my creative brain to create movement phrases. While I was not nearly as active as I used to be, my body was now up and moving. I started to notice a difference in my academic and cognitive abilities on the days I was more active. If I took the time to move and create, my words came to me at a quicker speed, I was less forgetful, and my typing was more precise. This became a small study for myself to truly discover if there is a link between my physical activity and cognitive abilities. The integration of mind and body helped me to care for myself on a different level. With the time taken to care for my body through dance and movement, my mind benefitted as well in retaining or rediscovering my cognitive abilities. From this experience, I learned the undeniable connection between the mind and the body and the role they play in working towards healing, whatever that may be.

With these personal experiences, I am hopeful that more research can be performed to garner support in that DMT can deepen the retention and repair of these cognitive abilities in cancer patients undergoing chemotherapy. There is a major theory to practice gap in DMT for oncology. I did not have access to a dance/movement therapist while I was in treatment, but from my research I can discern that the use of these skills would be more beneficial. The undeniable mind-body connection that was experienced during my treatment demonstrated the importance of both my own physical and mental health. In order to thrive in one area, I had to tend to the other. This small act in return improved my mood and quality of life. Being able to feel like "me" was powerful. The cyclical nature of the mind-body connection is a constant. As an individual with first-hand experience in the importance of incorporating movement to improve cognitive abilities, I have witnessed the mind-body connection that DMT inhabits, establishing its cruciality to this work and understanding of how movement can impact cognition after changes due to chemotherapy.

References

Berrol, C. F., Ooi, W. L., & Katz, S. S. (1997). Dance/Movement Therapy with Older Adults Who Have Sustained Neurological Insult: A Demonstration Project. *American Journal of Dance Therapy, 19*(2), 135-160. doi: 10.1023/A:1022316102961

Burzynska, A. Z., Jiao, Y., Knecht, A. M., Fanning, J., Awick, E. A., Chen, T., ... Kramer, A. F. (2017). White Matter Integrity Declined Over 6-Months, but Dance Intervention Improved Integrity of the Fornix of Older Adults. *Frontiers in Aging Neuroscience, 9*, 1-15. doi: 10.3389/fnagi.2017.00059

Campbell, K. L., Zadravec, K., Bland, K. A., Chesley, E., Wolf, F., & Janelsins, M. C. (2020). The Effect of Exercise on Cancer-Related Cognitive Impairment and Applications for Physical Therapy: Systematic Review of Randomized Controlled Trials. *Physical Therapy, 100*(3), 523–542. doi: 10.1093/ptj/pzz090

Campbell, K. L., Kam, J. W. Y., Neil-Sztramko, S. E., Ambrose, T. L., Handy, T. C., Lim, H. J., ... Boyd, L. A. (2017). Effect of aerobic exercise on cancer-associated cognitive impairment: A proof-of-concept RCT. *Psycho-Oncology, 27*, 53–60. doi: 10.1002/pon.4370

chemo brain. (2015). In The Editors of the American Heritage Dictionaries (Ed.), *The American Heritage Dictionary of Medicine* (2nd ed.). Boston, MA: Houghton Mifflin. Retrieved from http://ezproxyles.flo.org/login?url=https://search.credoreference.com/content/entry/hmmedicaldict/chemo_brain/0?institutionId=1429

Cohen, S. O., & Walco, G. A. (1999). Dance/Movement Therapy for Children and Adolescents with Cancer. *Cancer Practice, 7*(1), 34–42. doi: 10.1046/j.1523-5394.1999.07105.x

Deprez, S., Amant, F., Smeets, A., Peeters, R., Leemans, A., Hecke, W. V., Sunaert, S. (2012). Longitudinal Assessment of Chemotherapy-Induced Structural Changes in Cerebral White Matter and Its Correlation With Impaired Cognitive Functioning. *Journal of Clinical Oncology, 30*(3), 274–281. doi: 10.1200/jco.2011.36.8571

Fernandez, C. (2018, January 12). After Cancer At 18, I Learned 'Chemo Brain' Can Last Long Past Chemo. Retrieved March 2, 2020, from https://www.wbur.org/commonhealth/2018/01/12/chemobrain-can-last-past-chemo

Garner, D., & Erck, E. G. (2008). Effects of Aerobic Exercise and Resistance Training on Stage I and II Breast Cancer Survivors. *American Journal of Health Education, 39*(4), 200–205. doi: 10.1080/19325037.2008.10599039

Goodill, S. W. (2018). Accumulating Evidence for Dance/Movement Therapy in Cancer Care. *Frontiers in Psychology, 9*, 238–246. doi: 10.3389/fpsyg.2018.01778

International Expressive Arts Therapy Association. (n.d.). Who We Are. Retrieved April 28, 2020, from https://www.ieata.org/who-we-are

Kattenstroth, J.-C., Kalisch, T., Holt, S., Tegenthoff, M., & Dinse, H. R. (2013). Six months of dance intervention enhances postural, sensorimotor, and cognitive performance in elderly without affecting cardio-respiratory functions. *Frontiers in Aging Neuroscience, 5*, 1-16. doi: 10.3389/fnagi.2013.00005

Kesler, S. R., & Blayney, D. W. (2016). Neurotoxic Effects of Anthracycline- vs Nonanthracycline-Based Chemotherapy on Cognition in Breast Cancer Survivors. *JAMA oncology, 2*(2), 185–192. https://doi.org/10.1001/jamaoncol.2015.4333

Leszczynski, M. (2011). How Does Hippocampus Contribute to Working Memory Processing? *Frontiers in Human Neuroscience, 5*. doi: 10.3389/fnhum.2011.00168

Love, S. M., Love, E., & Lindsey, K. (2015). *Dr. Susan Loves breast book*. Boston, MA: Da Capo Lifelong.

Mackenzie, M. J., Carlson, L. E., Paskevich, D. M., Ekkekakis, P., Wurz, A. J., Wytsma, K., ... Culos-Reed, S. (2014). Associations between attention, affect and cardiac activity in a single yoga session for female cancer survivors: An enactive neurophenomenology-based approach. *Consciousness and Cognition, 27*, 129–146. doi: 10.1016/j.concog.2014.04.005

Madden, J. R., Mowry, P., Gao, D., Cullen, P. M., & Foreman, N. K. (2010). Creative Arts Therapy Improves Quality of Life for Pediatric Brain Tumor Patients Receiving Outpatient Chemotherapy. *Journal of Pediatric Oncology Nursing, 27*(3), 133–145. doi: 10.1177/1043454209355452

Mendelsohn, J. (1999). Dance/Movement Therapy with Hospitalized Children. *American Journal of Dance Therapy, 21*(2), 65–80. doi: 10.1023/a:1022152519119

Mo, C., Lin, H., Fu, F., Lin, L., Zhang, J., Huang, M., Chen, X. (2017). Chemotherapy-induced changes of cerebral activity in resting-state functional magnetic resonance imaging and cerebral white matter in diffusion tensor imaging. *Oncotarget, 8*(46), 81273–81284. doi: 10.18632/oncotarget.18111

Myers, J. S. (2009). Chemotherapy-Related Cognitive Impairment. *Clinical Journal of Oncology Nursing, 13*(4), 413–421. doi: 10.1188/09.cjon.413-421

Pietrangelo, A. (2018, June 26). Chemo Brain With Cancer Survivors Retrieved January 28, 2020, from https://www.healthline.com/health-news/chemo-brain-cancer-survivors#1

Quinlan, E., Robertson, S., & Fitchner, P. (2017). Caring for cancer survivors with the popular expressive arts. *Journal of Applied Arts & Health, 8*(1), 9–24. doi: 10.1386/jaah.8.1.9_1

Salerno, E. A., Rowland, K., Kramer, A. F., & Mcauley, E. (2019). Acute aerobic exercise effects on cognitive function in breast cancer survivors: a randomized crossover trial. *BMC Cancer, 19*(1), 1-9. doi: 10.1186/s12885-019-5589-1

Sturm, I., Baak, J., Storek, B., Traore, A., & Thuss-Patience, P. (2014). Effect of dance on cancer-related fatigue and quality of life. *Supportive Care in Cancer, 22*(8), 2241–2249. doi: 10.1007/s00520-014-2181-8

Tannock, I. F., Ahles, T. A., Ganz, P. A., & Dam, F. S. V. (2004). Cognitive Impairment Associated With Chemotherapy for Cancer: Report of a Workshop. *Journal of Clinical Oncology, 22*(11), 2233–2239. doi: 10.1200/jco.2004.08.094

Tortora, S. (2019). Children Are Born to Dance! Pediatric Medical Dance/Movement Therapy: The View from Integrative Pediatric Oncology. *Children, 6*(1), 14–41. doi: 10.3390/children6010014

Wefel, J. S., Lenzi, R., Theriault, R. L., Davis, R. N., & Meyers, C. A. (2004). The cognitive sequelae of standard-dose adjuvant chemotherapy in women with breast carcinoma. *Cancer, 100*(11), 2292–2299. doi: 10.1002/cncr.20272

Welling, A. (2019, March 18). What is Dance/Movement Therapy? Retrieved January 31, 2020, from https://adta.org/2014/11/08/what-is-dancemovement-therapy/

Witt, C.; Balneaves, L.; Cardoso, M.; Cohen, L.; Greenlee, H.; Johnstone, P.; Kucuk, O.; Mailman, J.; Mao, J. (2017). A comprehensive definition for integrative oncology. *J. Natl. Cancer Inst. Monogr. 52*, 3–8.

DANCING WITH CANCER

Dorrie Orchard

I have been dancing for more than twenty years and during this time have been treated for two different types of cancer; the first nineteen years ago, involved lymph node removal and bilateral mastectomies and the second last year, chemotherapy alongside radiotherapy across my pelvic area. Different parts of my body have been affected therefore but I found that there was always some physical piece of me that could still participate in dance and mentally, all of me could. Tragically, cancer targets both the body and the mind, therefore any response to it needs to do the same. Dance, flamenco in my case, has helped me immensely to get through both episodes of my illnesses, aiding my return to physical strength and to mental positivity. Before my surgery for breast cancer, I practised my steps in the corridor outside the ward but in slippers rather than nailed shoes. Although logistically, I could not attend class for some time, I continued to go through the choreography at home, pushing myself a little but not too much and keeping focused on the day I would return. This latest recent diagnosis came very unexpectedly. I live an hour and a half's train journey from class, so found it impossible during and immediately after treatment to be present. Luckily, I have been able to work from videos sent by my tutor who has wonderfully supported me throughout, giving me encouragement without pressure. I have practised footwork on my kitchen floor, mentally worked through the choreography while the radiotherapy machines were spinning around me, imagined myself dancing to the music played over the noise of the MRI scanner and got myself back to class before the summer term ended. The autumn term's classes are signed up for. My doctors seem intrigued by my dancing, recording in their communications that I keep very active dancing flamenco. Is this because I am seventy, I wonder? (This I mention merely to say that dance is for everyone, regardless of age or ability). I promised I would show them one day. It is easy to feel out of control with a cancer diagnosis as if your body has let you down and is at the disposal now of others. While medical help is essential, there is much you can do to aid your own recovery. Dancing allows you to move your body in any way that you wish. It allows you to reassume control of it. But there is more. While helping to build physical strength it also allows you to express those feelings that may be locked deep inside. Not everyone wishes to talk with words. The body can speak its own hurt, fear, sadness, hope or elation. For me personally, dancing is part of my identity, something I cannot do without, a non-negotiable. It helped me heal and has gifted me both strength and joy. Music, rhythm and dance are deeply inherent in us all. Small children naturally love to move and dance while music can often reach those that cannot respond to words. Check online for the video of Marta C. González, once a prima ballerina but by this time an elderly dementia patient, who listens to a recording of Swan Lake and remembers. She sits in a wheelchair and dances with her arms, back on stage in the starring role. That is the healing power of dance, the force that aided my own recovery.

DANCING WITH CANCER

Krisztina Kerek

Type of cancer: Left breast cancer. Three times negative. Grade 3. Invasive ductal carcinoma. CT and bone scan showed no distant metastases. I was diagnosed with breast cancer on 13/10/2020. I started my usual flamenco courses in September 2020. It was just after the first covid lockdown period. My treatments started shortly after diagnosis as they considered my status to be serious. I was treated at the Royal Marsden Hospital, Sutton and Chelsea.

My treatment was in four parts:

- Four months of chemotherapy
- Operation (mastectomy - an 8-hour operation)
- Radiotherapy (3 weeks)
- Post-operation medication (6 weeks)

When I started my chemotherapy treatment, I had my usual dancing courses and workshops in college. I did all of them, my weekly classes and workshops, Spanish Dance Society exam preparation, and Morley Flamenco Dance Ensemble performance course and I also performed in a professionally produced dance video as part of Morley Flamenco Dance Ensemble (*Lockdown Alegrias*). Then the second wave of the covid lockdown period started, towards the end of November 2020. We couldn't come to dance in the college anymore but we could still attend our dance courses online, which I was able to do (via video recordings of the live-streamed classes). At the beginning of my chemotherapy treatment, it was not very difficult to dance. Although, after the second round of chemotherapy, my body became slowly sensitive to movement. Under the lockdown, I followed dancing through videos as much as I could. I had lots of hospital appointments beyond my chemotherapy and other basic ongoing treatments. During the second part of my chemotherapy treatments, I was unable to do any strong movements at home as my haemoglobin level started going down, so I didn't have much strength to dance. Fortunately, it didn't last long as I always take lots of vitamins, which helped me to get my strength back. After chemotherapy, I had 6 weeks break before my operation. During this time the college was allowed to open up again and I attended some dance lessons in the studio. I went back to college and danced, just three weeks after my operation. The first lesson was Morley Flamenco Dance Ensemble (usually on Sundays), then ongoing workshops and weekly classes. I had to be careful with my movements, for example, bending, especially backwards, and stretching my body and arms. Otherwise, it was fine. Later on, post-operation medications caused my feet to start to swell up. These post-operation medications were basically too much for my body to cope with. Dance helped me to go through this hard period of my life but mainly, and most importantly, dance was not an escape from this illness. Instead, it gave me strength, psychologically, physically and mentally to reach my aims. I'm the sort of person who always has goals and I concentrate on those goals, knowing very strongly where I want to end up. That strength and belief help me to get through obstacles in my life. I do things which interest me, such as dancing and teaching the English language (I'm an EFL Teacher in the UK). Also, I have been doing some social work (when I need to), helping people who need help, and doing good deeds. These are things which cheer me up. I'm not concentrating on bad things; I'm trying to avoid crying or struggling as much as I can. In the hospital, right after diagnosis, they asked me what my aim is. I said: "I'd like to go through this as fast as possible. Please save my life". They did that. I followed instructions very strictly. I can say I received a very high level of care from the NHS. My medical practitioners advised me the following regarding moving and dancing: moving is allowed, just keep away from aggressive movements. I think I managed to look after myself very well. Finally, I am fully recovered and just need now to have yearly checks.

I strongly advise anyone who is in a similar situation to think and concentrate on positive things. Set goals in life and do interesting things, following whatever interests them rather than concentrating on the disease and its problems. Well, it is not easy but mind over matter. For me, it was so hard as the whole thing happened during the covid lockdown, so I couldn't travel back home to Hungary. I kept in touch with my parents through technology (e.g. right after my operation I rang them from the critical care unit after 6pm; that was a great relief) but I couldn't go to see them and they couldn't come to see me. However, I had lots of support from my flamenco dance friends. My teacher, Fenella, was pampering me through the Internet. While I was undergoing my chemotherapy treatment, I continued to do social work (working in care homes) where people were really helpful, including donating money for me, etc.

DANCING WITH CANCER

Marlena Sakala

Type of cancer: secondary breast cancer

- **Length and type of treatment**: chemotherapy - 6 cycles, around 5 months

- **How did you participate in dance activities during your treatment? In the studio / via Microsoft Teams / via videos of classes or a mixture of all 3?**
  A mixture of all 3, however in the studio was my favourite and I tried to be there as often as I could.

- **What were the benefits of dancing through your treatment, ie positivity/motivation, fitness, carrying on as normal, socialising, escaping through dance, or something else?**
  Learning flamenco during treatment gave me lots of joy and happiness, and also increased my energy level. I had the feeling of normality and the motivation to carry on. I was positive and also keen on doing other stuff. It also allowed me to escape from the negative thoughts as I had to focus, follow the routine and also listen to music and rhythms. It was like jumping into a different world and forgetting about the surreal things happening in my life.

- **What were the difficulties of dancing through your treatment and how did you overcome them or did you overcome them?**
  The only difficult thing for me was not being able to come to the studio sometimes. Luckily, I could participate in the class via Microsoft Teams although as I mentioned before being in the studio is my favourite form of learning flamenco.

- **What would you say to someone thinking of dancing through cancer treatment, based on your own experiences?**
  I would strongly recommend it as there are lots of benefits. It is a form of exercise, which is recommended during chemotherapy. However it is important to realise that chemotherapy weakens the body, so if you get too tired during the class, just sit down and have a rest, do not push yourself too much.

- **Did your doctors or any other medical practitioners comment on you dancing through your treatment?**
  I did not mention it to the doctors.

- **In hindsight, is there anything you would have done differently?**
  No, there is nothing I would do differently, I am very happy that I did not give up dancing when I received my diagnosis as it helped so much in different aspects of my life.

TAO TE CHING OF A VIBRANT DIET

Prof. Chris Palmer

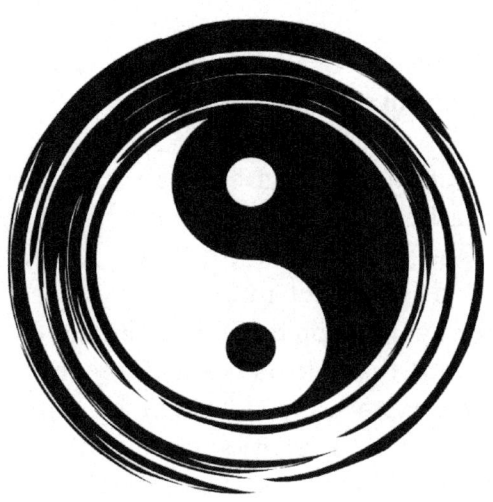

A vibrant diet which can aid the prevention, treatment and recurrence of cancer should provide us with the necessary energy sources to drive the processes within our cells but also provide vital nutrients such as vitamins and minerals. Food affects our mood, immune system, sleep, creativity, cognition, and recovery from injury or disease. Additionally, our nutrition should provide the phytochemicals obtained from plants to prevent cells from becoming pre-initiated for cancer and provide natural anti-inflammatory phytochemicals to reduce inflammation in the body which can cause or enhance other diseases such as cardiovascular disease, vascular dementia, diabetes and liver or pancreas inflammation. The body can be divided according to scientific principles into eleven different systems. These systems and their <u>major</u> functions are listed below.

Integumentary system	skin - acts as a barrier to the external environment
Skeletal system	provides support for the body to enable movement
Immune system	defence against microorganisms, parasites, and viruses
Muscular system	augments movement with the skeletal system
Lymphatic system	removes waste, prevents infection, regulates fluids
Respiratory system	provides oxygen to produce cellular energy
Digestive system	absorption of nutrients from food into the body

Nervous system   includes the mind, senses, coordination of movement
Endocrine system   hormones- communication between parts of the body
Cardiovascular system   pumps and supplies nutrients to all cells in the body
Urinary system   filters and removes waste from the blood
Reproductive systems   provide structures and mechanisms for reproduction

Homeostasis - maintaining an internal balance

The quality of your nutrition will have effects on all these systems which is important to maintain a healthy and vibrant life, in particular when you are undergoing or recovering from cancer treatment. However, each of these systems does not work by itself but through a process called "homeostasis" mediated by internal communication between cells and tissues. Homeostasis is a property of living systems that allows the maintenance and regulation of an organism as a whole. Homeostasis is a state that is maintained by the constant adjustment of biochemical and physiological pathways. For example, maintenance of blood pressure is important for the delivery of nutrients around the whole body via the blood vessels which branch through our body delivering oxygen, sugars, amino acids, and fats to every cell and taking away waste products. The regulation of blood pressure is accomplished through a series of fine adjustments to the hormonal, neuromuscular, and cardiovascular systems. These adjustments allow the maintenance of blood pressure needed for the body to function despite environmental changes and changes in a person's activity level and position. Your whole body is in a state of homeostasis where the body is a sum of its parts all working together in harmony. Not surprising then that one part of your body can affect another part. As such it is important during cancer treatment and recovery to treat the whole body not just the part affected but also to consider the effect on the mind and spirit.

Deficiencies in scientific thought concerning nutrition

It is both an advantage and a weakness of science to separate things into categories and systems. This is an analytical method and should not be utilized when trying to understand the whole person. As an example, I may as a scientist be able to describe the systems which make up your body in detail, but this would not allow me to understand you as a living being. Thus, the whole is much more than a sum of its parts. In fact, this separation has its origins in "European" philosophy to divide, conquer and ultimately understand the human body. This scientific analysis can only understand the human body to a degree as a separation of its constituent parts. The effects of this philosophy on civilization can be seen in religion, nature, science, philosophy, and metaphysics where there is a separation of mankind from an anthropomorphic God in the so-called "West". While traditionally in the "East" there is an inward-directed search for union with the whole. Therefore, creation can be seen as a fragmentation of the whole according to "traditional Western" thought, while "traditional Eastern" thought seeks a reunion with the cosmic "oneness" through an egoless life. We can see this in the writings of Descartes who said, "I think therefore I am" and thus the spirit/mind was cleaved from the body. Such thought processes have led us to "vandalize" the temple that is our body ignoring our intuition and the natural processes in our bodies. For example, high blood pressure and some cases of type 2 diabetes can be reversed without recourse to pills through diet modification and exercise. Note however this does not mean a rejection of the benefits of science but a re-joining of modern science with older traditional philosophies to come to a more enlightened understanding of our bodies and their needs.

Taoist philosophy

Science cannot define or explain everything, especially regarding complex systems such as our bodies. Science is useful however in understanding natural phenomena through isolation and separation. To fully understand the human body (as a whole) "Eastern" philosophy should be merged with modern-day science as according to the Tao Te Ching there are no simple answers to life's mysteries [Mitchell, 2006]. The Tao Te Ching is a Chinese classic text and one of the founding texts of Taoism, an ancient Chinese philosophical and religious tradition. The Tao Te Ching includes short verses regarding several central aspects of Taoism, such as action, the duality of nature, knowledge, and virtue [Mitchell, 2006]. Therefore according to the Tao Te Ching, it is important to realise that knowledge is not knowing and that both knowledge and intuition should be utilized when considering the fundamental process of taking care of our body. Food and activity can affect our physical energy, all organ systems, cognition, health, and mental state. It should therefore be realised that the concept that our bodies are just mechanical engines requiring fuel to power us is incomplete wisdom. A feature of Taoist philosophy is the concept of duality a Ying and Yang with both polarities being important in encompassing the whole [Mitchell, 2006]. Therefore, when it comes to cancer nutrition or any nutrition it is important to consider both the body, mind, and spirit. Ignoring any of these can lead to excessive dietary habits. For example, going on an extreme diet or a diet which avoids certain food groups you would think may be one way to become healthy, however, this negates the fact that this will affect your mind leading to cravings for food and possible weight fluctuations rather than weight loss in the long term. Additionally, it will affect your mood and may lead to depressive symptoms. Therefore, a diet regime could be described as having Yang principles and therefore is likely to fail. Although some short-term weight loss may be obtained, overall such a diet would be detrimental to your whole body's health. On the other hand, listening to intuition alone may lead to unhealthy diet choices as we "give in" to our cravings for "unhealthy" food especially given the bombardment of our visual senses with food adverts and the ease of pre-prepared or takeaway food. The fact is that neither is correct all the time balance must be achieved by taking on both principles. Therefore, nutrition should be modified without cutting out food groups, this is the Yang principle. Intuition, asking yourself what your body is telling you that you need to eat represents a Yin principle. Listen to your body and mind as a whole when determining your meal choices. Acknowledging that sometimes you will want to eat food which may be considered "unhealthy food" is a part of this concept but always returning to your centre afterwards without feeling guilty, rather than ignoring your intuition and sticking to a rigid diet plan. Although this writing may sound very transcendental, the Tao Te Ching is a philosophy which has lasted over 3000 years [Mitchell, 2006]. Science has given us technology capable of complex fabrications and advances in our lives and health while on the other hand destroying our natural environment and overall being detrimental to our health with increasing obesity, diabetes, abnormal diet conditions and metabolic disorders.

Conclusions

In a summary, to achieve wisdom both knowledge and intuition should be utilized when considering nutrition. Rather than focusing on an easy fix for cancer, we should remove the root causes of cancer. In one study, 50% of breast cancer patients were taking a multivitamin, but 70% of these individuals had an unhealthy BMI, one of the main risk factors for increased risk of breast cancer. The real focus should not be on supplements, but on eating a healthy diet focused on whole grains, vegetables, fruits, and legumes that will nourish your body with all the nutrients you need to prevent and treat cancer and other chronic diseases which are often prevalent in individuals with cancer. Drastically cutting down on calories, omitting or reducing food groups and eating bland food will result in mental stress and will not provide the nutrition needed to live a vibrant and productive life. A healthy body can be achieved in general by modification of nutrition to provide natural vitamins and minerals, lowering simple sugar consumption, avoiding unhealthy fats, increasing fibre, and eating foods which make you feel full and that satisfy your appetite. However, also realise that on some days we will want to eat "unhealthy foods", and rather than stick to a rigid regime build into our meals days when we can simply enjoy these types of food types without feeling guilty. In this way, the entire system of body will function in an optimum manner feeding the mind, body and spirit.

References

Mitchell S. Tao Te Ching: A New English Version. Harper Collins USA; 2006.

MICROBIOME, NUTRITION, CANCER, AND MENTAL HEALTH

Afshan Aghili

The human body is host to trillions of microorganisms which are mostly made up of bacterial cells [Sender et al., 2016]. These microorganisms are collectively known as the microbiome and are believed to play a role in many aspects of our health ranging from breaking down food to fighting illness. The quantity and diversity of microorganisms in the gut stretch from the stomach to the colon [Thursby and Juge, 2017]. There are variations in every person's microbiome which is influenced by genetics and factors such as diet, physical activity, illnesses, medication (in particular antibiotics) and other environmental exposures. The characteristics of a healthy microbiome are currently not properly understood and are the subject of rigorous research however, there is convincing scientific consensus that an imbalanced microbiome can be associated with several adverse health conditions including cancer (Vijay and Valdes, 2022).

In recent times, the actions of the microbiome and its influence on diseases such as cancer have become the subject of much research. In particular, its role in the treatment of cancer has indicated that modifications to the gut microbiome can affect cancer therapy [Chaput et al., 2017, Frankel et al., 2017, Gopalakrishnan et al., 2018]. It is widely accepted that our immune system plays a major role in cancer, its progression and its response to treatment [Chen and Mellman, 2017, Spitzer et al., 2017]. As the microbiota is made up of trillions of microbial cells, they have the ability to interact with numerous functions including our immunity functions [Synder et al., 2016]. The role of the microbiome and the immune system can be explained through the actions of the microbiota (microorganism) which take place at the site of the gut. The gut microbiota which inhabits the gastrointestinal (GI) tract provides fundamental health benefits by regulating our immune homeostasis. This close interaction with the immune system is thought to play a critical role in averting bacterial invasion and infection by recognising and attacking harmful bacteria thereby increasing immune response [Honda and Littman, 2016]. The cells in the intestine support the interaction with the immune system through the secretion of a mucus layer. In addition to this, there are a number of immune cells and beneficial lymphoid cells which are present underneath this mucosal layer. These lymphoid cells which are related to the gut form the biggest part of the immune system thereby incurring beneficial immune responses. Further evidence of the importance of the microbiota at the gut level comes from models involving mice with severely defective immunity when devoid of intestinal microbiota and lacking the protective mucus layer [Spiljar et al., 2017]. The homeostatic balance of the intestinal microbiota is therefore an important contributor to the immune system. Consequently, any alterations to the composition or functions of the intestinal microbiota can result in reductions in microbial diversity and increases in pathogenic bacteria causing a condition known as dysbiosis [Bien et al., 2013, Knights et al., 2013, Frosali et al., 2015, Levy et al., 2017]. This imbalance in the microbial equilibrium which results in dysbiosis has been associated with increased risk of several pathological conditions such as obesity, diabetes, neurodegenerative diseases and cancers as well as inflammatory bowel diseases such as Crohn's Disease and Ulcerative Colitis.

Colorectal cancer (CRC) which is the third most common cancer globally and one of the leading causes of mortality has been associated with impaired gut microbiota composition [Xi and Xu 2020, Ferlay et al., 2012]. Whilst the precise cause of CRC is not fully understood, genetic and environmental factors have been indicated in its aetiology. In particular, sedentary lifestyle, smoking and diets high in fat, rich in processed and red meat, low intake of fibre, excessive alcohol consumption, and obesity have been implicated in worsening the composition of the gut microbiota [Xi and Xu 2020, Nakatsu et al., 2015]. Recent research has shown that the gut microbiota can alter the progression of colorectal cancer through the production of metabolites which cause inflammation and damage to the DNA resulting in tumour progression [Dzutsev et al., 2014]. Patients with CRC have been shown to have dysbiosis of gut microbiota with reductions in beneficial bacterial species and increases in harmful pro-inflammatory pathogens.

Various studies have demonstrated that carcinogenicity is strongly attributed to microbial dysbiosis. A review of the latest evidence indicates that diet plays a critical role in the risk of developing CRC. It appears that the regulation of the gut microbiota through diets high in fibre accompanied with polyunsaturated fatty acids, polyphenols and probiotics may be associated with lowering the risk of CRC and even improved response to cancer therapy when used in addition to conventional treatment. Hence modification of the gut microbiome through dietary intake can be an encouraging strategy for the prevention, progression and treatment of CRC. Other forms of carcinogenesis such as gastric cancer are understood to involve bacterial infections [Polk and Peek 2010]. Gastric cancer is characterised as inflammation-associated cancer. Infections caused by the bacteria known as *Helicobacter pylori* (*H. pylori*) is considered to be a major risk factor in its development [Diaz et al., 2018]. It appears that infections caused by *H. pylori* stimulate inflammation and immune responses leading to precancerous lesions which can progress to intestinal metaplasia, then dysplasia and finally gastric cancer [Diaz et al., 2018]. Therefore, eradicating *H. pylori* could be a preventative strategy to combat gastric cancer [Doorakkers et al., 2016].

Pancreatic ductal adenocarcinoma (PDAC) is the most common type of pancreatic cancer and is considered to be one of the most fatal cancers worldwide. Known risk factors such as smoking, chronic pancreatitis, obesity and type 2 diabetes are estimated to be responsible for under half of all pancreatic cancer cases. In addition to this, pathogenic microorganisms associated with gut microbiota also play a role in pancreatic carcinogenesis via increased cancer-associated inflammation [Wang and Li, 2015, Zambirinis, 2014]. *Other risk factors include H. pylori,* infections which may also play a part in pancreatic cancer production through dysregulation of pancreatic cellular processes and increased inflammation [Manes et al., 2003]. Liver cancer is believed to be influenced by the pathogens produced by the microbiota in the GI tract through the hepatic portal system. The role of the liver in neutralising toxins from intestinal microbes can become impaired due to gut microbial dysbiosis leading to liver cancer [Ohtani, 2015]. This process involves bile acids which regulate the gut microbiome causing DNA damage as well as accelerated inflammation [Payne et al., 2007, Ridlon et al., 2014, Louis et al., 2014]. Oesophageal cancer (EC) is characterised by a malignant tumour of the upper digestive tract and is one of the most common cancers globally [Smyth et al., 2017]. Whilst the exact cause of EC is unknown, like other cancers, genetic and environmental factors such as smoking and increased alcohol consumption play a key role in the formation and progression of EC [Lichtenstein et al., 2000]. More recent studies have shown that drinking very hot tea may also be associated with an increased risk of EC [Kamangar et al., 2018]. Mounting evidence has shown that patients with EC display changes in their microbial composition. Therefore, it appears that once again mechanisms related to cancer development such as inflammation and impaired immunity are closely linked to the gut microbiota [Zou et al., 2021].

Nutrition and Gut Health

It is evident that gut microbiota can exert a powerful influence on cancers of the GI tract. Therefore, improving gut health through diet is now the subject of intense research. It is well established that the immune system can be stimulated by our microbiota which can break down toxic compounds. Consuming plant-based foods containing complex carbohydrates such as starches and fibre can help increase the amount and diversity of the microbes in the gut. For example, dietary fibre can only be broken down and fermented by the microbiota in the colon. The result of the fermentation process is the production of short-chain fatty acids (SCFA) which lowers the pH of the colon making the environment acidic and thereby preventing the growth of harmful bacteria. In addition to this, SCFA may benefit the host by stimulating the activity of the immune system as well as controlling normal blood levels of cholesterol and glucose [den Besten et al., 2013].

Prebiotics

Foods which can increase SCFA are referred to as prebiotics and include complex carbohydrates and fibre such as resistant starches, inulin, gums, pectins and fructo-oligosaccharides and galacto-oligosaccharides. Prebiotics can improve our immunity by increasing the population of protective bacteria. Studies have shown that prebiotics can also reduce the number of harmful bacteria. Also, prebiotics can generate immunity molecules, known as cytokines [Steed and Macfarlane, 2009] Prebiotics can be obtained by consuming: Jerusalem artichokes, asparagus, garlic, onions, leeks, bananas, and seaweed. Generally, good sources of prebiotics include plant-based foods such as vegetables, dandelion greens, fruits, legumes and whole grains (oat and barley).

Probiotics

Probiotics are referred to foods that naturally contain microbiota or supplements which contain live active bacteria. Best sources of naturally occurring probiotics can be found in natural bio-live yoghurts and other fermented foods including:

- Kefir (fermented milk)
- Kombucha (fermented tea)
- Miso (fermented soybean paste)
- Kimchi (fermented vegetables)
- Sauerkraut (fermented cabbage)
- Tempeh (fermented soybean paste)

A number of studies have suggested that probiotics may reduce the risk of certain GI cancers by improving the gut microbiota. However, there is disagreement on the beneficial effects of probiotics on cancer and a mechanism for their antitumour properties is yet to be fully understood. The main effect of probiotics is believed to be their role in maintaining the homeostasis of the colon and their involvement in regulating the pH and bile acids. It is proposed that in the future, probiotics may be used in the prevention of cancer and its treatment [Jia et al., 2017].

Synbiotics

This refers to a combination of probiotic bacteria and prebiotics produced to work together (synergistically) in the digestive tract. The main purpose of these is to support the survival of probiotics in the colon, stimulate the growth of probiotics and improve the microbiota by increasing its microbial composition. However, the beneficial actions of synbiotics are still under research and much of the evidence comes from laboratory studies. Further research on their actions in the human body is still needed to make recommendations for their use [Iannitti and Palmieri, 2010, Rafter et al., 2007].

Dance and Gut Health

Most of the cancers reviewed in this chapter have implicated low physical activity as one of the risk factors for their development. The question is can dance improve microbial species, increase microflora diversity, and improve gut health? Whilst, there are limited studies on the effects of dance on gut microbiota, the evidence suggests that both nutrition and exercise can enhance the beneficial microbial species. It appears that increased physical activity can improve the microbiota's responsive to both homeostatic and physiological regulations [Bermon et al., 2015].

To date, the evidence suggests that physical activity can exert positive influences on the GI tract such as reducing the stool transit time thereby reducing the length of time pathogens would be in contact with the GI tract [Bermon et al., 2015]. Exercise can incur important protective effects by reducing the risk of colon cancer, and other inflammatory bowel diseases [Peters et al., 2001]. Furthermore, exercise may protect the intestine and prevent inflammation even in the presence of high-fat diets [Campbell et. al., 2016]. Ordinarily, intake of a high-fat diet and low physical activity has been shown to result in inflammation and impaired form and function of the intestine.

Further evidence that exercise is beneficial to gut health comes from studies conducted by Estaki et al., 2016 where faecal samples were examined and found to be closely associated with cardiorespiratory fitness. The results also illustrated that cardiorespiratory fitness was correlated with increased gut microbial diversity regardless of diet. Furthermore, fit individuals such as dancers are believed to have a microbiome rich in bacterial species such as *Clostridiales, Roseburia, Lachnospiraceae*, and *Erysipelotrichaceae*, which can increase SCF production and improve gut health. In light of these findings, exercise such as dance could be potentially used as an additional form of treatment for diseases related to dysbiosis.

Microbiome and Mental Health

There is mounting evidence that the gut microbiota plays a vital role in our regulation of metabolic, endocrine and immune functions. More recent evidence suggests that the gut microbiota is also involved in our neurochemical pathways. The two-way communication between the central nervous system and gut microbiota is known as the gut-brain axis [Carabotti et al., 2015]. However, the exact mechanism for this bidirectional communication between the gut and the brain is not fully understood. This bidirectional communication is thought to be transmitted via pathways including:

- the vagus nerve which connects the brain to the colon [Carabotti et al., 2015]
- the immune system [Carabotti et al., 2015]
- the hypothalamic-pituitary-adrenal (HPA) axis [Mudd et al., 2017]
- tryptophan metabolism which has the ability to synthesise neurotransmitters and produce as SCFA with neuroactive properties [O'Mahony et al., 2015, Calvani et al., 2018, Dalile et al., 2019]

Our understanding so far indicates that SCFAs which are metabolites produced by the fermentation of fibre in the colon play a major role in neuro-immunoendocrine regulation thereby affecting the brain and behaviour. It appears that these SCFA are closely linked with neurotransmitters and brain-derived neurotrophic factor (BDNF). Emerging evidence suggests that neurotrophic factors can build neurons and aid in the synthesis of serotonin. In addition, BDNF supports neuroplasticity which means the brain remains flexible and resilient. Overall, it is believed that the combined actions of the SCFAs and BDNF can affect cognitive behaviour, emotional behaviour and brain disorders [Savignac et al., 2013, Kim et al., 2009]. Further proof that the gut microbiota influences mental health comes from animal studies where it has been shown that emotional behaviour in mice is altered when there are changes in the gut microbiome [Cryan and Dinan, 2012] and similarly depressive disorders in humans are associated with changes of the gut microbiome [Kelly et al., 2016]. Furthermore, in studies where faecal matter from humans suffering from depression has been transferred into mice, depressive symptoms have been observed in the mice. Research suggests that gut microbiota is an important driver in the bidirectional communications between the gut and the nervous system and it can regulate brain chemistry, and response to stress, anxiety and memory. However, these effects tend to depend on specific bacterial strains indicating that certain probiotic strains may be used as additional innovative strategies to treat neurological disorders [Carabotti et al., 2015]. These findings have important implications for the role of improving gut health to prevent and treat depressive symptoms such as low mood and anxiety. However, further research is needed to fully understand the role of nutrition on the brain. Overall, it is exciting to acknowledge that in the near future, it may be possible to consider dietary interventions as one of the therapies to reduce the symptoms of depressive disorders.

In general, research into interactions between microorganisms and tumours has shaped our understanding of the involvement of microbiota and chronic disease. The evidence suggests that imbalances in microbiota can cause inflammation and dysregulation of the immune system, leading to genetic impairment and disease development. In future, it may be viable to use the microbiota as a screening tool to detect microbial activity and dysbiosis. This could lead to treating cancer and lowering the harmful effects of cancer treatment by modifying the levels of microorganisms. Ultimately, nutrition appears to play a critical role in maintaining a healthy gut microbiome and it has the potential to be used as a therapeutic strategy to modify the composition and function of the gut microbiome. Understanding the composition of a healthy microbiome will be a key tool in manipulating the microbiome to improve health.

References:

Sender R., Fuchs S., Milo R. Revised Estimates for the Number of Human and Bacteria Cells in the Body. PLoS Biol. 2016; 14(8): e1002533. doi: 10.1371/journal.pbio.1002533

Thursby E., Juge N., Introduction to the human gut microbiota. Biochem J. 2017 1; 474(11): 1823–1836. doi: 10.1042/BCJ20160510

Vijay A., Vlades A., Role of the gut microbiome in chronic diseases: a narrative review. Eur J of Clin Nutr **76**, 489–501 (2022). doi.org/10.1038/s41430-021-00991-6

N. Chaput, P. Lepage, C. Coutzac, E. Soularue, K. LeRoux, C. Monot, L. Boselli, E. Routier, L. Cassard, M. Collins, et al. Baseline gut microbiota predicts clinical response and colitis in metastatic melanoma patients treated with ipilimumab Ann Oncol. 2017 1;28(6):1368-1379. doi: 10.1093/annonc/mdx108

A.E. Frankel, L.A. Coughlin, J. Kim, T.W. Froehlich, Y. Xie, E.P. Frenkel, A.Y. Koh Metagenomic shotgun sequencing and unbiased metabolomic profiling identify specific human gut microbiota and metabolites associated with immune checkpoint therapy efficacy in melanoma patients Neoplasia, 19 (2017), pp. 848-855

V. Gopalakrishnan, C.N. Spencer, L. Nezi, A. Reuben, M.C. Andrews, T.V. Karpinets, P.A. Prieto, D. Vicente, K. Hoffman, S.C. Wei, et al. Gut microbiome modulates response to anti-PD-1 immunotherapy in melanoma patients. Science, 359 (2018), pp. 97-103

D.S. Chen, I. Mellman. Oncology meets immunology: the cancer-immunity cycle Immunity, 39 (2013), pp. 1-10

M.H. Spitzer, Y. Carmi, N.E. RetickerFlynn, S.S. Kwek, D. Madhireddy, M.M. Martins, P.F. Gherardini, T.R. Prestwood, J. Chab on, S.C. Bendall, et al. Systemic immunity is required for effective cancer immunotherapy. Cell, 168 (2017), pp. 487-502.e15

A. Snyder, V. Makarov, T. Merghoub, J. Yuan, J.M. Zaretsky, A. Desrichard, L.A. Walsh, M.A. Postow, P. Wong, T.S. Ho, et al. Genetic basis for clinical response to CTLA-4 blockade in melanoma. N. Engl. J. Med., 371 (2014), pp. 2189-2199

K. Honda, D.R. Littman. The microbiota in adaptive immune homeostasis and disease. Nature, 535 (2016), pp. 75-84

M. Spiljar, D. Merkler, M. Trajkovski. The immune system bridges the gut microbiota with systemic energy homeostasis: focus on TLRs, mucosal barrier, and SCFAs Front. Immunol., 8 (2017), p. 1353

M. Levy, A.A. Kolodziejczyk, C.A. Thaiss, E. Elinav Dysbiosis and the immune system. Nat. Rev. Immunol., 17 (2017), pp. 219-232

Bien J, Palagani V, Bozko P, et al. The intestinal microbiota dysbiosis and *Clostridium difficile* infection: is there a relationship with inflammatory bowel disease? Ther Adv Gastroenterol. 2013;6:53–68.

Knights D, Lassen K, Xavier R. Advances in inflammatory bowel disease pathogenesis: linking host genetics and the microbiome. Gut. 2013;62(10):1505–10.

Frosali, D. Pagliari, G. Gambassi, R. Landolfi, F. Pandolfi, R. Cianci. How the intricate interaction among toll-like receptors, microbiota, and intestinal immunity can influence gastrointestinal pathology J. Immunol. Res., 2015 (2015), p. 489821

Polk DB, Peek RM. Helicobacter pylori: gastric cancer and beyond. Nat Rev Cancer 2010;10:40314 doi:10.1038/nrc2857

Diaz P, Vladerrama MV, Bravo J and Quest AFG. Helicobacter pylori and Gastric Cancer: Adaptive Cellular Mechanisms Involved in Disease Progression. Front. Microbiol 2018. Sec. Infectious Agents and Disease https://doi.org/10.3389/fmicb.2018.00405

Xi Y and Xu P. Global colorectal cancer burden in 2020 and projections to 2040. Transl Oncol., 2021;14(10): 101174 https://doi.org/10.1016/j.tranon.2021.101174

Ferlay J., Soerjomataram I., Dikshit R., Eser S., Mathers C., Rebelo M., Parkin N.M., Forman D., Bray F. Cancer incidence and mortality worldwide: Sources, methods and major patterns in Globocan 2012. Int. J. Cancer. 2014;136:359–386. doi: 10.1002/ijc.29210.

Nakatsu G., Li X., Zhou H., Sheng J., Wong S.H., Wu W.K., Ng S.C., Tsoi H., Dong Y., Zhang N., et al. Gut mucosal microbiome across stages of colorectal carcinogenesis. Nat. Commun. 2015;6:8727. doi: 10.1038/ncomms9727.

Doorakkers E., Lagergren J., Engstrand L., Brusselaers N. Eradication of Helicobacter pylori and gastric cancer: a systematic review and meta-analysis of cohort studies. J Natl Cancer Inst. 2016;108:djw132.

Louis P., Hold G.L., Flint H.J. The gut microbiota, bacterial metabolites and colorectal cancer. Nat Rev Microbiol. 2014;12:661–672.

Wang C., Li J. Pathogenic microorganisms and pancreatic cancer. Gastrointest Tumors. 2015;2:41–47.

Zambirinis C.P., Pushalkar S., Saxena D., Miller G. Pancreatic cancer, inflammation, and microbiome. Cancer J. 2014;20:195–202.

Manes G., Balzano A., Vaira D. *Helicobacter pylori* and pancreatic disease. JOP. 2003;4:111–116.

Ohtani N. Microbiome and cancer. Semin Immunopathol. 2015;37:65–72.

Payne C.M., Weber C., Crowley-Skillicorn C., Dvorak K., Bernstein H., Bernstein C. Deoxycholate induces mitochondrial oxidative stress and activates NF-kappaB through multiple mechanisms in HCT-116 colon epithelial cells. Carcinogenesis. 2007;28:215–222.

Ridlon J.M., Kang D.J., Hylemon P.B., Bajaj J.S. Bile acids and the gut microbiome. Curr Opin Gastroenterol. 2014;30:332–338.

Louis P., Hold G.L., Flint H.J. The gut microbiota, bacterial metabolites and colorectal cancer. Nat Rev Microbiol. 2014;12:661–672.

Smyth EC, Lagergren J, Fitzgerald RC, Lordick F, Shah MA, Lagergren P, et al.. Oesophageal Cancer. Nat Rev Dis Primers (2017) 3:17048. doi: 10.1038/nrdp.2017.48.

Lichtenstein P, Holm NV, Verkasalo PK, Iliadou A, Kaprio J, Koskenvuo M, et al.. Environmental and Heritable Factors in the Causation of Cancer–Analyses of Cohorts of Twins From Sweden, Denmark, and Finland. N Engl J Med (2000) 343(2):78–85. doi: 10.1056/NEJM200007133430201

Kamangar F, Freedman ND. Hot Tea and Esophageal Cancer. Ann Internal Med (2018) 168(7):519–20. doi: 10.7326/M17-3370

Zou J, Sun S, Xiao X, Yang Y, Mao C, et al., Gut Microbiata for Esophageal Cancer: Role in Carcinogenesis an dClinical Implications. Front. Oncol., (2021) Sec. Gastrointestinal Cancers doi: 10.3389/fon.2021.717242

den Besten G, Eunen K, Groen A, et al., The role of short-chain fatty acids in the interplay between diet, gut microbiota, and host energy metabolism. *J Lipid Res.* 2013 Sep; 54(9): 2325–2340

Steed H., Macfarlane S. Prebiotics and Probiotics Science and Technology. Springer; New York, NY, USA: 2009. Mechanisms of prebiotic impact on health; pp. 135–161.

Jia W, Xie G, Jia W. Bile acid–microbiota crosstalk in gastrointestinal inflammation and carcinogenesis. Nat Rev Gastroenterol Hepatol. 2017

Iannitti T, Palmieri B. Therapeutical use of probiotic formulations in clinical practice. Clin Nutr. 2010;29:701–25. doi: 10.1016/j.clnu.2010.05.004.

Rafter J, Bennett M, Caderni G, Clune Y, Hughes R, Karlsson PC, et al. Dietary synbiotics reduce cancer risk factors in polypectomized and colon cancer patients. Am J Clin Nutr. 2007;85:488–96.

Bermon S., Petriz B., Kajeniene A., Prestes J., Castell L., Franco O. L. The microbiota: an exercise immunology perspective. *Exercise Immunology Review*. 2015;21:70–79.

Peters H. P. F., De Vries W. R., Vanberge-Henegouwen G. P., Akkermans L. M. A. Potential benefits and hazards of physical activity and exercise on the gastrointestinal tract. *Gut*. 2001;48(3):435–439. doi: 10.1136/gut.48.3.435.

Campbell S. C., Wisniewski P. J., Noji M., et al. The effect of diet and exercise on intestinal integrity and microbial diversity in mice. *PLoS ONE*. 2016;11(3):1–17. doi: 10.1371/journal.pone.0150502.e0150502

Estaki M., Pither J., Baumeister P., et al. Cardiorespiratory fitness as a predictor of intestinal microbial diversity and distinct metagenomic functions. *The FASEB Journal*. 2016;30(1):1027–1035.

Carabotti M., Scirocco A., Severi C. The gut -brain axis: interactions between enteric microbiota, central and enteric nervous system. Ann Gastroenterol. 2015;28(2):203-209

Mudd AT, Berding K, Wang M, Donovan SM, Dilger RN. Serum cortisol mediates the relationship between fecal Ruminococcus and brain N-acetylaspartate in the young pig. Gut Microbes. (2017) 8:589–600. 10.1080/19490976.2017.1353849

O'Mahony SM, Clarke G, Borre YE, Dinan TG, Cryan JF. Serotonin, tryptophan metabolism and the brain-gut-microbiome axis. Behav Brain Res. (2015) 277:32–48. 10.1016/j.bbr.2014.07.027

Calvani R, Picca A, Lo Monaco MR, Landi F, Bernabei R, Marzetti E. Of microbes and minds: a narrative review on the second brain aging. Front Med. (2018) 5:53. 10.3389/fmed.2018.00053

Dalile B, Van Oudenhove L, Vervliet B, Verbeke K. The role of short-chain fatty acids in microbiota–gut–brain communication. Nat Rev Gastroenterol Hepatol. (2019) 16:461–78. 10.1038/s41575-019-0157-3

Savignac HM, Corona G, Mills H, Chen L, Spencer JPE, Tzortzis G, et al.. Prebiotic feeding elevates central brain derived neurotrophic factor, N-methyl-d-aspartate receptor subunits and d-serine. Neurochem Int. (2013) 63:756–64. 10.1016/j.neuint.2013.10.006

Kim HJ, Leeds P, Chuang DM. The HDAC inhibitor, sodium butyrate, stimulates neurogenesis in the ischemic brain. J Neurochem. (2009) 110:1226–40. 10.1111/j.1471-4159.2009.06212.x

Cryan JF, Dinan TG., Mind-altering microorganisms: the impact of the gut microbiota on brain and behaviour. *Nat Rev Neurosci.* 2012;13:701-12. doi:10.1038/nrn3346 pmid:22968153.

Kelly JR, Borre Y, O'Brien C, et al. Transferring the blues: depression-associated gut microbiota induces neurobehavioural changes in the rat. *J Psychiatr Res* 2016;82:109-18. doi:10.1016/j.jpsychires.2016.07.019 pmid:27491067.

NUTRITION AND CANCER

What to eat to prevent, augment the treatment of and stop the reoccurrence of cancer?

Professor Christopher Palmer, Dr Ebru Aydar and Eliz Arter

Despite advances made in cancer treatment for certain types of cancer, the fact is that the rate of cancer is increasing particularly for individuals who follow a Western dietary pattern. [Steck and Murphy, 2020]. There are good studies linking diet with the occurrence of breast, colon, and prostate cancer [Donaldson, 2004].

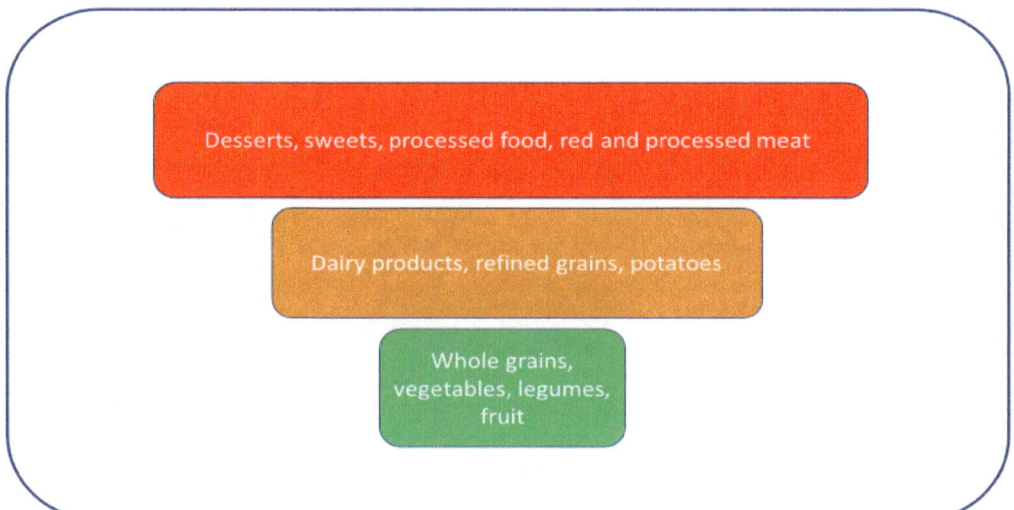

A typical Western diet is top heavy with a preponderance of sugar, processed food and meat products

The fact is that many cancers that occur have their roots in lifestyle or environment [Anand et al., 2008]. The role of nutrition on cancer incidence multi-factorial and complex which is a reason some studies may be contradictory.

Cancer is a product of sequential changes to our DNA which over time turn a normal cell into an invasive cell capable of spreading to other parts of our body (this is termed metastasis). These changes to our DNA are a result of both external and internal factors. One of the most important external factors is the nutrition which we supply to our cells which can either promote or inhibit the stages involved in transforming a normal cell into a cancerous one. Over thirty years ago the links between diet and cancer were investigated with a finding that more than a third of cancers are associated with dietary factors [Doll and Peto, 1981]. Furthermore, it is now clear that approximately 67% of colorectal cancers may be prevented by dietary changes [Block et al., 1992; Goon et al., 2022]. We are born with the genes that we inherited from our parents. However, the fact is that your DNA can be modified throughout your lifetime which can alter the pattern of expression of genes either involved in promoting or inhibiting cancer. Moreover, nutrition plays a significant part in how our DNA is modified. For example, in one study, after three months following a switch to a plant-based diet over 450 cancer genes were down-regulated and 48 cancer-inhibiting genes were up-regulated regarding prostate cancer [Ornish et al., 2008].

Mutagens and cancer

Mutation of our DNA is the root cause of the initiation of cancer. You will be surprised to know that on average every day the body suffers thousands of changes to its DNA.

Some of these changes will start a cell on its path to becoming cancerous ("pre-initiation"). The steps for a cell to become cancerous are many, however, every day some of the cells in our body become "pre-initiated" for cancer. The body supplied with the correct nutrients can disable these cells very effectively [Lee et al, 2013]. The early stages of most cancers are a result of changes in genes involved in the ability of cells to divide. This can often be powered by increases in growth hormones in the body resulting in a small colony of abnormal cells - a tumour, particularly for hormone-dependent cancers such as breast and prostate cancer. Further mutational changes can result in cells becoming invasive and eventually metastasizing to other parts of the body.

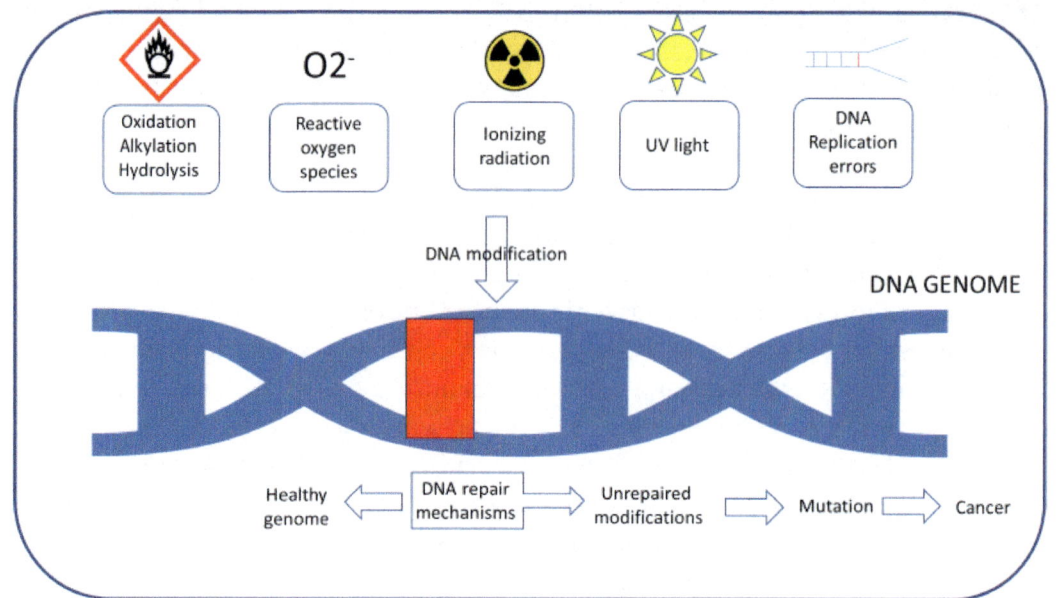

Your DNA is subjected to numerous modifications every day which are corrected by repair mechanisms in your cells. If these are not corrected then they can result in a permanent modification to our genetic code

Animal-based foods and cancer

Many studies indicate that people who eat a diet with more animal-based foods rather than fruits, and vegetables have a considerably higher risk of cancer. For example, one study indicated that women with a high number of plants in their diet are 3.5 times less likely to be diagnosed with pre-cancerous cervical lesions, and the risk of head, neck, and bladder cancers was reduced compared to people who ate diets that contained more meat, fat, and junk food [Barchitta et al., 2019]. However, it should be noted that people who eat more vegetables may have other cancer-modifying life habits. An issue with animal proteins, in particular, is that they are often high in signalling molecules that resemble our own bodies' molecules. An example is oestrogen which is present in all vertebrate animal products, and which can act to increase the growth of breast and ovarian cancers [Persson, 2000]. Note that circulating levels of oestrogen are much lower in people who consume a plant-based diet [Harmon et al., 2014]. The link between dairy consumption and cancer is still inconsistent [World cancer fund research report, 2018) but the fact is that dairy milk contains a cocktail of hormones and growth factors that can in theory promote cancer growth. In a recent report consumption of dairy products by Chinese people was linked to an increased risk of cancer [Kakkora et al., 2022]. However, it should be noted that dairy products such as cheese and yoghurt have many beneficial health aspects including providing calcium, vitamin D and probiotic activity which may lower cancer risk. One study implies that high milk consumption, especially high/whole-fat milk, was associated with higher cancer mortality, whereas fermented milk consumption was associated with lower cancer mortality, and this was particularly evident in females [Jin and Je, 2022]. Despite the inconsistency growth factors and hormones whether externally or internally derived are important for the promotion of many cancers. One of the most important is Insulin growth factor-1 (IGF-1). While IGF-1 is vital when we are growing up, levels should decrease once we reach adulthood. Studies indicate that men with high levels of IGF-1 have a 4.3-fold increased risk of prostate cancer compared to those with low levels [Stattin et al., 2004].

Soya products and cancer

Initial poorly controlled trials looking at the effect of soya products on diet indicated that they might promote cancer. The fact is that people have been eating and drinking soya products for thousands of years with populations consuming a traditional Chinese diet having one of the lowest risks of cancer incidence. People have postulated that soya and other beans contain phytoestrogens which mimic the effect of cancer-promoting oestrogens in our bodies.

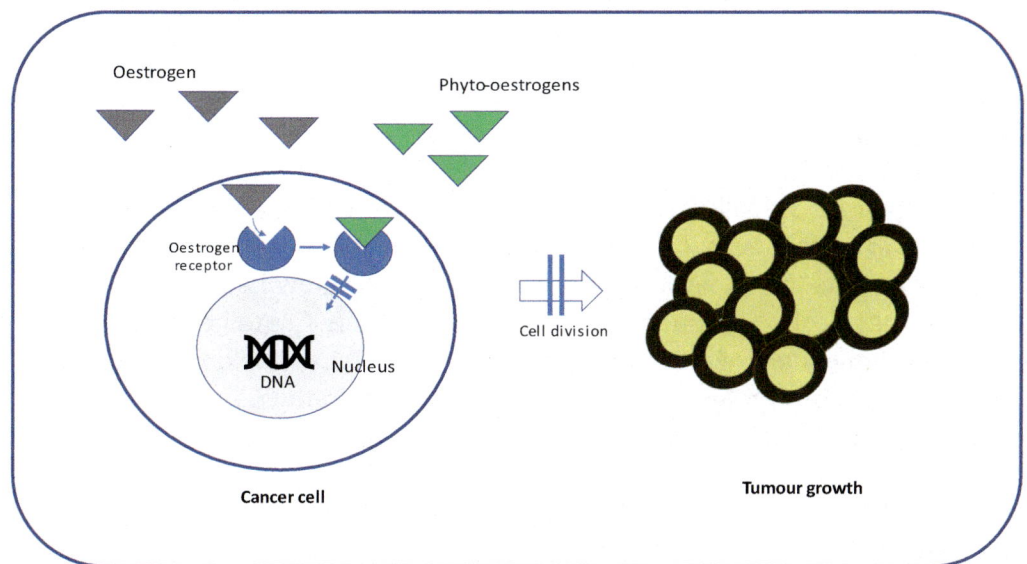

Phytoestrogens can prevent more potent oestrogens produced by the body from binding to the oestrogen receptor and promoting the growth of cancer cells to form a tumour

However, research indicates that these phytoestrogens bind to the cell's oestrogen receptors with far less affinity and may help to prevent the far stronger human oestrogens from binding [Gómez-Zorita et al., 2020]. The soya phytoestrogen isoflavone has been shown to lower the risk of prostate cancer [Sugiyama et al., 2013]. Studies have indicated that soya may be associated with better survival for breast cancer patients [Chi et al., 2013; for a review see Messina, 2016].

Pesticides and cancer

Pesticide residues are present in a variety of foods [Tudi et al., 2021]. There is increasing evidence that individuals who are exposed to high amounts of pesticides in an occupational setting have a higher risk of cancer [Lewis-Mikhael et al, 2016]. However, the risk of low levels of these chemicals in our food over a lifetime has not been proven. Although, it is feasible that over time they can accumulate to high levels capable of causing abnormalities in humans. The switch to an entirely organic diet may be expensive unless you can grow your produce. The Pesticide Action Network indicates that the plant foods with the highest residues are barley, oats and wheat, grapefruit, clementines, mandarins and satsumas, strawberries, pre-packed salad, grapes, lemons, peaches and nectarines, pears, spinach, chilli peppers, apples, blackberries and blueberries [www.pan-uk.org]. Therefore, as a start, if consuming these types of produce switch to an organic version and wash all vegetables and fruit well before consuming.

Anti-cancer diet

We often hear of so-called "superfoods" which are endowed with miraculous capabilities. The fact is that no one food can prevent cancer. However, there are dietary habits that can reduce our risk. There are a few people who can eat whatever they desire and not get cancer. In part, this is due to genetics in a few very lucky individuals. For the rest of us, the following guidelines should be followed. This diet is relevant for people who wish to reduce the risk of cancer, during treatment and to prevent the re-occurrence of cancer.

- Reduce refined sugar (sucrose, glucose, fructose)
- Eat "real" food, cook your own food
- Take time to eat well
- Eat complex carbohydrates by switching to a whole-grain variety
- Eat less red meat and replace it with some fish or other protein alternatives

- Eat more nuts and seeds (if not allergic)
- Reduce unhealthy trans fats and replace them with healthier oils such as olive oil
- Consume more omega-3 oils (found in fish and nuts/seeds)
- Eat more beans and lentils (full of fibre and phytochemicals)
- Reduce whole milk consumption but consume alternative food sources of calcium such as cheese, yogurt, tofu, dark leafy greens, almonds, dried figs, butternut squash, broccoli, and white beans
- Eat more probiotic food
- Avoid preserved meats
- Consume a wide variety of plant-based foods
- Reduce or eliminate alcohol consumption
- Eat less fried food
- Reduce consumption of barbecued foods
- Reduce or eliminate highly processed foods

It is difficult to determine a particular food benefit unless the studies are undertaken over a long period and with a significant amount of people. Additionally, the benefits of a particular food are dependent on the subject's nutritional background and diet. Since cancer occurs more frequently in older people there is a trend to eat unhealthy food in our younger years and then subsequently become healthier in our older years or after a health-threatening event. However, the timeframe is important, the effects are not immediate so what you ate ten or twenty years ago is likely to have a more relevant effect. Thus, our diet during our childhood and adolescent years affects the risk of cancer in our adult years [Mahabir, 2013]. However, as indicated by one study even a short-term switch to a healthier diet can affect genes involved in preventing cancer [Ornish et al, 2009].

The benefits of phytochemicals

Phytochemicals are an extraordinary, varied group of chemicals derived from plants. Additionally, cooking plants can produce further variants of phytochemicals by conjugation (joining together of chemicals). Many cancer-treating drugs have been discovered in plants which remain a vital source for the discovery of new anticancer treatments. Phytochemicals are not essential nutrients to humans, but they do have health benefits although research is still being undertaken to clarify this. The main problem is that plants contain thousands of different phytochemicals which may have synergistic effects and may have effects on health only on a long-term basis. Additionally, cultivation, harvesting and cooking methods may alter the levels and types of phytochemicals within plants. This can result in ambivalent outcomes when attempting to decipher their effects on health. In total, there has been over 25,000 phytochemicals discovered and, in most cases, these phytochemicals are concentrated in colourful parts of plants like fruits, vegetables, nuts, legumes, and whole grains, etc. Eating a diet high in fruits, vegetables, grains, legumes, has long-term health benefits, but there is little evidence that taking dietary supplements of non-nutrient phytochemicals extracted from plants similarly benefits health. Phytochemicals can be divided into several groups (see the figure below). Phytochemicals have a range of pharmacological bioactivities and are used for their aromatic qualities and play a role in traditional herbal remedies. Based on their chemical structures, polyphenols can be divided into different subgroups and exhibit a tremendous antioxidant activity as well as other health benefits. Epidemiological evidence indicates that a diet rich in antioxidant fruits and vegetables significantly reduces the risk of many oxidative stress related diseases such as cancers, diabetes and cardiovascular [Rudrapal et al., 2022]. There is no recommended dietary allowance for phytochemicals. Eat a variety of foods, including plenty of fruits and vegetables, to ensure you are getting adequate amounts in your diet.

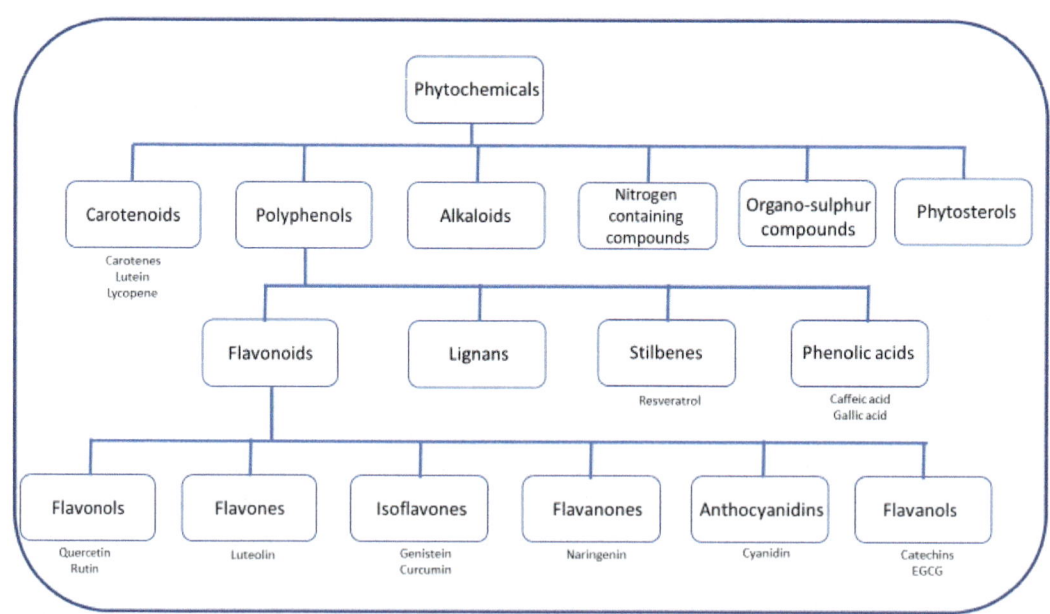

There are many different types of phytochemicals found in plants. Major groups are listed with relevant examples shown below some boxes

Cancer is characterized by uncontrolled cell growth and dedifferentiation. The features of cancer cells include "tuning out" from signals of proliferation and differentiation, overcoming cell apoptosis (cell death), gaining the ability to migrate, and promoting angiogenesis (formation of new blood vessels). This occurs by sequential genetic mutations in cell proliferation genes, DNA repair genes, tumour suppressor genes, oncogenes, and genes involved in apoptosis and migration turning a normal cell over time into a metastatic cell capable of spreading around the body. As you can see carcinogenesis (cancer-forming process) is a complex process and includes multiple events. Phytochemicals are varied in their function and can target these events in multiple manners.

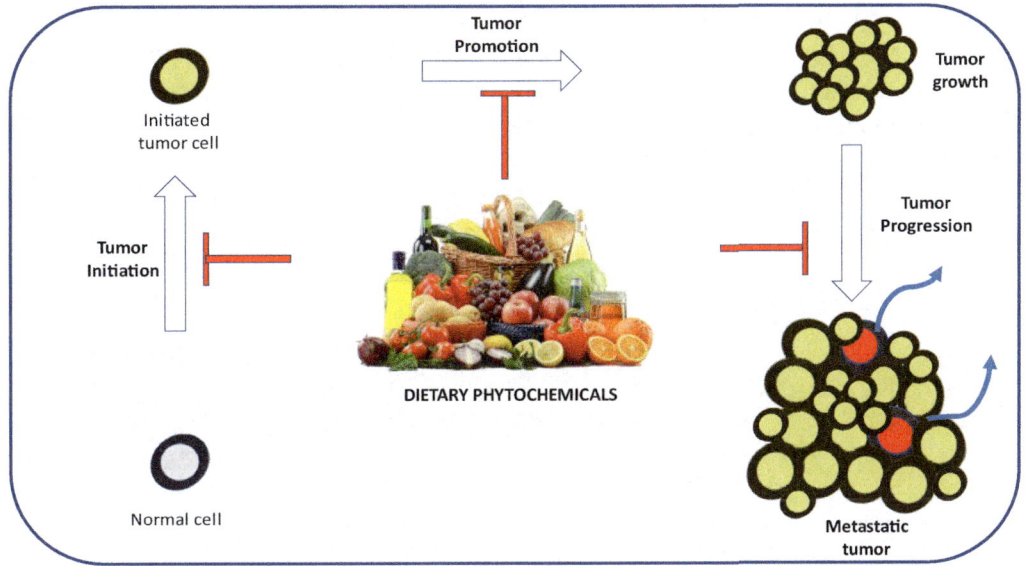

Phytochemicals are chemically varied and can affect many different stages in the transformation of a normal cell into a metastatic cell

The exact mechanism by which phytochemicals perform anticancer functions is still a topic of research. They exert a wide and complex range of actions on nuclear and cytosolic factors in a cancer cell as listed below [Golovinskaia and Chin-Kun Wang, 2021; Rajabi et al., 2021; Almatroodi et al., 2021; Ma et al., 2021].

- Absorption of reactive oxygen species (ROS)
- Promotion of antioxidant enzymes
- Suppression of malignant transformation of an initiated pre-cancerous cell
- Blocking the metabolic conversion of a pro-carcinogen

- Modulation of cellular and signalling events involved in the growth, invasion, and metastasis of cancer cells
- Promotion of apoptosis (cell death)
- Modulation of signals involved in the cell cycle (which controls cell proliferation)
- Blocking of angiogenesis (forming new blood vessels)
- Reduction of the activities of enzymes involved in DNA modification
- Blocking signalling events involved in cancer initiation and progression

It would be difficult to identify one individual plant which is capable of performing all these activities hence the need to consume a variety of plant-derived food. Phytochemicals which have been implicated in prevention of cancer are shown below along with examples of foods which contain those named phytochemicals.

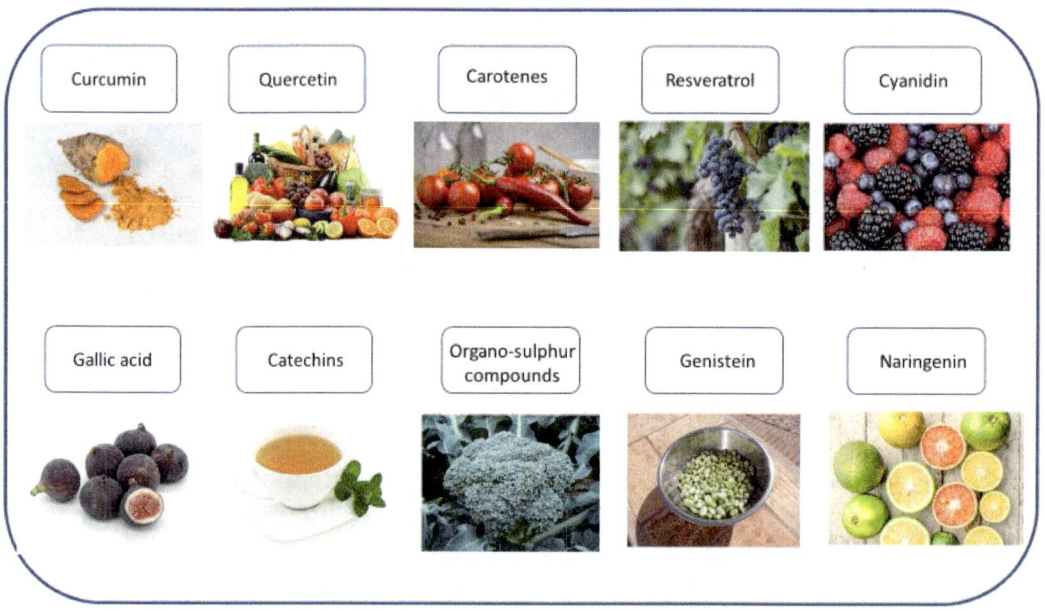

Phytochemicals which have been implicated in prevention of cancer are shown along with examples of foods which contain those named phytochemicals

Over-supplementation and cancer

There is now good evidence that having a balanced healthy diet can result in a lower risk of cancer. However, there is also now building evidence that obtaining vitamins, phytochemicals and minerals through pills may increase the risk of cancer due to the risk of over-supplementation [Martinez et al, 2012]. However, more research needs to be performed on this subject. While there are legitimate medical reasons for taking supplements, these should be discussed with your medical practitioner. Additionally, phytochemical supplements taken at a high concentration may have toxic effects on the liver [Schmidt et al, 2005]. Note that supplements are considered food rather than medicine as such they are not governed by the strict regulations regarding the effectiveness of medicines.

Cancer and being overweight

It has been unequivocally shown that being overweight is a leading factor in the development of cancer [Avgerinos et al, 2019]. Therefore for a person wishing to reduce their risk of cancer or recurrence, the primary objective should be to lose weight. However, it is important to maintain muscle mass. A combination of physical activity and nutritional change is an ideal way to reduce weight while maintaining muscle mass. This does not mean that we need to start running marathons or go on a restrictive diet. The middle road is more likely to prove effective in the long term. Often incorporating moderate exercise in your daily routine such as going for a walk can lower cancer risk considerably. Cooking your food using a variety of plants can provide a range of cancer-fighting nutrients. In general, it is better not to rely on supplements but to obtain cancer-preventing nutrients from natural sources. The reason being is that supplementation may lead to overly high levels of vitamins and minerals in the body which may increase the risk of cancer [Martinez et al, 2012]. Additionally, supplements in particular those that act as antioxidants can flood the body with high levels of a few particular antioxidants (such as in a multi-vitamin pill). As a result, the body's system of dealing with cancer-causing oxidants is compromised as antioxidants are converted to oxidants by electron transfer, and the body's enzymes whose job it is to detoxify oxidants are overloaded. Additionally, while so-called "superfoods" may have a role to play in cancer prevention it is better to consume a diet containing a wide variety of plants rather than overreliance on one food type. Make gradual switches to your diet and remove or reduce some of the riskier foods in your diet. Finally, consider changing to organic sources of food. Ultimately for the majority of people, it is better to first concentrate on losing weight as obesity and being overweight is the third highest cause of cancer and may be a factor in cancer reoccurrence [Avgerinos et al., 2019]. However, losing weight may be difficult but not impossible due to the legion of misinformation available from internet gurus and fad diets. It has been scientifically proven that diets over a year are not sustainable for the majority of people [Ge et al, 2020]. Once a person finishes a diet then often the lost weight is regained resulting in yo-yo weight loss which can be psychologically difficult. It should be noted that diets which omit certain food groups can lead to food cravings and discontinuation of the diet resulting in psychological effects such as guilt. Better to moderate food intake by changing to a nutrition plan with more fruit and vegetables, reducing simple sugars, eating whole grain products and combining with physical activity to slowly lose weight. If you are underweight, then it is better to consult with a dietitian. Ways to gain weight when you are underweight are given below.

- Consume food more frequently. Eat several small meals during the day rather than a few large meals which rapidly fill you up
- Change your diet to foods containing more nutrients
- Consume nutrients in liquid forms such as smoothies and shakes
- Snack frequently during the day
- Immediately after finishing physical activity consume a post-activity snack consisting of carbohydrate and protein
- Stick to a meal plan prescribed by a trained dietitian but allow an occasional treat. However, still be mindful of excess sugar and fat

The benefits of Mediterranean food and medicinal food in terms of cancer are summarized below.

The Mediterranean diet

The concept and the health benefits of the 'Mediterranean diet' were first described by Keys and Grande in the early 1960s after studying dietary patterns in Greece and Southern Italy where olive growing was abundant. A similar diet is also found in other countries within the region including Spain, France, and Portugal [Davis et al., 2015; Martinez-González and Sánchez-Villegas, 2004; Trichopoulou et al., 2014]. In their 'Seven Countries Study, Keys and his colleagues came up with an important conclusion that low incidences of heart disease could be correlated to the low intake of saturated fats in these countries [Trichopoulou et al., 2014]. However, it should be noted that correlation is not evidence of causation [Malhotra, 2013], and although the link between saturated fat and cardiovascular disease remains tentative and the original study has limitations the Mediterranean diet approach has gained a lot of interest. The main characteristics of the Mediterranean diet include high consumption of whole grains, legumes, fruits, vegetables, and nuts, low consumption of meat with more fish and white meat (such as chicken) than red or processed meat - and low to moderate consumption of dairy foods with low-fat cheese and yoghurt preferred more. Alcohol consumption is moderate and usually in the form of wine with meals. One of the distinctive components of a typical Mediterranean diet is the use of olive oil, particularly extra virgin olive oil, as it is rich in 'beneficial' monounsaturated fats. It is the main source of fat in this dietary pattern compared to saturated fats which mainly come from animal foods. It is thought that, in addition to the high consumption of plant foods, the higher proportion of olive oil to animal fat is responsible for the prevention of chronic diseases including coronary heart disease, obesity and cancer. It must also be noted that the Mediterranean diet includes mostly locally and seasonally grown foods with minimal processing and few sweets [Bach-Faig et al., 2011; Boucher, 2017; Trichopoulou et al., 2014]. The beneficial effects of the Mediterranean diet in terms of cancer incidence are likely due to the high contents of antioxidants and anti-inflammatory nutrients in plants which have a protective effect [Augimeri and Bonofiglio, 2021]. Omega-3 oil, found in fish, and in nuts (almonds, walnuts, and pumpkin seeds) is thought to slow down cancer cell proliferation, angiogenesis, and metastasis [Mentella et al, 2019]. Additionally, fibre, calcium and a regular intake of garlic may represent protective elements reducing cancer risk [Nicastro et al, 2015; Galas et al, 2013]. A low intake of meat and alcohol contributes to a reduction of risk for colorectal cancer [Tan and Chen, 2016]. Finally, there is a psychophysical aspect to the Mediterranean diet encompassing a variety of food cultivation and preparation practises with meal time as a fundamental part of the daily routine [de la Torre-Moral et al, 2021].

Medicinal cooking and functional foods

Processed low-variety and nutritionally poor foods which many people consume are convenient and flavoursome but in the long-term are detrimental to our health. In modern life, we have lost the connection between the cultivation and preparation of food and the eventual consumption of food. As a result, food consumption has become dysfunctional, and we no longer reap the many benefits which are associated with these activities. Hippocrates who is thought to be the founder of rational modern medicine stated, "Let food be thy medicine and medicine be thy food". The concept of "functional foods" which supply both nutritional and therapeutic value dates back 4000 years to China. In the early Zhou dynasty (1100-221 BC) the imperial palace court appointed a nutritionist to examine the medicinal properties of food [Chinese State Council Information Office, 2016]. More recently the Functional Food Science in Europe project, stated that: "A food can be regarded as functional if it is satisfactorily demonstrated to affect beneficially one or more target functions in the body, beyond adequate nutritional effects, thus either improving general physical conditions or/and decreasing the risk of the generation of diseases" [Contor, 2001]. Note that there is some crossover with plant-derived pharmaceuticals which are specially formulated and developed to treat, cure, or prevent disease, [Contor, 2001]. Although pharmaceuticals generally have higher potency or biological activity compared to the phytochemicals normally consumed in the diet and functional foods exert physiological effects only after long-term use [Veeresham, 2012]. Plants contain thousands of chemicals (Phytochemicals) that can be found as bioactive components in foods. However, only a small number have been isolated and identified [Cao et al., 2017]. The types of phytochemicals include coumarins, flavonoids, polyphenols, carotenoids, indoles, isoflavones, lignans, catechins, phenolic acids, stilbenoids, isothiocyanates, saponins, procyanidins, phenylpropanoids, anthraquinones, ginsenosides, and so on [Xiao and Bai, 2019]. The great biodiversity of phytochemicals is a unique resource for the discovery of new functional foods [Sen and Samanta, 2015). Additionally, the cooking and processing of foods can provide new subsets of dietary phytochemicals by the formation of new conjugates and intermediates. However, this area of research is riddled with low-quality clinical trials and as a result many of the conclusions are inconclusive and or difficult to interpret. Every week new research is touted online stating the amazing health benefits of some new "superfood". Any such claims should be treated with suspicion and care. The reason for this is multifactorial but includes the following:

- Low subject numbers in trials
- Varying methods in the cultivation and preparation of food as a result the levels of active ingredients may be inconsistent
- Inconsistencies in study design
- Variations in the length of studies with few longer-term studies
- Differences between subjects in terms of absorption of food into the bloodstream
- Synergistic effects of ingredients in food
- Variations in subject groups with different effects seen in groups with different nutritional status
- Lack of mechanistic understanding

Regarding functional foods, the quality of clinical data is often unreliable leading to inconclusive outcomes. However, it is clear that, in particular, plant-derived foods contain a variety of phytochemicals that may be beneficial to health over a long-term period. Therefore, it is recommended to include in the diet a variety of foods particularly fruits, nuts, and vegetables and to supplement those foods with a variety of herbs and spices. However, believing that one superfood is the "be-all" of human nutrition or cancer prevention/treatment would be misguided.

Nutrition during cancer treatment

It may be challenging to maintain nutrition and eat well during cancer treatment. However, it is important to maintain a healthy weight and consume food which is nutritious to provide all the vitamins, minerals and phytochemicals to support your body. Additionally, it is vital to drink plenty of water. It may be that your cancer treatment can cause changes in your appetite and weight resulting in weight gain or weight loss. Although small changes are not a problem, drastic changes should be avoided as they are an indication you are not getting sufficient nutrition to support your needs. Essential nutrients such as protein, carbohydrates and fats should be present in your diet as well as vitamins, minerals and phytochemicals. Loss of muscle mass may be a danger so it is vital to consume protein-rich foods and to be as active as possible. Consulting a dietician may be beneficial to create an eating plan for you. In general, the same guidelines outlined above in the anti-cancer diet should be followed. Additionally foods which boost cognitive function, mental health, the immune system, the digestive system, and promote consistent sleep as described in previous chapters should be consumed. To date the evidence supporting the utility of vitamins or minerals to treat cancer is weak. Many promising *in vitro* experiments have been carried out to evaluate the effect of individual phytochemicals on cultured (lab grown) cancer cells. However, to date many of these experiments have not been performed in clinical trials on humans. As such while a promising direction of research, it requires further confirmation before any conclusive statements can be made. Although the effect of plant based diets on the occurrence of cancer are conclusive the effect on cancer survival are less clear. However, there is indication that higher intake of plant-based foods was associated with improved prognosis in cancer survivors. For colorectal cancer survival, a better prognosis was observed for a high intake of whole grains and fibre. For breast cancer survival, a higher intake of fruit, vegetable and fibre and a moderate intake of soy/isoflavone were associated with beneficial outcomes. A higher vegetable fat intake was related to improved prognosis in prostate cancer survivors. Emerging evidence suggests benefits of postdiagnosis plant-based diets on prognosis in cancer survivors.

However, given the high heterogeneity between studies, further research in cancer survivors, considering clinical factors (e.g. treatment, stage) and methodological aspects (e.g. timing of dietary assessment), is needed [for a review Hardt et al, 2022]. Of note high dietary intake of soy isoflavones was associated with lower risk of recurrence among post-menopausal patients with breast cancer positive for oestrogen and progesterone receptor and those who were receiving anastrozole as endocrine therapy [Kang et al, 2010].

Countering inflammatory pathways that contribute to cancer-related symptoms

Common cancer and cancer treatment side effects include anorexia, cachexia, depression, fatigue, anxiety, neuropathic pain, cognitive impairment, sleep disorders and confusion. There is evidence that dysregulation of inflammatory pathways contributes to the expression of these symptoms. Cancer patients have been found to have higher levels of proinflammatory cytokines such as interleukin-6 [Kumar, 2021]. Cytokines are a type of protein that is made by certain immune and non-immune cells. Some cytokines stimulate the immune system (pro-inflammatory) and others slow it down (anti-inflammatory). Certainly it is known that phytochemicals such as genistein, curcumin, resveratrol, lycopene, and epigallocatechin gallate can modulate inflammatory pathways [Ricker and Haas, 2017] especially in regards to chronic disease.

Treatment side effects and nutrition

It is often the case that cancer treatment causes side effects such as diarrhoea, nausea and vomiting, mouth sores, and changes in the way things taste. These may make it difficult to eat and drink. Here are some basic tips to ensure you get adequate nutrition.

- If water does not taste good, get more liquid in foods and other drinks
- If food tastes bland, try adding some flavourful herbs and spices
- If your mouth is sore, avoid too much acid, such as lemon or other citrus, or spicy heat, such as cayenne or other hot peppers
- Eat several small meals instead of 3 large meals each day
- To maintain protein levels try fish, eggs, cheese, beans, nuts, tofu, or high-protein smoothies or shakes
- If you have a strange taste in your mouth, suck on mints or lemon drops, chew gum, or try fresh citrus fruits

References

Almatroodi SA, Alsahli MA, Almatroudi A, Verma AK, Aloliqi A, Allemailem KS, Khan AA, Rahmani AH. Potential Therapeutic Targets of Quercetin, a Plant Flavonol, and Its Role in the Therapy of Various Types of Cancer through the Modulation of Various Cell Signaling Pathways. Molecules. 2021 Mar 1;26(5):1315. doi: 10.3390/molecules26051315.

Augimeri G, Bonofiglio D. The Mediterranean Diet as a Source of Natural Compounds: Does It Represent a Protective Choice against Cancer? Pharmaceuticals (Basel). 2021 Sep 11;14(9):920. doi: 10.3390/ph14090920.

Avgerinos KI, Spyrou N, Mantzoros CS, Dalamaga M. Obesity and cancer risk: Emerging biological mechanisms and perspectives. Metabolism. 2019 Mar;92:121-135. doi: 10.1016/j.metabol.2018.11.001.

Anand P, Kunnumakkara AB, Sundaram C, Harikumar KB, Tharakan ST, Lai OS, Sung B, Aggarwal BB. Cancer is a preventable disease that requires major lifestyle changes. Pharm Res. 2008 Sep;25(9):2097-116. doi: 10.1007/s11095-008-9661-9.

Bach-Faig A, Berry EM, Lairon D, Reguant J, Trichopoulou A, Dernini S, Medina FX, Battino M, Belahsen R, Miranda G, Serra-Majem L; Mediterranean Diet Foundation Expert Group. Mediterranean diet pyramid today. Science and cultural updates. Public Health Nutr. 2011 Dec;14(12A):2274-84. doi: 10.1017/S1368980011002515.

Barchitta M, Maugeri A, Li Destri G, Basile G, Agodi A. Epigenetic Biomarkers in Colorectal Cancer Patients Receiving Adjuvant or Neoadjuvant Therapy: A Systematic Review of Epidemiological Studies. Int J Mol Sci. 2019 Aug 6;20(15):3842. doi: 10.3390/ijms20153842.

Block G, Patterson B, Subar A. Fruit, vegetables, and cancer prevention: a review of the epidemiological evidence. Nutr Cancer. 1992;18(1):1-29. doi: 10.1080/01635589209514201.

Boucher JL. Mediterranean Eating Pattern. Diabetes Spectr. 2017 May;30(2):72-76. doi: 10.2337/ds16-0074.

Chi F, Wu R, Zeng YC, Xing R, Liu Y, Xu ZG. Post-diagnosis soy food intake and breast cancer survival: a meta-analysis of cohort studies. Asian Pac J Cancer Prev. 2013;14(4):2407-12. doi: 10.7314/apjcp.2013.14.4.2407.

Chinese state council information offfice. Traditional Chinese Medicine in China [Internet]. China's State Council Information Office issues a white paper on the development of traditional Chinese medicine (TCM) in China. 2016. Available from: http://www.china.org.cn/node 7247529/content_40621689.htm

Contor L. Functional Food Science in Europe. Vol. 11, Nutrition, metabolism, and cardiovascular diseases : NMCD. Netherlands; 2001. p. 20–3.

Cao H, Chai TT, Wang X, Morais-Braga MFB, Yang JH, Wong FC, Wang R, Yao H, Cao J, Cornara L, Burlando B, Wang Y, Xiao J, Coutinho HDM. Phytochemicals from fern species: potential for medicine applications. Phytochem Rev. 2017;16(3):379-440. doi: 10.1007/s11101-016-9488-7.

Davis C, Bryan J, Hodgson J, Murphy K. Definition of the Mediterranean Diet; a Literature Review. Nutrients. 2015 Nov 5;7(11):9139-53. doi: 10.3390/nu7115459.

de la Torre-Moral A, Fàbregues S, Bach-Faig A, Fornieles-Deu A, Medina FX, Aguilar-Martínez A, Sánchez-Carracedo D. Family Meals, Conviviality, and the Mediterranean Diet among Families with Adolescents. Int J Environ Res Public Health. 2021 Mar 3;18(5):2499. doi: 10.3390/ijerph18052499.

Doll R, Peto R. The causes of cancer: quantitative estimates of avoidable risks of cancer in the United States today. J Natl Cancer Inst. 1981 Jun;66(6):1191-308.

Donaldson MS. Nutrition and cancer: a review of the evidence for an anti-cancer diet. Nutr J. 2004 Oct 20;3:19. doi: 10.1186/1475-2891-3-19.

Galas A, Augustyniak M, Sochacka-Tatara E. Does dietary calcium interact with dietary fiber against colorectal cancer? A case-control study in Central Europe. Nutr J. 2013 Oct 4;12:134. doi: 10.1186/1475-2891-12-134.

Ge L, Sadeghirad B, Ball GDC, da Costa BR, Hitchcock CL, Svendrovski A, Kiflen R, Quadri K, Kwon HY, Karamouzian M, Adams-Webber T, Ahmed W, Damanhoury S, Zeraatkar D, Nikolakopoulou A, Tsuyuki RT, Tian J, Yang K, Guyatt GH, Johnston BC. Comparison of dietary macronutrient patterns of 14 popular named dietary programmes for weight and cardiovascular risk factor reduction in adults: systematic review and network meta-analysis of randomised trials. BMJ. 2020 Apr 1;369:m696. doi: 10.1136/bmj.m696.

Golovinskaia O, Wang CK. Review of Functional and Pharmacological Activities of Berries. Molecules. 2021 Jun 25;26(13):3904. doi: 10.3390/molecules26133904.

Gómez-Zorita S, González-Arceo M, Fernández-Quintela A, Eseberri I, Trepiana J, Portillo MP, et al. Influence of isoflavone intake and equol-producing intestinal flora on prostate cancer risk. Antioxidants (Basel, Switzerland). 2021 Jun;10(1):1–4.

Harmon BE, Morimoto Y, Beckford F, Franke AA, Stanczyk FZ, Maskarinec G. Oestrogen levels in serum and urine of premenopausal women eating low and high amounts of meat. Public Health Nutr. 2014 Sep;17(9):2087-93. doi: 10.1017/S1368980013002553.

Hardt L, Mahamat-Saleh Y, Aune D, Schlesinger S. Plant-Based Diets and Cancer Prognosis: a Review of Recent Research. Curr Nutr Rep. 2022 Dec;11(4):695-716. doi: 10.1007/s13668-022-00440-1.

Jin S, Je Y. Dairy Consumption and Total Cancer and Cancer-Specific Mortality: A Meta-Analysis of Prospective Cohort Studies. Adv Nutr. 2022 Aug 1;13(4):1063-1082. doi: 10.1093/advances/nmab135.

Kakkoura MG, Du H, Guo Y, Yu C, Yang L, Pei P, Chen Y, Sansome S, Chan WC, Yang X, Fan L, Lv J, Chen J, Li L, Key TJ, Chen Z; China Kadoorie Biobank (CKB) Collaborative Group. Dairy consumption and risks of total and site-specific cancers in Chinese adults: an 11-year prospective study of 0.5 million people. BMC Med. 2022 May 6;20(1):134. doi: 10.1186/s12916-022-02330-3.

Kang X, Zhang Q, Wang S, Huang X, Jin S. Effect of soy isoflavones on breast cancer recurrence and death for patients receiving adjuvant endocrine therapy. CMAJ. 2010 Nov 23;182(17):1857-62. doi: 10.1503/cmaj.091298.

Kumar NB. The Promise of Nutrient-Derived Bioactive Compounds and Dietary Components to Ameliorate Symptoms of Chemotherapy-Related Cognitive Impairment in Breast Cancer Survivors. Curr Treat Options Oncol. 2021 Jun 10;22(8):67. doi: 10.1007/s11864-021-00865-w.

Lee JH, Khor TO, Shu L, Su ZY, Fuentes F, Kong AN. Dietary phytochemicals and cancer prevention: Nrf2 signaling, epigenetics, and cell death mechanisms in blocking cancer initiation and progression. Pharmacol Ther. 2013 Feb;137(2):153-71. doi: 10.1016/j.pharmthera.2012.09.008.

Lewis-Mikhael AM, Bueno-Cavanillas A, Ofir Giron T, Olmedo-Requena R, Delgado-Rodríguez M, Jiménez-Moleón JJ. Occupational exposure to pesticides and prostate cancer: a systematic review and meta-analysis. Occup Environ Med. 2016 Feb;73(2):134-44. doi: 10.1136/oemed-2014-102692.

Ma L, Zhang M, Zhao R, Wang D, Ma Y, Li A. Plant Natural Products: Promising Resources for Cancer Chemoprevention. Molecules. 2021 Feb 10;26(4):933. doi: 10.3390/molecules26040933.

Mahabir S. Association between diet during preadolescence and adolescence and risk for breast cancer during adulthood. J Adolesc Health. 2013 May;52(5 Suppl):S30-5. doi: 10.1016/j.jadohealth.2012.08.008.

Malhotra A. Saturated fat is not the major issue. BMJ. 2013 Oct;347:f6340.

Martínez-González MA, Sánchez-Villegas A. The emerging role of Mediterranean diets in cardiovascular epidemiology: monounsaturated fats, olive oil, red wine or the whole pattern? Eur J Epidemiol. 2004;19(1):9-13. doi: 10.1023/b:ejep.0000013351.60227.7b.

Martínez ME, Jacobs ET, Baron JA, Marshall JR, Byers T. Dietary supplements and cancer prevention: balancing potential benefits against proven harms. J Natl Cancer Inst. 2012 May 16;104(10):732-9. doi: 10.1093/jnci/djs195.

Mentella MC, Scaldaferri F, Ricci C, Gasbarrini A, Miggiano GAD. Cancer and Mediterranean Diet: A Review. Nutrients. 2019 Sep 2;11(9):2059. doi: 10.3390/nu11092059.

Messina M. Impact of Soy Foods on the Development of Breast Cancer and the Prognosis of Breast Cancer Patients. Forsch Komplementmed. 2016;23(2):75-80. doi: 10.1159/000444735. Epub 2016 Apr 12.

Ornish D, Magbanua MJ, Weidner G, Weinberg V, Kemp C, Green C, Mattie MD, Marlin R, Simko J, Shinohara K, Haqq CM, Carroll PR. Changes in prostate gene expression in men undergoing an intensive nutrition and lifestyle intervention. Proc Natl Acad Sci U S A. 2008 Jun 17;105(24):8369-74. doi: 10.1073/pnas.0803080105.

Persson I. Estrogens in the causation of breast, endometrial and ovarian cancers - evidence and hypotheses from epidemiological findings. J Steroid Biochem Mol Biol. 2000 Nov 30;74(5):357-64. doi: 10.1016/s0960-0760(00)00113-8.

Rajabi S, Maresca M, Yumashev AV, Choopani R, Hajimehdipoor H. The Most Competent Plant-Derived Natural Products for Targeting Apoptosis in Cancer Therapy. Biomolecules. 2021 Apr 3;11(4):534. doi: 10.3390/biom11040534.

Ricker MA, Haas WC. Anti-Inflammatory Diet in Clinical Practice: A Review. Nutr Clin Pract. 2017 Jun;32(3):318-325. doi: 10.1177/0884533617700353. Epub 2017 Mar 28. PMID: 28350517.

Rudrapal M, Khairnar SJ, Khan J, Dukhyil AB, Ansari MA, Alomary MN, Alshabrmi FM, Palai S, Deb PK, Devi R. Dietary Polyphenols and Their Role in Oxidative Stress-Induced Human Diseases: Insights Into Protective Effects, Antioxidant Potentials and Mechanism(s) of Action. Front Pharmacol. 2022 Feb 14;13:806470. doi: 10.3389/fphar.2022.806470

Schmidt M, Schmitz HJ, Baumgart A, Guédon D, Netsch MI, Kreuter MH, Schmidlin CB, Schrenk D. Toxicity of green tea extracts and their constituents in rat hepatocytes in primary culture. Food Chem Toxicol. 2005 Feb;43(2):307-14. doi: 10.1016/j.fct.2004.11.001.

Sen T, Samanta SK. Medicinal plants, human health and biodiversity: a broad review. Adv Biochem Eng Biotechnol. 2015;147:59-110. doi: 10.1007/10_2014_273.

Stattin P, Rinaldi S, Biessy C, Stenman UH, Hallmans G, Kaaks R. High levels of circulating insulin-like growth factor-I increase prostate cancer risk: a prospective study in a population-based nonscreened cohort. J Clin Oncol. 2004 Aug 1;22(15):3104-12. doi: 10.1200/JCO.2004.10.105.

Steck SE, Murphy EA. Dietary patterns and cancer risk. Nat Rev Cancer. 2020 Feb;20(2):125-138. doi: 10.1038/s41568-019-0227-4.

Sugiyama Y, Masumori N, Fukuta F, Yoneta A, Hida T, Yamashita T, Minatoya M, Nagata Y, Mori M, Tsuji H, Akaza H, Tsukamoto T. Influence of isoflavone intake and equol-producing intestinal flora on prostate cancer risk. Asian Pac J Cancer Prev. 2013;14(1):1-4. doi: 10.7314/apjcp.2013.14.1.1.

Tan J, Chen YX. Dietary and Lifestyle Factors Associated with Colorectal Cancer Risk and Interactions with Microbiota: Fiber, Red or Processed Meat and Alcoholic Drinks. Gastrointest Tumors. 2016 Sep;3(1):17-24. doi: 10.1159/000442831.

Trichopoulou A, Martínez-González MA, Tong TY, Forouhi NG, Khandelwal S, Prabhakaran D, Mozaffarian D, de Lorgeril M. Definitions and potential health benefits of the Mediterranean diet: views from experts around the world. BMC Med. 2014 Jul 24;12:112. doi: 10.1186/1741-7015-12-112.

Tudi M, Daniel Ruan H, Wang L, Lyu J, Sadler R, Connell D, Chu C, Phung DT. Agriculture Development, Pesticide Application and Its Impact on the Environment. Int J Environ Res Public Health. 2021 Jan 27;18(3):1112. doi: 10.3390/ijerph18031112.

Veeresham C. Natural products derived from plants as a source of drugs. J Adv Pharm Technol Res. 2012 Oct;3(4):200-1. doi: 10.4103/2231-4040.104709.

Xiao J, Bai W. Bioactive phytochemicals. Crit Rev Food Sci Nutr. 2019;59(6):827-829. doi: 10.1080/10408398.2019.1601848

PLANT-BASED DIETS AND CANCER PREVENTION

Dr Dee Bhakta

As you have read in previous chapters, the causes of cancer are complex and it is difficult to pin down exactly what causes cancer in the individual. We know diet is important but risk will vary depending on factors such as genetic vulnerability, the environment you live in and the other lifestyle choices you make. I add this caveat because I had the pleasure, as part of my research, to interview hundreds of wonderful women who had recently been treated for cancer and it was sad to see that many were filled with guilt regarding their previous dietary habits. Food should not be about guilt. It is essential to nourish our bodies adequately but food is also more than this, as cooking and communal eating in a convivial atmosphere brings joy to our lives, it helps our mental well-being, social cohesion and improves our overall quality of life. Individual foods should not be labelled as "clean", "unclean", "unhealthy" or even "superfoods". It should always be about moderation and balance.

The chance of developing cancer in the UK, during our lifetime is now one in two (NHS, 2023a). Fortunately, the survival rate for most cancers is improving with earlier diagnosis and better treatment and is now considered by many health organisations as a chronic condition such as heart disease and type 2 diabetes. Similarly, like all chronic conditions we may be able to change our risk by modifying our behaviour. The purpose of this chapter is to summarise and bring together all the evidence for plant-based diets and cancer prevention and provide some sensible guidance.

Definition of a plant-based dietary pattern

Plant-based diets are dietary patterns that have a higher consumption of foods derived from plants. This does not mean the total exclusion of meat and meat products, rather that most of the foods consumed are chosen from plant sources. It is commonly defined as a dietary pattern which is high in vegetables, fruits, wholegrains, unsaturated fats, and omega-3 fats and low in red and processed meats, trans fats, and sugar-sweetened beverages. Traditional food systems which are largely plant-based and include a variety of foods such as the Mediterranean Diet have been shown to have a lower risk of some cancers (Dinu et al., 2017). The reduction in cancer risk differs between those who have adopted a vegetarian diet as a lifestyle choice (Keys et al., 2014) rather than those who have been life-long vegetarians (dos Santos Silva, 2002) as this may depend on the level of restriction of animal products (Craig et al., 2021). It is also important to bear in mind that people who choose to follow a vegetarian lifestyle tend to exercise more, are less likely to smoke and come from a high socioeconomic group, factors which can help reduce the risk cancer independent of dietary intake.

Following a healthy plant-based dietary pattern

A large study (Li et al., 2018) followed participants for thirty-five years to see if adhering to five positive lifestyle-related behaviours: never smoking; maintaining a healthy weight; regularly exercise; consuming alcohol only in moderation; and consuming a healthy plant-based diet, improved life expectancy. The study found that the risk of dying from cancer was lower by sixty five percent compared to individuals who did not follow these five lifestyle behaviours. These positive lifestyle behaviours are encompassed in the current dietary recommendations for cancer prevention (WRCF, 2023):
- Be a healthy weight
- Eat a diet rich in wholegrains, vegetables, fruit and beans
- Limit consumption of "fast foods", sugar sweetened beverages and other processed foods high in fat or sugars
- Limit consumption of red and processed meat
- Limit alcohol consumption
- Do not use supplements for cancer prevention
- After a cancer diagnosis: follow the recommendations if you can

Maintaining a healthy weight

Plant-based diets encourage weight loss (Turner-McGrievy et al., 2017) as they are high in fibre and nutrient-dense. Obesity is a risk factor for thirteen different cancers (Kitahara et al., 2014) so therefore maintenance of a healthy weight is important. Fat mass is metabolically active and the higher risk of cancer could potentially be related to fat cells producing increased levels of oestrogen, leptin, insulin and insulin-like growth factor-1, all of which have been implicated in the aetiology of cancer (Friedenreich et al., 2021).

Plant-based diets are rich in wholegrains, vegetables, fruit and beans

Wholegrains (such as oats, wholemeal bread, brown rice, wholewheat pasta), peas, beans and legumes are excellent sources of fibre, phytochemicals and butyrate levels, all of which we know from previous chapters can reduce the risk of cancer. We also know that a well-planned plant-based diet, one that contains a variety of vegetables and fruit of different colours provides a naturally high intake of vitamins, minerals and phytochemicals, which regulate antioxidant and anti-inflammatory processes. Furthermore, vegetables such as onions, cauliflower, tomatoes, green tea and wholegrains contain plant bioactive substances such as sulphur compounds, carotenoids, and polyphenols which are also protective.

Limit "fast foods", sugar sweetened beverages and other processed foods high in fat or sugars

There is strong evidence that diets that contain greater amounts of "fast foods", sugar sweetened beverages and other processed foods high in fat, starches or sugars as in a "Western type" diet are causes of weight gain, overweight and obesity (WRCF, 2023). These types of foods tend to be high in saturated fat, energy dense but poor in nutrient quality. There is much confusion about sugar and cancer. It is recommended that we all cut down our intake of refined sugar (SACN, 2015) to lower the risk of obesity. Some have advocated a low carbohydrate diet to reduce cancer risk or improve cancer treatment and / or prevent recurrence. However, following severely restricted diets with low amounts of carbohydrates leads to imbalance and could damage health by eliminating foods that are good sources of fibre, vitamins and phytochemicals (Seidelmann et al., 2018, Shah et al., 2022).

Limit consumption of red and processed meat

There is strong evidence that processed meat (such as bacon, salami and sausages) and to a certain extent red meat is associated with cancer, particularly colon cancer (WRCF, 2023). Clear mechanisms of action have been identified. Haem, found naturally in red and processed meat can damage cells and can cause bacteria in the body to produce harmful chemicals which can increase the risk of cancer (Bastide et al., 2011). Nitrates and nitrites are added to processed meat to keep them fresher for longer. When they are eaten, they produce N-nitroso compounds which are well-known to cause cancer (Chazelas et al., 2021). Furthermore, when meat is cooked at high temperatures, which includes grilling or barbecuing they can release chemicals such as heterocyclic amines and polycyclic amines which can damage cells in the bowel (PHE, 2008). However, it is important to note that animal food sources make an important contribution to some nutrients in the UK diet. For example, vitamin B_{12} and vitamin D are naturally absent from most plant foods, although they may be present in fortified foods such as breakfast cereals, fat spreads and alternative dairy products. Long chain omega-3 fats are found in highest amounts in oily fish although vegetarian supplements made from algae are available (BDA, 2023) and iodine is found in highest amounts in seafood, dairy foods and eggs (Eveleigh et al., 2020). Dairy foods are also important contributors to most people's calcium intake. Furthermore, iron and zinc are more easily absorbed from animal than plant foods. For example, phytates found in plant foods, such as wholegrains and beans, reduce zinc absorption (Foster et al., 2013). The UK government currently recommends that people who eat a lot of meat should cut down to 70g or less of red and processed meat per day (NHS, 2023b).

There is now a growing worldwide movement to switch to more plant-based diets to reduce the impact of climate change, improve animal welfare, minimize agricultural land use, alleviate hunger, potentially save lives and ultimately save the planet (Willett et al., 2019). A new healthy eating strategy has also been devised (EAT-Lancet Commission, 2021) with most of the energy and nutrients derived from plant-based foods. However, this is not so simple – some fruit and vegetable consumption can still lead to a higher water, land and carbon footprint and perhaps we may need to rely more on local produce that is in season. It is also important to ensure that a population transition to more plant-based diets also considers the nutritional needs of all individuals (Hemler & Hu, 2019, Magkos, *et al.*, 2020).

Limit alcohol consumption

There is convincing evidence that alcohol can increase the risk for several cancers. This is linked to the ethanol content found in beer, wine and spirits. When the body breaks down ethanol it forms acetaldehyde which may damage DNA and proteins (Bofetta & Hashibe, 2006). Alcohol also increases oxidative stress, damages healthy cells, increase oestrogen levels and can lower absorption of important nutrients in the diet.

Aim to meet your nutritional needs through diet alone, not supplements

Conventional advice recommends that all nutrient requirements for cancer prevention should be met by diet alone and not dietary supplements. There is plenty of evidence that shows a varied plant-based dietary pattern can provide all your daily requirements for health (Melina et al., 2016) and there are many bioactive compounds found in plant foods that have yet to be identified so consuming these in their natural form as much as possible is favourable for overall health. In fact, there is strong evidence that high dose beta-carotene supplements may increase the risk of lung cancer in some people (ATBC Cancer Prevention Group, 1994). It is important however, to note that some individuals or group may have specific requirement, for example Vitamin B^{12} (Gisling et al., 2010), iron and folic acid supplements during pregnancy (NHS, 2023c) and Vitamin D for the UK population during the winter months (SACN, 2016). Some vulnerable groups may require Vitamin D supplements for the whole year. During cancer treatment you may be prescribed specific nutritional supplementation to aid your progress and it is important to heed medical advice at this time.

Cancer survivorship and dietary guidelines

Congratulations, you have got through it. It is important to celebrate this success with food you enjoy and only restrict items that you find difficult to manage. It may take some time for you to get back to your normal diet or you may have to make some permanent modifications. You may be medically advised to gain or lose weight, depending on your individual condition. Whatever is necessary, it's still about your quality of life. You may choose to follow a plant-based dietary pattern because the evidence suggests that it may help decrease the risk of recurrence of some cancers and improve life expectancy (Schwedhelm et al., 2016, Shah et al., 2022), but it is also important to listen to your intuition. In the end, it's about balance, you need to nourish your body adequately so that you can embrace life and live a vibrant life!

References

Alpha-Tocopherol, Beta Carotene Cancer Prevention Study Group. The effect of vitamin E and beta carotene on the incidence of lung cancer and other cancers in male smokers. N Engl J Med. 1994 Apr 14;330(15):1029-35. doi: 10.1056/NEJM199404143301501. PMID: 8127329.

Bastide N, Fabrice H.F. Pierre, Denis E. Corpet; Heme Iron from Meat and Risk of Colorectal Cancer: A Meta-analysis and a Review of the Mechanisms Involved. *Cancer Prev Res (Phila)* 1 February 2011; 4 (2): 177–184. https://doi.org/10.1158/1940-6207.CAPR-10-0113

Boffetta P, Hashibe M. Alcohol and cancer. Lancet Oncol. 2006 Feb;7(2):149-56. doi: 10.1016/S1470-2045(06)70577-0. PMID: 16455479.

Bouvard V, Loomis D, Guyton KZ, Grosse Y, Ghissassi FE, Benbrahim-Tallaa L, Guha N, Mattock H, Straif K; International Agency for Research on Cancer Monograph Working Group. Carcinogenicity of consumption of red and processed meat. Lancet Oncol. 2015 Dec;16(16):1599-600. doi: 10.1016/S1470-2045(15)00444-1. Epub 2015 Oct 29. PMID: 26514947.

BDA (2023) Vegetarian, vegan, and plant-based diet: Food Fact Sheet, https://www.bda.uk.com/resource/vegetarian-vegan-plant-based-diet.html (accessed 4.04.23)

Carbohydrate and Health Report (2015), Scientific Advisory Committee on Nutrition Public Health England. https://www.gov.uk/government/publications/sacn-carbohydrates-and-health-report

Craig WJ, Mangels AR, Fresán U, Marsh K, Miles FL, Saunders AV, Haddad EH, Heskey CE, Johnston P, Larson-Meyer E, Orlich M. The Safe and Effective Use of Plant-Based Diets with Guidelines for Health Professionals. Nutrients. 2021 Nov 19;13(11):4144. doi: 10.3390/nu13114144. PMID: 34836399; PMCID: PMC8623061.

Dinu M, Abbate R, Gensini GF, Casini A, Sofi F (2017) Vegetarian, vegan diets and multiple health outcomes: A systematic review with meta-analysis of observational studies, *Critical Reviews in Food Science and Nutrition*, 57:17, 3640-3649, doi: 10.1080/10408398.2016.1138447

Dos Santos Silva I, Mangtani, P, McCormack, V, Bhakta, D, Sevak, L, McMichael, AJ (2002). Lifelong vegetarianism and risk of breast cancer: a population-based case-control study among South Asian migrant women living in England. *International Journal of Cancer*, 99 (2). pp. 238-244. ISSN 0020-7136 DOI: https://doi.org/10.1002/ijc.10300

E Chazelas, F Pierre, N Druesne-Pecollo, S Gigandet, B Srour, I Huybrechts, C Julia, E Kesse-Guyot, M Deschasaux-Tanguy, M Touvier, Nitrites and nitrates from food additives and cancer risk: results from the NutriNet-Santé cohort, *European Journal of Public Health*, Volume 31, Issue Supplement_3, October 2021, ckab165.244, https://doi.org/10.1093/eurpub/ckab165.244

EAT-Lancet Commission Summary Report (2019), https://eatforum.org/content/uploads/2019/07/EAT-Lancet_Commission_Summary_Report.pdf (accessed April 2023)

Eveleigh ER, Coneyworth LJ, Avery A, Welham SJM (2020). Vegans, Vegetarians, and Omnivores: How Does Dietary Choice Influence Iodine Intake? A Systematic Review. *Nutrients*. May 29;12(6):1606. doi: 10.3390/nu12061606.

Foster M, Chu A, Petocz P, Samman S (2013). Effect of vegetarian diets on zinc status: a systematic review and meta-analysis of studies in humans. *J Sci Food Agric*. Aug 15;93(10):2362-71. doi: 10.1002/jsfa.6179.

Friedenreich CM, Ryder-Burbidge C, McNeil J. Physical activity, obesity and sedentary behavior in cancer etiology: epidemiologic evidence and biologic mechanisms. Mol Oncol. 2021 Mar;15(3):790-800. doi: 10.1002/1878-0261.12772. Epub 2020 Aug 18. PMID: 32741068; PMCID: PMC7931121.

Gilsing AM, Crowe FL, Lloyd-Wright Z, Sanders TA, Appleby PN, Allen NE, Key TJ (2010). Serum concentrations of vitamin B12 and folate in British male omnivores, vegetarians and vegans: results from a cross-sectional analysis of the EPIC-Oxford cohort study. *Eur J Clin Nutr*. Sep;64(9):933-9. doi: 10.1038/ejcn.2010.142.

Hemler EC, Hu FB. Plant-Based Diets for Personal, Population, and Planetary Health. Adv Nutr. 2019 Nov 1;10(Suppl_4): S275-S283. doi: 10.1093/advances/nmy117.

https://www.ahajournals.org/doi/full/10.1161/CIRCULATIONAHA.117.032047

https://www.wcrf.org/diet-activity-and-cancer/risk-factors/obesity-weight-gain-and-cancer/accessed 28/10/22

Kitahara CM, Flint AJ, Berrington de Gonzalez A, Bernstein L, Brotzman M, MacInnis RJ, Moore SC, Robien K, Rosenberg PS, Singh PN, Weiderpass E, Adami HO, Anton-Culver H, Ballard-Barbash R, Buring JE, Freedman DM, Fraser GE, Beane Freeman LE, Gapstur SM, Gaziano JM, Giles GG, Håkansson N, Hoppin JA, Hu FB, Koenig K, Linet MS, Park Y, Patel AV, Purdue MP,

Schairer C, Sesso HD, Visvanathan K, White E, Wolk A, Zeleniuch-Jacquotte A, Hartge P. Association between class III obesity (BMI of 40-59 kg/m2) and mortality: a pooled analysis of 20 prospective studies. PLoS Med. 2014 Jul 8;11(7):e1001673. doi: 10.1371/journal.pmed.1001673. PMID: 25003901; PMCID: PMC4087039.

Li Y, Pan A, Wang DD, Liu X, Dhana K, Franco OH, Kaptoge S, Di Angelantonio E, Stampfer M, Willett WC, Hu FB. Impact of Healthy Lifestyle Factors on Life Expectancies in the US Population. Circulation. 2018 Jul 24;138(4):345-355. doi: 10.1161/CIRCULATIONAHA.117.032047. Erratum in: Circulation. 2018 Jul 24;138(4):e75. PMID: 29712712; PMCID: PMC6207481.

Magkos F, Tetens I, Bügel SG, Felby C, Schacht SR, Hill JO, Ravussin E, Astrup A (2020). A perspective on the transition to plant-based diets: a diet change may attenuate climate change, but can it also attenuate obesity and chronic disease risk? *Adv Nutr.* Jan 1;11(1):1-9. doi: 10.1093/advances/nmz090.

Melina V, Craig W, Levin S (2016). Position of the Academy of Nutrition and Dietetics: Vegetarian Diets. *J Acad Nutr Diet.* Dec;116(12):1970-1980. doi: 10.1016/j.jand.2016.09.025.

NHS (2023a), Cancer https://www.nhs.uk/conditions/cancer/ (accessed 04.04.23)

NHS (2023b), Vitamins, supplements and nutrition during pregnancy. https://www.nhs.uk/pregnancy/keeping-well/vitamins-supplements-and-nutrition/ (accessed 04.04.23)

NHS (2023c) Red meat and the risk of bowel cancer https://www.nhs.uk/live-well/eat-well/food-guidelines-and-food-labels/red-meat-and-the-risk-of-bowel-cancer/#:~:text=But%20eating%20a%20lot%20of,your%20risk%20of%20bowel%20cancer. (accessed 05.04.23)

PHE (2008) Public Health England: Polycyclic aromatic hydrocarbons, P. T. Department, England (2008)

Schwedhelm C, Boeing H, Hoffmann G, Aleksandrova K, Schwingshackl L. Effect of diet on mortality and cancer recurrence among cancer survivors: a systematic review and meta-analysis of cohort studies. Nutr Rev. 2016 Dec;74(12):737-748. doi: 10.1093/nutrit/nuw045. PMID: 27864535; PMCID: PMC5181206.

Seidelmann SB, Claggett B, Cheng S, Henglin M, Shah A, Steffen LM, Folsom AR, Rimm EB, Willett WC, Solomon SD. Dietary carbohydrate intake and mortality: a prospective cohort study and meta-analysis. Lancet Public Health. 2018 Sep;3(9):e419-e428. doi: 10.1016/S2468-2667(18)30135-X. Epub 2018 Aug 17. PMID: 30122560; PMCID: PMC6339822.

Shah UA, Iyengar NM. Plant-Based and Ketogenic Diets As Diverging Paths to Address Cancer: A Review. *JAMA Oncol.* 2022;8(8):1201–1208. doi:10.1001/jamaoncol.2022.1769

Timothy J Key, Paul N Appleby, Francesca L Crowe, Kathryn E Bradbury, Julie A Schmidt, Ruth C Travis, Cancer in British vegetarians: updated analyses of 4998 incident cancers in a cohort of 32,491 meat eaters, 8612 fish eaters, 18,298 vegetarians, and 2246 vegans, *The American Journal of Clinical Nutrition*, Volume 100, Issue suppl_1, July 2014, Pages 378S–385S, https://doi.org/10.3945/ajcn.113.071266

Turner-McGrievy G, Mandes T, Crimarco A. A plant-based diet for overweight and obesity prevention and treatment. J Geriatr Cardiol. 2017 May;14(5):369-374. doi: 10.11909/j.issn.1671-5411.2017.05.002. PMID: 28630616; PMCID: PMC5466943.

Vitamin D and health report (2016). The Scientific Advisory Committee on Nutrition (SACN) recommendations on vitamin D. Public Health England.

Willett W, Rockström J, Loken B, Springmann M, Lang T, & Vermeulen S & Garnett T, Tilman D, Declerck F, Wood A, Jonell, M, Clark M, Gordon L, Fanzo J, Hawkes C, Zurayk R, Rivera, J, Vries W, Sibanda L, Murray C. (2019). Food in the Anthropocene: the EAT–Lancet Commission on healthy diets from sustainable food systems. The Lancet. 393. 10.1016/S0140-6736(18)31788-4.

World Cancer Research Fund (2023), Cancer Prevention Programme https://www.wcrf.org/diet-activity-and-cancer/cancer-prevention-recommendations/ (accessed 05.04.23)

EFFECT OF MICRONUTRIENTS ON COGNITIVE FUNCTION, MENTAL HEALTH, AND SLEEP

Dr Ebru Aydar and Prof Christopher Palmer

Chemobrain refers to the cognitive impairment that can occur after cancer treatment. It's not limited to people who get chemotherapy (surgery and radiation can also contribute), but it's more noticeable if you had chemotherapy. Symptoms may include decreased short-term memory, problems finding words, short attention span, and difficulty concentrating and multitasking. There is some evidence that inflammation may contribute to chemobrain [Rao et al., 2022] and cancer patients have higher levels of proinflammatory cytokines [Gupta et al, 2011]. The nuclear factor (NF)-κB is a major mediator of inflammatory pathways and as such it is possible that nutritional agents such as curcumin, genistein, resveratrol, epigallocatechin gallate and lycopene which are able to target this nuclear factor may aid in alleviating chemobrain [Gupta et al, 2011]. Certainly it is known that cognitive brain function can be aided by micronutrients with anti-inflammatory activity [Wärnberg et al., 2009]. Therefore it is recommended to ensure that your diet contains a significant amount of phytochemicals in a natural form in order to provide a sufficient level of anti-inflammatory compounds.

Micronutrients such as vitamins and minerals play vital roles in several basic metabolic pathways that are needed for neuronal functions which in turn, result in effects on cognitive functioning, although the exact mechanisms are poorly understood. All the B vitamins (except folate) are involved in at least one and often more steps in the production of ATP within cells and as such an adequate supply of each B vitamin is required for adequate functioning of the energy-production system and maintaining brain structures in all people but particularly critical in infancy and childhood [For a review see Tardy et al., 2020]. The vitamins B1, B5, B6, B9, and C are precursors for the synthesis of neurotransmitters which play the role of chemical messengers between nerve cells. Additionally, vitamins B3 and B5, Iron, Magnesium, and Zinc play important roles in neurotransmission. Cognitive impairment may occur in people with very low dietary intakes of vitamin B1 [Gibson et al., 2016] and long-term vitamin B3 deficiency can lead to neurological symptoms, including depression and loss of memory [Mikkelsen et al., 2016]. Additionally, a higher intake of B vitamins throughout young adulthood is associated with better cognitive function in midlife [Qin et al., 2017].

Iron

If iron is not provided adequately then it will be preferentially utilized for the production of red blood cells rather than the brain and can lead to impairment in both motor and cognitive function in children [Radlowski and Johnson, 2013]. The negative effects of iron-deficiency anaemia are lasting and negatively impact academic performance [Grantham-McGregor and Ani, 2001].

Zinc and Magnesium

Other important minerals include zinc, which is vital for brain development, playing an essential role in neurogenesis (formation of new nerve cells), and synaptogenesis (formation of new connections between nerve cells) [Golub et al., 1995]. Magnesium is essential for learning and memory. Low magnesium levels are linked to many neurological diseases, including migraines, depression, and epilepsy [Kirkland et al., 2018].

Carotenoids

Carotenoids are a type of pigment found in leafy vegetables, pumpkins, carrots, corn, tomatoes, salmon, lobster & shrimp, and consumption of which are correlated with higher cognitive test scores within the visual-spatial domain [Davinelli et al., 2021]. Lutein is specifically related to cognitive measures of executive function including memory, self-motivation, language, and learning and improves temporal processing in young adults which refers to the processing of acoustic stimuli such as speech and music [Stringham et al., 2019].

Omega-3

Omega-3 fatty acids are a type of polyunsaturated fat that occur in three different forms in food.

- Docosahexaenoic acid (DHA) and Eicosapentaenoic acid (EPA) are found mainly in oily fish, such as salmon and mackerel.

- Alpha-linolenic acid (ALA) can be found mainly in green vegetables (Brussels sprouts, spinach, and kale), vegetable oils (canola or soybean), nuts (walnuts), and seeds (flaxseeds and pumpkin seeds).

*Note that the body has a limited capacity of converting ALA to EPA.

Omega-3 fats are especially important for building cellular membranes in all parts of the body but particularly important for the sensitive cells in the brain which provide cognitive function. Additionally, they have antioxidant and anti-inflammatory effects and may protect the brain from deterioration [Dyall, 2015]. The evidence for eating naturally occurring omega-3 provided by food is reasonable in terms of sustaining cognitive abilities. A systematic review revealed that consumption of seafood during childhood resulted in neurocognitive benefits [Hibbeln et al., 2019].

Polyphenols

Polyphenols are a class of mostly natural organic chemicals containing large multiples of phenol units. Polyphenol-rich products have benefits for brain function, particularly in early age, providing acute cognitive benefits. [Ammar et al., 2020]. Flavonoids are a type of polyphenols found in plants. Flavonoids, especially anthocyanins (a type of pigment found particularly in blackberry, raspberry, blueberries, purple corn, and red cabbage) have an effect on the brain cells associated with memory and neuronal function, mainly attributed to an increase of cerebral blood flow [Salehi et al., 2020]. This results in an improvement in cognitive capacities, shown particularly in animal studies and with flavonoid-enriched diets containing grape, pomegranate, strawberry, blueberry, cocoa, and pure flavonoids, such as quercetin [Waheed Janab et al., 2020]. A region of the hippocampus (found in the brain) that is involved in memory appears to be susceptible to improvement in old and young by consumption of polyphenol-rich foods, especially flavonoids. This may be due to the modulation of nitric oxide signalling which affects endothelial cells, which line blood vessels, and improves the supply of blood to the brain [Duarte et al., 2014]. Dark chocolate and cocoa powder contain a significant amount of flavonoids. The flavonoids in chocolate accumulate in the areas of the brain that deal with learning and memory [Nehlig, 2013]. In one study including over 900 people, those who ate chocolate more frequently performed better in a series of mental tasks, including some involving memory, than those who rarely ate it [Crichton et al., 2016]. Choline is an important micronutrient that your body uses to create acetylcholine, a neurotransmitter that helps regulate mood and memory. One study found lower risk of dementia and improved cognitive performance with dietary choline consumption [López-Sobaler et al, 2021]. Adequate amounts of choline can be found in beef, liver, scallops, salmon, chicken, and cod. Vegetarians can get choline in eggs and milk products.

Nutrition and mental well-being

Nutrition not only has a role in cognitive ability but also in depression and mood. While there is no diet plan which is proven to treat depression, it is apparent that a nervous system supplied with adequate nutrition is less prone to depression [Rao et al., 2008]. It should be noted also that depression itself may lead to poor nutrition. Carbohydrates may have a calming effect as they are linked to the production of serotonin - a mind boosting chemical in the brain and low serotonin activity may be linked to cravings for carbohydrates especially during winter months when lack of sunshine may increase seasonal affective disorders. In this instance, complex carbohydrates are preferred over simple sugars. Depression can also be influenced by genetics, stress, environment, sleep and mood disorders so it is difficult to assess the role that nutrition plays. However, a short discussion on the benefits of some key nutrients which may improve mood is provided.

Vitamin B

In a systematic review and meta-analysis there appears to be evidence for the benefit of B vitamin supplementation for healthy and at-risk populations for stress, but not for depressive symptoms or anxiety. Supplementation of the diet with B vitamins particularly benefit populations who are at risk due to poor nutrient status or poor mood status [Young et al., 2019]. However, there is a danger of over-supplementation therefore it is recommended to obtain B vitamins if possible, from natural sources.

Vitamin D

Receptors for vitamin D can be found throughout the body including the brain. Research has found that people with low levels of vitamin D have a greater likelihood of depression [Milaneschi et al., 2014]. Additionally, people with depression symptoms in particular in reference to seasonal affective disorder improved overall when vitamin D levels increased [Penckofer et al., 2010; Melrose, 2015]. Note that vitamin D can be obtained from food and from sunlight exposure via the skin.

Selenium

There appears to be a link between low mood and selenium. However, the benefits of selenium supplements are not clear and may have a detrimental effect if over-supplementation occurs [Wang et al., 2018].

Omega-3

There are links between societies that do not eat enough omega-3 and the rates of depressive disorders [Grosso et al., 2014]. However, supplementation with fish oils has not been conclusively proven to improve depressive disorders [Wolters et al., 2021]. The consumption of oily fish containing omega-3 is recommended to improve cognitive ability however these types of fish may contain high levels of mercury so care should be taken in selecting the types and sources of fish.

Flavonoids

Researchers have linked the consumption of flavonoids in young people with decreased risk of developing depression, [Khalid et al., 2017] especially anthocyanins (a type of pigment found particularly in blackberry, raspberry, blueberries, purple corn, and red cabbage). Dark chocolate contains substances such as caffeine, theobromine and N-acetyl ethanolamine thought to be able to provide a feel-good effect. However, the levels in chocolate are low and it is unclear if they can provide a physiological response. Although, dark chocolate contains significant amounts of flavonoids which may boost brain health and support mood regulation. It is recommended to select a brand of chocolate with a high cocoa content and thus a lower sugar content.

Nutrients influence many cognitive functions such as both immediate and working memory, selective and sustained attention, processing of visual-spatial information, temporal processing, and mood. Overall, it is better to obtain micronutrients such as vitamins from natural sources as the value of supplements generally has not been proven.

Nutrition to improve sleep

Getting the right amount of sleep is very important due to its restorative effects on the body and its role in memory formation. Generally, a meal with less fibre, more saturated fat and sugar is linked with poorer quality sleep [St-Onge et al.,

2016]. Also, diets that lack calcium, magnesium, and vitamins A, C, D, and E are correlated with poorer sleep [Ikonte et al., 2019]. Levels of the hormone melatonin are related to sleep quality. Melatonin regulates your internal clock and signals when it is time to sleep. Food with significant amounts of melatonin include cherries, eggs, milk, almonds, pistachios, and walnuts. Additionally, food such as turkey and bananas contain the amino acid tryptophan which increases melatonin production (Peuhkuri et al., 2012). It is recommended not to drink beverages containing caffeine before sleeping, rather chamomile tea can reduce stress and anxiety thus aiding sleep.

References

Ammar A, Trabelsi K, Boukhris O, Bouaziz B, Müller P, M Glenn J, Bott NT, Müller N, Chtourou H, Driss T, Hökelmann A. Effects of Polyphenol-Rich Interventions on Cognition and Brain Health in Healthy Young and Middle-Aged Adults: Systematic Review and Meta-Analysis. J Clin Med. 2020 May 25;9(5):1598. doi: 10.3390/jcm9051598.

Crichton GE, Elias MF, Alkerwi A. Chocolate intake is associated with better cognitive function: The Maine-Syracuse Longitudinal Study. Appetite. 2016 May 1;100:126-32. doi: 10.1016/j.appet.2016.02.010.

Davinelli S, Ali S, Solfrizzi V, Scapagnini G, Corbi G. Carotenoids and Cognitive Outcomes: A Meta-Analysis of Randomized Intervention Trials. Antioxidants (Basel). 2021 Feb 2;10(2):223. doi: 10.3390/antiox10020223.

Duarte J, Francisco V, Perez-Vizcaino F. Modulation of nitric oxide by flavonoids. Food Funct. 2014 Aug;5(8):1653-68. doi: 10.1039/c4fo00144c.

Dyall SC. Long-chain omega-3 fatty acids and the brain: a review of the independent and shared effects of EPA, DPA and DHA. Front Aging Neurosci. 2015 Apr 21;7:52. doi: 10.3389/fnagi.2015.00052.

Gibson GE, Hirsch JA, Fonzetti P, Jordan BD, Cirio RT, Elder J. Vitamin B1 (thiamine) and dementia. Ann N Y Acad Sci. 2016 Mar;1367(1):21-30. doi: 10.1111/nyas.13031.

Golub MS, Keen CL, Gershwin ME, Hendrickx AG. Developmental zinc deficiency and behavior. J Nutr. 1995 Aug;125(8 Suppl):2263S-2271S. doi: 10.1093/jn/125.suppl_8.2263S.

Grantham-McGregor S, Ani C. A review of studies on the effect of iron deficiency on cognitive development in children. J Nutr. 2001 Feb;131(2S-2):649S-666S; discussion 666S-668S. doi: 10.1093/jn/131.2.649S.

Grosso G, Galvano F, Marventano S, Malaguarnera M, Bucolo C, Drago F, Caraci F. Omega-3 fatty acids and depression: scientific evidence and biological mechanisms. Oxid Med Cell Longev. 2014;2014:313570. doi: 10.1155/2014/313570.

Gupta SC, Kim JH, Kannappan R, Reuter S, Dougherty PM, Aggarwal BB. Role of nuclear factor κB-mediated inflammatory pathways in cancer-related symptoms and their regulation by nutritional agents. Exp Biol Med (Maywood). 2011 Jun 1;236(6):658-71. doi: 10.1258/ebm.2011.011028.

Hibbeln JR, Spiller P, Brenna JT, Golding J, Holub BJ, Harris WS, Kris-Etherton P, Lands B, Connor SL, Myers G, Strain JJ, Crawford MA, Carlson SE. Relationships between seafood consumption during pregnancy and childhood and neurocognitive development: Two systematic reviews. Prostaglandins Leukot Essent Fatty Acids. 2019 Dec;151:14-36. doi: 10.1016/j.plefa.2019.10.002.

Ikonte CJ, Mun JG, Reider CA, Grant RW, Mitmesser SH. Micronutrient Inadequacy in Short Sleep: Analysis of the NHANES 2005-2016. Nutrients. 2019 Oct 1;11(10):2335. doi: 10.3390/nu11102335.

Khalid S, Barfoot KL, May G, Lamport DJ, Reynolds SA, Williams CM. Effects of Acute Blueberry Flavonoids on Mood in Children and Young Adults. Nutrients. 2017 Feb 20;9(2):158. doi: 10.3390/nu9020158.

Kirkland AE, Sarlo GL, Holton KF. The Role of Magnesium in Neurological Disorders. Nutrients. 2018 Jun 6;10(6):730. doi: 10.3390/nu10060730.

López-Sobaler AM, Lorenzo Mora AM, Salas González MªD, Peral Suárez Á, Aparicio A, Ortega RMª. Importancia de la colina en la función cognitiva [Importance of choline in cognitive function]. Nutr Hosp. 2021 Jan 13;37(Spec No2):18-23. Spanish. doi: 10.20960/nh.03351.

Melrose S. Seasonal Affective Disorder: An Overview of Assessment and Treatment Approaches. Depress Res Treat. 2015;2015:178564. doi: 10.1155/2015/178564.

Milaneschi Y, Hoogendijk W, Lips P, Heijboer AC, Schoevers R, van Hemert AM, Beekman AT, Smit JH, Penninx BW. The association between low vitamin D and depressive disorders. Mol Psychiatry. 2014 Apr;19(4):444-51. doi: 10.1038/mp.2013.36.

Nehlig A. The neuroprotective effects of cocoa flavanol and its influence on cognitive performance. Br J Clin Pharmacol. 2013 Mar;75(3):716-27. doi: 10.1111/j.1365-2125.2012.04378.x.

Penckofer S, Kouba J, Byrn M, Estwing Ferrans C. Vitamin D and depression: where is all the sunshine? Issues Ment Health Nurs. 2010 Jun;31(6):385-93. doi: 10.3109/01612840903437657.

Peuhkuri K, Sihvola N, Korpela R. Diet promotes sleep duration and quality. Nutr Res. 2012 May;32(5):309-19. doi: 10.1016/j.nutres.2012.03.009.

Qin B, Xun P, Jacobs DR Jr, Zhu N, Daviglus ML, Reis JP, Steffen LM, Van Horn L, Sidney S, He K. Intake of niacin, folate, vitamin B-6, and vitamin B-12 through young adulthood and cognitive function in midlife: the Coronary Artery Risk Development in Young Adults (CARDIA) study. Am J Clin Nutr. 2017 Oct;106(4):1032-1040. doi: 10.3945/ajcn.117.157834.

Radlowski EC, Johnson RW. Perinatal iron deficiency and neurocognitive development. Front Hum Neurosci. 2013 Sep 23;7:585. doi: 10.3389/fnhum.2013.00585.

Rao V, Bhushan R, Kumari P, Cheruku SP, Ravichandiran V, Kumar N. Chemobrain: A review on mechanistic insight, targets and treatments. Adv Cancer Res. 2022;155:29-76. doi: 10.1016/bs.acr.2022.04.001.

Rao TS, Asha MR, Ramesh BN, Rao KS. Understanding nutrition, depression and mental illnesses. Indian J Psychiatry. 2008 Apr;50(2):77-82. doi: 10.4103/0019-5545.42391.

Salehi B, Selamoglu Z, Sevindik M, Fahmy NM, Al-Sayed E, El-Shazly M, Csupor-Löffler B, Csupor D, Yazdi SE, Sharifi-Rad J, Arserim-Uçar DK, Arserim EH, Karazhan N, Jahani A, Dey A, Azadi H, Vakili SA, Sharopov F, Martins N, Büsselberg D. Achillea spp.: A comprehensive review on its ethnobotany, phytochemistry, phytopharmacology and industrial applications. Cell Mol Biol (Noisy-le-grand). 2020 Jun 25;66(4):78-103.

St-Onge MP, Roberts A, Shechter A, Choudhury AR. Fiber and Saturated Fat Are Associated with Sleep Arousals and Slow Wave Sleep. J Clin Sleep Med. 2016 Jan;12(1):19-24. doi: 10.5664/jcsm.5384.

Stringham JM, Johnson EJ, Hammond BR. Lutein across the Lifespan: From Childhood Cognitive Performance to the Aging Eye and Brain. Curr Dev Nutr. 2019 Jun 4;3(7):nzz066. doi: 10.1093/cdn/nzz066.

Tardy AL, Pouteau E, Marquez D, Yilmaz C, Scholey A. Vitamins and Minerals for Energy, Fatigue and Cognition: A Narrative Review of the Biochemical and Clinical Evidence. Nutrients. 2020 Jan 16;12(1):228. doi: 10.3390/nu12010228.

Waheed Janabi AH, Kamboh AA, Saeed M, Xiaoyu L, BiBi J, Majeed F, Naveed M, Mughal MJ, Korejo NA, Kamboh R, Alagawany M, Lv H. Flavonoid-rich foods (FRF): A promising nutraceutical approach against lifespan-shortening diseases. Iran J Basic Med Sci. 2020 Feb;23(2):140-153. doi: 10.22038/IJBMS.2019.35125.8353.

Wang J, Um P, Dickerman BA, Liu J. Zinc, Magnesium, Selenium and Depression: A Review of the Evidence, Potential Mechanisms and Implications. Nutrients. 2018 May 9;10(5):584. doi: 10.3390/nu10050584.

Wärnberg J, Gomez-Martinez S, Romeo J, Díaz LE, Marcos A. Nutrition, inflammation, and cognitive function. Ann N Y Acad Sci. 2009 Feb;1153:164-75. doi: 10.1111/j.1749-6632.2008.03985.x.

Wolters M, von der Haar A, Baalmann AK, Wellbrock M, Heise TL, Rach S. Effects of n-3 Polyunsaturated Fatty Acid Supplementation in the Prevention and Treatment of Depressive Disorders-A Systematic Review and Meta-Analysis. Nutrients. 2021 Mar 25;13(4):1070. doi: 10.3390/nu13041070.

Young LM, Pipingas A, White DJ, Gauci S, Scholey A. A Systematic Review and Meta-Analysis of B Vitamin Supplementation on Depressive Symptoms, Anxiety, and Stress: Effects on Healthy and 'At-Risk' Individuals. Nutrients. 2019 Sep 16;11(9):2232. doi: 10.3390/nu11092232.

NUTRITION AND THE IMMUNE SYSTEM

Prof Chris Palmer

Nutrition is vital for the efficiency of the immune system. Food consists of both macronutrients (proteins, fats and carbohydrates) and micronutrients (vitamins and minerals) and all play a role in our overall health and immune response. All components of the immune system are composed of proteins including cells, cytokines, antibodies. Overconsumption or underconsumption of proteins can affect mucosal barrier defences, innate and adaptive immunity [Chandra, 1992; Woodward, 1998; Li et al., 2007] and will result in higher susceptibility to both bacterial and viral infection. Sugars or carbohydrates are utilised for energy production. However, high blood sugar can result in altered inflammatory responses. Low blood sugar, on the other hand, increases cortisol, which exhibits immunosuppressive activity.

The impact of dietary polyunsaturated fatty acids (PUFAs) on the immune system has been investigated for decades, with special focus on the omega-3 PUFAs α-linolenic acid (ALA), eicosapentaenoic acid (EPA), and docosahexaenoic acid (DHA). ALA is found in nuts and seeds whereas EPA and DHA are the main components of fish oil [Gutiérrez et al, 2019]. Dietary unsaturated fatty acids play a role in immune function and give rise to metabolites referred to as n-3 or n-6 eicosanoids (prostaglandins and leukotrienes). Generally, n-6 eicosanoids are pro-inflammatory whereas n-3 eicosanoids are more anti-inflammatory. Overall a balance is important with a ratio of 3:1 seen as ideal. Generally, ALA, DHA, and EPA exert an inhibitory effect on the activation of immune cells from both the innate and the adaptive branch. Interestingly, some specific immune functions are promoted by dietary omega-3 fatty acids in specific immune cell types, i.e., phagocytosis by macrophages and neutrophils or Treg differentiation, suggesting that omega-3 fatty acids do not act as unspecific immune-repressors [for a review see Gutiérrez et al, 2019].

Vitamin D is vital for the immune system and induces both positive and negative effects on innate and adaptive immunity [Lucas et al., 2014]. Vitamin D can be obtained from sunlight and food sources but during the winter a supplement may be necessary. Vitamin E induces natural killer cell activity, exerts an anti-inflammatory effect on cytokine production [Lee and Han, 2018]. Vitamin A is vital for mucosal defences; with reference to the gut, it supports barrier integrity and immune hypo-responsiveness (tolerance). In addition, Vitamin A also exerts an anti-inflammatory effect via suppression of pro-inflammatory cytokines, whilst inducing anti-inflammatory cytokines such as IL-10 [Hall et al., 2011;

Sirisinha, 2015]. Vitamin C can contribute to innate defence by enhancing phagocytic clearance, neutrophil activity, NK activity, anti-viral (interferon) production and mucosal barrier integrity. It also has a positive influence on adaptive immunity [Carr and Maggini, 2017].

Certain mineral micronutrients also exhibit immunomodulatory activity; these include zinc, iron and selenium. All of these minerals have a positive effect on innate immunity, where they are capable of boosting NK, neutrophil and macrophage functions. In addition, these minerals also maintain B cell antibody production and cell-mediated immunity. Thus, these minerals are important in primary recognition and defence against pathogens and induction of anti-viral and anti-tumour responses [Cunningham-Rundles et al., 2005]. A variety of phytochemicals have been tested to investigate their immune modulating characteristics. These include amongst others curcumin, piperidine, cinermaldehyde, probiotics, allicin and quercertin. Generally these phytochemicals have anti-inflammatory properties. Since inflammation appears to be a side effect of chemotherapy these phytochemicals may have value in alleviating these side effects [Sahin et a.,, 2021]. Additionally, the role of probiotic bacteria in the gastrointestinal tract in the production of immune boosting metabolites is discussed in a previous chapter.

Avoiding colds and flu

Cancer treatments can weaken the immune system leaving a person susceptible to respiratory infections. Most colds and cases of flu are caused by viruses that infect our respiratory tract. While in a healthy person they represent little more than a few days off training they may be more serious for those with a weakened immune system or undergoing cancer-related treatments. Factors associated with a weakened immune system include:

- Poor sleep
- Poor nutrition
- Excess alcohol
- Excess dietary fat
- Smoking
- Psychological stress
- Intense physical activity

Since these viruses spread through contact via coughs, sneezes, and hand-to-face transmission it is important to maintain good hygiene particularly when on public transport. This should be part of a good handwashing regime. However, it is impossible to avoid all sources of viruses therefore we can enhance our immune system through nutrition as listed below:

Adequate vitamins - vitamins are important for the functioning of the immune system [Calder et al., 2020]

Supply of minerals - such as zinc, iron, and selenium; zinc can be found in whole grain products, iron can be found in legumes, tofu, and green vegetables, selenium is found in mushrooms, and nuts (especially Brazil nuts). *Note can be combined with foods containing vitamin C to boost absorption*

Phytonutrients - can have anti-viral properties. For example, ginger has anti-viral properties [Chang et al., 2013]

Fibre - found in whole plant foods can benefit the bacteria living in our digestive system which produce short-chain fatty acids which boost our immune system [Arpaia et al., 2013].

Note that taking massive amounts of vitamin C (above 500 mg) has not been proven to affect the chance of getting flu or cold in most people. However, it has been proven effective for athletes undertaking intense training in sub-artic conditions [Douglas et al., 2007]. Therefore, in the winter months during the cold season, it may be beneficial to eat foods with more vitamin C such as citrus fruits and red peppers. Taking excessive vitamin C has been proven effective in reducing the course of a cold infection by an average of half a day in adults and by one day in children [Douglas et al., 2007]. Additionally, chewing on a raw cube of ginger or making a ginger tea may be beneficial in preventing viral infections. At least, some chemicals found in ginger have anti-viral activity when applied to *in vitro* cultures of cells [Chang et al., 2013]. Additionally, it was deduced that adherence to the Mediterranean diet may be associated with a lower risk of COVID-19 [Perez-Araluce et al., 2021].

Nutrition and the lymph system

The lymph system acts as a drainage and filtering system consisting of vessels, ducts, nodes, and glands. Blood flows from your heart along arteries and capillaries delivering about twenty litres of nutrients to the cells of the body. Cellular waste products and around seventeen litres of fluid return to the heart via the veins. The remaining three litres is collected by the lymphatic system in the form of a colourless liquid called the lymph fluid which eventually returns to the blood circulation via the lymph vessels. Lymph fluid contains proteins, minerals, fats, nutrients, damaged cells, cancer cells and foreign invaders (bacteria, viruses, etc). The lymphatic system is often neglected in terms of scientific research however it has a very important role to play in the body including:

- Regulation of fluid levels in the body
- Absorption of fats from the gastrointestinal tract
- Production and storage of white blood cells that can destroy foreign invaders such as bacteria, viruses, parasites and fungi

Lymph nodes are oval glands that filter out damaged and cancer cells. There are around six thousand lymph nodes in your body connected by lymphatic vessels to form an interconnecting network. The lymphatic vessels drain excess fluid from cells and tissues. Lymph vessels drain into ducts that connect to the subclavian vein, which returns lymph to your bloodstream just below the collarbone. The spleen is the largest lymph organ located on your left side under the ribs and functions to filter and store blood and produces white blood cells that fight infection or disease. Other major parts of the body with lymphatic functions include the thymus, tonsils and adenoids, bone marrow, Peyer's patches and the appendix. Despite many websites boasting of ways to detox your lymph system, there is no scientific evidence that any food, tea, juice, or supplement can perform this act. The lymph system is generally able to take care of itself in most cases as long as we eat a healthy diet and exercise regularly. Since the lymph system plays an important role in the immune system the same nutrition which is recommended for optimizing the functioning of the immune system should be applied to the lymph system.

References

Arpaia N, Campbell C, Fan X, Dikiy S, van der Veeken J, deRoos P, Liu H, Cross JR, Pfeffer K, Coffer PJ, Rudensky AY. Metabolites produced by commensal bacteria promote peripheral regulatory T-cell generation. Nature. 2013 Dec 19;504(7480):451-5. doi: 10.1038/nature12726.

Carr AC, Maggini S. Vitamin C and Immune Function. Nutrients. 2017 Nov 3;9(11):1211. doi: 10.3390/nu9111211.

Calder PC, Carr AC, Gombart AF, Eggersdorfer M. Optimal Nutritional Status for a Well-Functioning Immune System Is an Important Factor to Protect against Viral Infections. Nutrients. 2020 Apr 23;12(4):1181. doi: 10.3390/nu12041181.

Chandra RK. Protein-energy malnutrition and immunological responses. J Nutr. 1992 Mar;122(3 Suppl):597-600. doi: 10.1093/jn/122.suppl_3.597.

Chang JS, Wang KC, Yeh CF, Shieh DE, Chiang LC. Fresh ginger (Zingiber officinale) has anti-viral activity against human respiratory syncytial virus in human respiratory tract cell lines. J Ethnopharmacol. 2013 Jan 9;145(1):146-51. doi: 10.1016/j.jep.2012.10.043.

Cunningham-Rundles S, McNeeley DF, Moon A. Mechanisms of nutrient modulation of the immune response. J Allergy Clin Immunol. 2005 Jun;115(6):1119-28; quiz 1129. doi: 10.1016/j.jaci.2005.04.036.

Douglas RM, Hemilä H, Chalker E, Treacy B. Vitamin C for preventing and treating the common cold. Cochrane Database Syst Rev. 2007 Jul 18;(3):CD000980. doi: 10.1002/14651858.CD000980.pub3. Update in: Cochrane Database Syst Rev. 2013;1:CD000980.

Gutiérrez S, Svahn SL, Johansson ME. Effects of Omega-3 Fatty Acids on Immune Cells. Int J Mol Sci. 2019 Oct 11;20(20):5028. doi: 10.3390/ijms20205028.

Hall JA, Grainger JR, Spencer SP, Belkaid Y. The role of retinoic acid in tolerance and immunity. Immunity. 2011 Jul 22;35(1):13-22. doi: 10.1016/j.immuni.2011.07.002.

Lee GY, Han SN. The Role of Vitamin E in Immunity. Nutrients. 2018 Nov 1;10(11):1614. doi: 10.3390/nu10111614.

Li P, Yin YL, Li D, Kim SW, Wu G. Amino acids and immune function. Br J Nutr. 2007 Aug;98(2):237-52. doi: 10.1017/S000711450769936X.

Lucas RM, Gorman S, Geldenhuys S, Hart PH. Vitamin D and immunity. F1000Prime Rep. 2014 Dec 1;6:118. doi: 10.12703/P6-118.

Perez-Araluce R, Martinez-Gonzalez MA, Fernández-Lázaro CI, Bes-Rastrollo M, Gea A, Carlos S. Mediterranean diet and the risk of COVID-19 in the 'Seguimiento Universidad de Navarra' cohort. Clin Nutr. 2022 Dec;41(12):3061-3068. doi: 10.1016/j.clnu.2021.04.001.

Sahin TK, Bilir B, Kucuk O. Modulation of inflammation by phytochemicals to enhance efficacy and reduce toxicity of cancer chemotherapy. Crit Rev Food Sci Nutr. 2021 Sep 16:1-15. doi: 10.1080/10408398.2021.1976721.

Sirisinha S. The pleiotropic role of vitamin A in regulating mucosal immunity. Asian Pac J Allergy Immunol. 2015 Jun;33(2):71-89.

Woodward B. Protein, calories, and immune defenses. Nutr Rev. 1998 Jan;56(1 Pt 2):S84-92. doi: 10.1111/j.1753-4887.1998.tb01649.x.

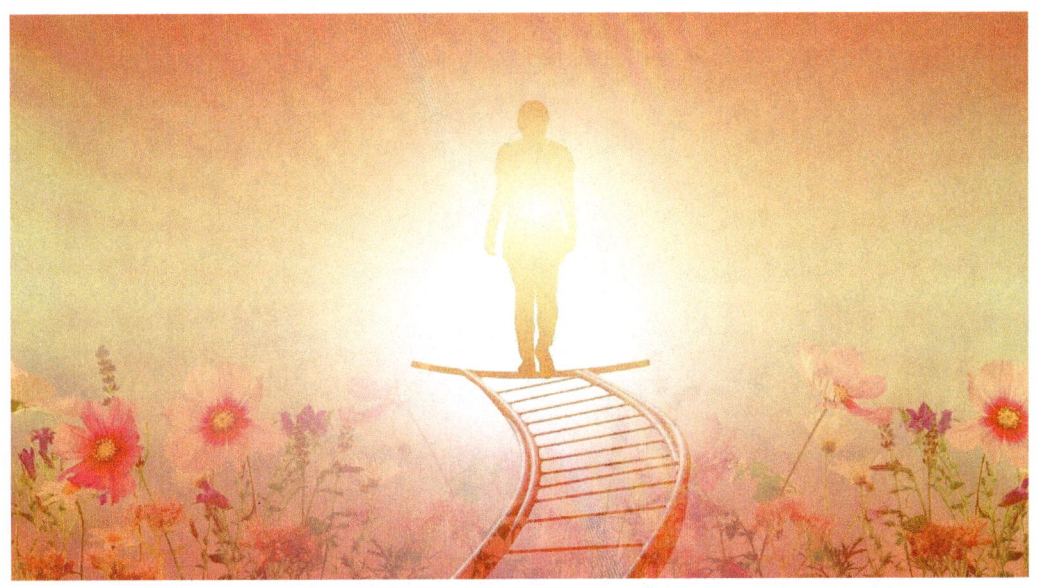

The pathway to hope is within yourself.

Printed in Great Britain
by Amazon

24529329R00076

SEO の教科書

検索エンジン最適化

Yahoo!・Google 対策から、SEM 併用・ブログ向け SEO まで

ドラゴンフィールド株式会社
吉村 正春

A TEXTBOOK OF SEARCH ENGINE OPTIMIZATION

秀和システム

●注意
・本書は著者が独自に調査した結果を出版したものです。内容については万全を期して作成しておりますが、その影響に関しての責任は負いかねます。
・本書に記載されている会社名、商品名などは、一般に各社の商標または登録商標です。本文中では、TMおよびRは省略いたしました。
・本書に記載されているURLなどは、予告なく変更されることがあります。
・本書の全部または一部について、著者権法の定める範囲を超え、出版元から文書による承諾を得ずに無断で複写、複製、転載することを禁じます。

まえがき

☐ 誰もが検索する時代になった

　最近、「××で検索」と検索キーワードを表示させる広告が増えてきました。
　これは、それは取りも直さず、ユーザーの検索リテラシーの高まりを反映しているといえるでしょう。近年、ユーザーの検索に対するリテラシーは、数年前とは比較にならないほど向上しました。「ネットで検索する」ということがどういうことなのか知らない人は、もはやいないのではないでしょうか。
　検索エンジンの影響度は、確実に大きくなっています。
　そして、それに応じて、検索エンジンは日々変化を遂げています。Yahoo!やGoogle、MSNなど大手検索エンジンも新サービスも次々とリリースしていますし、それは他の検索エンジンも同様です。サービスの形態も多様化し、Googleは地図情報までも検索サービスの領域に組み込んでいます。

☐ SEOに取り組まなければスタートラインにも立てない

　こうした変化に伴って、あらゆるビジネスで検索エンジン対策——すなわちSEOの重要性が高まってきています。
　SEOという言葉が認知され（いわゆる「キャズムの壁」を越えて）、LPO、ロングテールといったSEOから派生した言葉も、IT業界では一般的に認知されるようになりました。
　また、様々なSEO支援ツールがリリースされており、それらのツールを駆使することにより、従来よりも格段に効果的にSEO作業を進められるようになりました。
　例えば、SEOにおいてキーワード選定は重要なフローです。この選定作業は、オーバーチュアのキーワードアドバイスツールを使うことが定番でしたが、同様のサービスが各検索サービスから提供され始めています。Yahoo!は組み合わせ検索キーワードを閲覧できる「関連検索ワード」、Googleは「Google Trend」と任意のキーワードの人気を時間軸で表示するサービスを始めました。米Microsoftは「adCenter Labs」で、「任意のキーワードに続けてユーザーがどんなキーワードで検索しているかを検索ボリュームや割合で表示するツール」などを提供しています。
　現在のSEOは、これらのサービスを複合的に使うことにより、より精度の高いキーワードを選定することが求められているのです。
　もはや、単にSEOをしていれば勝てる時代は終わったといえるでしょう。求められ

ているのは、いかにSEOを使いこなしているか、そのレベルです。

「SEOをしなければスタートラインにすら立てない」時代になっているといっても過言ではないでしょう。

☐ ブログにもSEOは必要になった

そして、ウェブ業界には、もう一つの大きな変化がありました。いわゆるウェブ2.0と呼ばれるサービスの出現です。

中でも、その代表格とされるのが「ブログ」でしょう。そして、このブログの普及も、SEOに大きな影響を与えています。

現在は「一億総ブロガー時代」が到来し、ユーザーの嗜好は、情報を捜すだけではなく、ブログを使って積極的に情報発信することにシフトしてきました。ブロガーの中には、積極的にアフィリエイトなどで収益を生み出している方も少なくありません。このような個人ブログの参入によって、検索結果画面の縄張り争いは熾烈を極めています。ビッグキーワードからスモール（ニッチ）キーワードへと主戦場は移り、成果を挙げられるのはどのキーワードなのかとキーワードの金脈を探しに明け暮れている方も多いと聞きます。

これほどブログが普及すると、検索エンジンと相性が良いはずのブログといえど、どれだけSEOを意識しているかどうかで、その後の検索エンジン結果への反映度が変わってきます。

ブログはテンプレートと呼ばれるひな型にコンテンツを当て込んで、ウェブページを生成していきますが、このテンプレートは必ずしもSEOを意識されたものではありませんので、ブログのSEOではテンプレートの修正は必須です。また、ブログはプラグインの導入によって、機能を拡張することができますが、SEO効果が期待できるものや、回遊率向上や直帰率抑制に効果があるものなども存在します。これらをうまく導入することで、SEOや更新性に優れたブログを実現できます。

SEOにも、新しい波が訪れているのです。

☐ ウェブ2.0時代のSEOの基本図書

前著『SEOで検索エンジンもユーザーも味方に付けるホームページ改造術』が出たのが、2005年1月。おかげさまで、第4刷を発行するまで可愛がっていただきました。近所の書店で平積みされている姿を見かける度に、感謝の念がふつふつと湧いてきます。本当にありがとうございました。

しかし、それから2年が経ち、Yahoo!が検索結果画面を刷新してYST主体になったり、大手企業がGoogle八分を受けたり、と細々とした修正だけでは間に合わないほど、あまりにも検索エンジン業界の変化は早く大きなものでした。

こうした状況を鑑みて、SEOの基本を伝える本として、最新の情報を反映させてあらためて書き下ろしたのが、本書です。

この本では、通常のSEOの範疇であるhtmlのチューニングや、SEMに触れつつ、ブログをベースにしたSEOをご紹介していきます。

　特にブログについては、前著でも「Movable Type」については多少触れましたが、静的ページを生成する「Movable Type」を取り上げるならば、動的ページを生成するブログツールの代表格「WordPress」を取り上げないわけにはいかないだろうということで、本著では両方のブログツールでできるSEOを紹介しています。

　ウェブ2.0時代のSEOの基本図書として、本書が前著同様、みなさまの検索エンジン対策のお役に立ち、愛される存在となることを、心より祈っております。

2007年3月

ドラゴンフィールド株式会社　吉村 正春

まえがき ・・・・・・・・・・・・・・・・・・・3

　❏誰もが検索する時代になった
　❏SEOに取り組まなければスタートラインにも立てない
　❏ブログにもSEOは必要になった
　❏ウェブ2.0時代のSEOの基本図書

第1章　SEOの現状と基本

1 検索エンジンを取り巻く現状 ・・・・・・・・・20

　❏ユーザーの検索エンジン依存度は高まるばかり
　❏SEOをしなければスタートラインには立てない

2 SEOをしないとどうなるのか？ ・・・・・・・23

　❏ユーザーが出会う5つのハードル
　❏SEOの作業フロー

3 キーワードの重要性 ・・・・・・・・・・・・・25

　❏キーワードの争奪戦が始まっている
　❏ユーザーニーズにフィットしたキーワードを探そう
　❏ページ内容とキーワードは一致させなければ意味がない

4 内部要素と外部要素 ・・・・・・・・・・・・・・27

☐SEOを構成する2つの要素
☐htmlを調整する内部要素対策
☐被リンクを確保する外部要素対策

5 SEOの効果測定 ・・・・・・・・・・・・・・・・29

☐検索エンジンスパムには気を付けよう
☐目先の数字に一喜一憂しない

6 ブログとSEOの関係 ・・・・・・・・・・・・・31

☐もともと相性が良いブログもSEO対策が必要
☐ウェブ2.0の変化に対応するために

第2章　キーワード選定

1 キーワード選定 ・・・・・・・・・・・・・・・・・36

☐「どんなキーワードでも上位表示」を目指しては成果は出ない
☐適切なキーワードを選定するための5つの方法

2 アクセスログからユーザーニーズを探る ・・・・・・37

☐検索窓にはユーザーのニーズが反映される
☐アクセスログ解析の3つの種類

3 競合サイト調査からキーワードを選ぶ・・・・・・・・・・39

　　□競合サイトのキーワードを調査する

4 ツールを使ってみよう・・・・・・・・・・・・・・40

　　□代表的な無料ツールは？
　　□オーバーチュアのキーワードアドバイスツールを使う
　　□Google Trendを使う
　　□Googleウェブマスターツールを使う
　　□BIGLOBEの指標からキーワードの激戦度を探る

5 複合キーワードを狙う・・・・・・・・・・・・・45

　　□90％のユーザーは複合キーワードを使っている
　　□ツールを使って複合キーワードを探す

6 キーワードに対応するランディングページを用意する・・・47

　　□LPO（ランディングページ最適化）とは何か
　　□ランディングページの有無で成果は大きく変わる
　　□検索キーワードにユーザーニーズは宿る
　　□デザインやナビゲーションも重要

第3章 htmlの最適化

1 内部要素のSEO ・・・・・・・・・・・・・・52

□検索エンジンが理解しやすいhtmlを書こう
□SEOに関係するタグは？

2 <title>要素におけるSEO ・・・・・・・・・54

□検索エンジンにもユーザーにも最重要な<title>タグ
□タイトルは30字以内で付けよう！
□<title>タグで気を付けるその他のこと

3 <meta>タグのSEO ・・・・・・・・・・・57

□検索エンジンにだけ働きかける特殊なタグ
□本当に必要な<meta>タグは4つだけ
□<charset>で文字コードを指定する
□<description>で説明文を伝える
□<keywords>でキーワードを明示する
□<robots>で検索エンジンの振る舞いを指示する

4 <hX>タグのSEO ・・・・・・・・・・・61

□タイトルと並んで重要な見出しタグ
□<h1>には<title>と近似の内容を入れよう
□文章構造に見合った見出しタグを使おう

5 <a>タグのSEO ・・・・・・・・・・・63

- □アンカーテキストとリンク先の内容を一致させよう
- □相互リンクの書式を徹底させよう
- □リンクスパムを防止するための<nofollow>属性

6 <strong>タグと<em>タグ ・・・・・・・・65

- □論理タグと視覚タグ
- □強調したいキーワードだけに適用する

7 画像に<alt>属性を付ける ・・・・・・・・・67

- □<alt>属性で検索エンジンに画像情報を伝える

8 <acronym>タグと<abbr>タグ ・・・・・・68

- □略称を定義できるタグ

9 キーワードの出現頻度 ・・・・・・・・・・・69

- □キーワードの出現頻度と近接度
- □表記は統一させよう

10 サイドメニューの配置 ・・・・・・・・・・71

- □検索エンジンは<body>直後のテキストを重要視する
- □CSSで、<body>直下にメインコンテンツを持ってくる

11 CSSとJavaScriptの外部化・・・・・・・・・・73

　　□外部化することの2つのメリット

12 サブドメインの活用・・・・・・・・・・・・74

　　□サブドメインを使う3つのメリット
　　□サブドメイン間のリンクは外部リンクとして扱われる
　　□検索結果にすべて表示される
　　□エイジングフィルタ対策になる
　　□サブドメインを使う注意点
　　□サブドメイン対応のブログサービス

13 サイトマップの役割・・・・・・・・・・・・78

　　□ユーザーだけでなく検索エンジンも利用する案内板
　　□内部リンクの充実にも効果的

第4章　制作後の告知活動

1 外部要素のSEO・・・・・・・・・・・・・・82

　　□内部要素だけではSEO効果は8割減
　　□自力で被リンクを獲得しよう

2 検索エンジンへのサイト登録・・・・・・・・・・・・84

❏Googleウェブマスターツールを使ってみよう
❏アカウントを取得してURLを登録する
❏認証作業で、登録したサイトの持ち主であることを証明する
❏サイト構造を記したxmlファイルをアップロードする
❏注意すべき設定
❏Yahoo! Site Explorerへの登録
❏ディレクトリ型検索エンジンに登録される

3 エイジングフィルタ対策・・・・・・・・・・・・・89

❏立ち上げから半年は検索エンジンに表示されない!?
❏情報を小出しにして更新頻度を高めよう
❏SEMやサブドメインを併用することでチャンスロスを抑える

4 SEMの併用・・・・・・・・・・・・・・・・・・91

❏SEOとの使い分けがますます重要になったSEM
❏SEMなら検索結果順位をコントロールできる
❏キーワード単位で効果測定ができるのもメリット
❏重要性を増していくSEM

5 検索エンジン以外の外部リンクを確保する ・・・・・・・・95

❏外部リンクを確実に獲得する3つの方法
❏プレスリリースを流す
❏メールマガジンを発行する
❏Wikipediaに会社情報を登録する
❏ソーシャルブックマークに登録する

第5章　検索エンジンスパム

1 検索エンジンスパムとはなにか？　・・・・・・・・・100

- ☐ 過度のSEOにはペナルティがある
- ☐ 検索エンジンスパムの種類

2 コンテンツスパムの手法　・・・・・・・・・・・・102

- ☐ 代表的な3つの手法
- ☐ 見えない文字を使う
- ☐ キーワードの詰め込み
- ☐ <noflames>タグや<noscript>タグにキーワードやアンカーテキストを埋める

3 リンクスパムの手法　・・・・・・・・・・・・・104

- ☐ 代表的な6つの手法
- ☐ 隠しリンク
- ☐ リダイレクト
- ☐ ドアウェイページ
- ☐ リンクファーム
- ☐ トラックバックスパム・コメントスパム
- ☐ リファラースパム

4 ユーザビリティ的に避けるべき行為・・・・・・・・・・108

　　　□代表的な4つのNG手法と回避策
　　　□文字を画像にしてあるページ
　　　□Flash、JavaScriptをページ移動用の手段にする
　　　□フレームを使ったページ
　　　□動的ページ生成

第6章　効果測定と調整

1 効果測定の必要性・・・・・・・・・・・・・・・116

　　　□PDCAサイクルを回そう
　　　□効果測定の4つの手法

2 SEO TOOLSで効果を測定する・・・・・・・・・118

　　　□複数の検索エンジンを横断的にチェックするツール群
　　　□SEOアクセス解析ツール
　　　□SEOアクセス解析履歴
　　　□順位チェックツール

3 Google AdSenseで効果を測定する・・・・・・・121

　　　□検索エンジンはキーワードを適切に判断しているか？

4 Google Analyticsでアクセスログを分析する・・・・122

　　　□アクセスログデータの4つのポイント

5 SEMの効果を測定する ・・・・・・・・・・・・・124

　　□SEMではキーワード単位での効果測定が求められる
　　□自動ツールを活用しよう
　　□ウェブサイト オプティマイザーを使ったA/B スプリットテスト

第7章　ブログツールのSEO

1 SEOの視点から見たブログのメリット ・・・・・・・128

　　□ブログと検索エンジンが好相性の理由
　　□内部リンクが作りやすい
　　□被リンクを得られやすい
　　□CSSとhtmlの分離が実現されている
　　□SEO対応のページが量産できるのがブログのメリット

2 どのブログツールを使うか？ ・・・・・・・・・・・131

　　□サーバー設置型のMovable TypeかWordPressがお勧め
　　□Movable Typeの5つのメリット
　　□WordPressの4つのメリット
　　□いずれもSEO仕様のチューニングは必至

3 \<title\>タグのチューニング ・・・・・・・・・・・137

　　□個別の記事タイトルを表示させる

4 <meta>タグのチューニング ・・・・・・・・・・・・・138

- ❏<keywords>と<description>のチューニングが必要
- ❏<keywords>のチューニング
- ❏<description>のチューニング
- ❏検索エンジンに拾われないページを作る
- ❏不要な<meta>タグは削除しておこう

5 <hX>タグのチューニング ・・・・・・・・・・・・141

- ❏見出しとして機能するようにしよう

6 パーマリンクの設定 ・・・・・・・・・・・・・・142

- ❏パーマリンクの重要性
- ❏Movable Typeでのパーマリンク設定
- ❏WordPressでのパーマリンク設定

7 パンくずリストを作ろう ・・・・・・・・・・・・145

- ❏トップページ以外のページに来たユーザーに現在地を教える

8 RSSフィードの設定 ・・・・・・・・・・・・・・146

- ❏検索エンジンにもRSSを読んでもらおう
- ❏RSSには概要だけ書くのがお勧め

9 更新作業が終わった後にやること ・・・・・・・・・・147

- ❏PingサーバーにPingを打つ
- ❏Googleウェブマスターツールを使う
- ❏ソーシャルブックマークしてもらう

10 プラグインでSEO仕様にパワーアップさせる ・・・・・・151

- ❏SEOに有効なプラグインはたくさんある
- ❏画像アップロード時に<alt>属性を追加するプラグイン
- ❏関連記事を表示するプラグイン
- ❏自動的に文中リンクするプラグイン
- ❏コンテンツを拡充するプラグイン
- ❏スパム対策するプラグイン
- ❏テキスト要素のデザイン性を崩さずにSEO対策をするツール

あとがき ・・・・・・・・・・・・・・・・・・・・・・・157

- ❏本書を全面的に書き下ろした理由
- ❏SEOとオリコンチャートの類似点
- ❏支えてくれた人に感謝を込めて

SEO「検索エンジン最適化」の教科書

第 **1** 章

SEOの現状と基本

SEOは「やって当たり前」の時代に何をすべきか？

1.1 検索エンジンを取り巻く現状

◻ ユーザーの検索エンジン依存度は高まるばかり

　SEOをテーマにした書籍が数多く発行され、IT系雑誌でもごく当たり前にSEO特集が組まれるようになりました。もちろん本著を手に取った方は、SEOに多少なりとも知識を持っていると推測しますが、SEOはここ数年で一挙に市民権を獲得した感があります。

　SEOが市民権を得ていることは、各種のアンケート結果からも明らかです。

　オプトが2006年3月下旬、18歳以上のネットユーザーを対象にして実施した調査によると、検索結果の閲覧ページ数は平均で3.6ページであることが分かりました。1ページに表示される検索結果はデフォルトで20件ですので、実際にアクセスするかどうかは置いといて、1回の検索で70～80くらいのサイトをユーザーは視認している計算になります。

　また、もしニーズに合致しないページしか検索されなかった場合は、「キーワードを替えて」「キーワードを追加して再検索する」ユーザーは90％を超えます。

　このデータからも、ネットユーザーが検索エンジンを重要視していることがよく分かります。

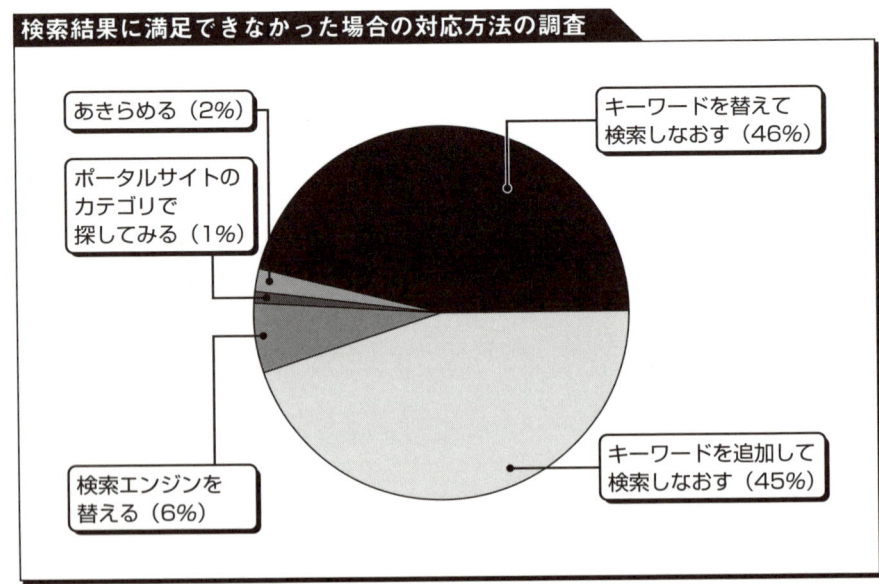

検索結果に満足できなかった場合の対応方法の調査

この調査で注目すべきは「あきらめる」と回答したユーザーはわずか2％しかいなかったこと。ユーザーは検索エンジンに依存していることを示唆しています。「検索エンジンに補足されないページは、ウェブに存在しないのも同じ」といっても過言ではありません。

もちろん、検索エンジン以外の手段で情報に辿り着くユーザーもいます。お気に入りから直接やってきたり、掲示板の書き込み、ブログのトラックバックやコメント、ソーシャルブックマーク（→P149参照）、RSSリーダーなど、その経路は多岐に渡るものの、対策が打てる経路もありますので、それらのユーザーを取りこぼすことなく、サイトに誘導することも重要です。

しかし、もっとも重要なのが、検索エンジンからの経路であることは、間違いがありません。

以前、マーケティング用語として、AIDMAがいわれていました。Attention（注意喚起）→Interest（興味）→Desire（購買欲求）→Memory（記憶）→Action（購入）という、ユーザーの行動パターンを表したものです。

ところがウェブの発達により、今はAISASに移行したといわれています。Attention（注意喚起）→Interest（興味）→Search（検索）→Action（購入）→Share（情報共有）と、興味を持ったユーザーはまず検索して調べることから行動を始めます。

検索エンジンからの経路を、太く確実なものにするSEOは、もはやウェブビジネスを行う上で必須といえるでしょう。

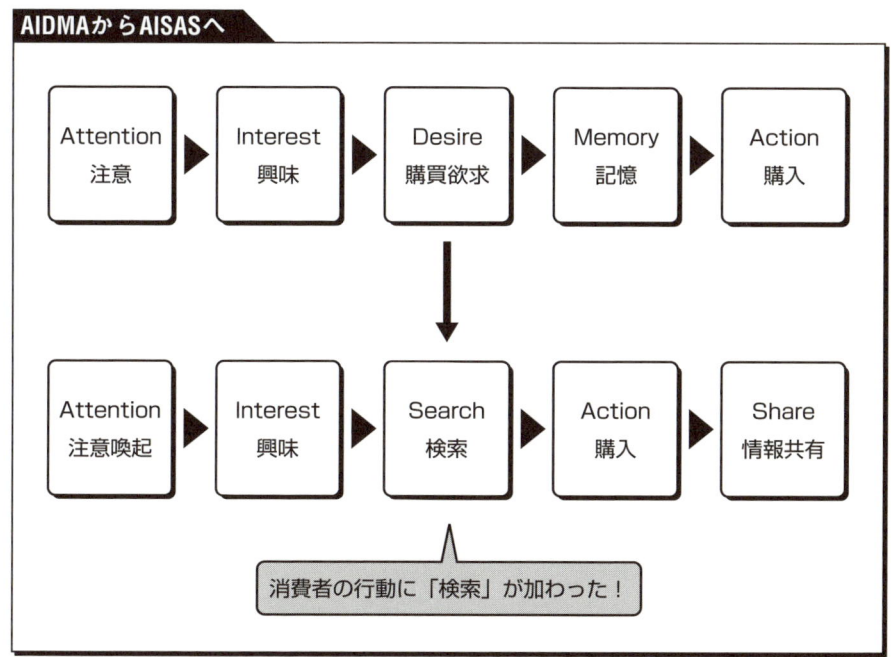

AIDMAからAISASへ

□SEOをしなければスタートラインには立てない

　当然ながら、このような状況に対応して、企業のSEOに対する意識も変わってきています。

　日経BPコンサルティングが2005年7月、企業サイトのウェブマスターを対象に実施したアンケートによると、「SEO対策を現在実施している」（52.0％）、「現在、過去とも実施したことはないが、将来検討したい」（27.2％）という結果が出ました。つまり約8割の企業は（程度の差はあるものの）SEOを意識しているということです。

　既にそのアンケート実施日から1年以上が経過していることを考えれば、SEOに対する認知度はさらに上昇し、「SEOはやるべきこと」から「SEOは当然やっておくべきこと」に意識はスライドしていると考えるのが妥当でしょう。

　ということは、SEOをしなければ、8割の企業サイトに後れを取ることになります。SEOをしていないということは、それほどのハンデを抱えることを意味するのです。そして、SEOをして、はじめて他の企業サイトと同じスタートラインに立ったといえるのです。

　ただし、SEOを施したウェブサイトでも、「検索結果の上位に表示されなかった」「検索エンジンからの誘導が増えなかった」などの不満を抱えているところが少なくありません。8割の企業がSEOを視野に入れている現状では、普通にSEOを行ったとしても検索順位が上がりにくくなっているのも当然です。

　そのため、ライバルサイトと差を付けるためには、今の検索エンジンのトレンドに合ったSEOを施す必要があります。加えて、さらに検索結果上位を狙うための「＋α」要素が必要になっています。

　今は、SEOの是非を問う次元から、どのウェブサイトもSEOをやっていることを前提として、「その中からいかに抜きん出るか」ということに議論のテーマは移っているのです。

1-2 SEOをしないとどうなるのか？

□ ユーザーが出会う5つのハードル

　前節で説明したように、検索エンジンはネットユーザーの行動に強く影響を与えます。では、SEOに取り組まないと、どうなるのでしょうか？　ユーザーの行動をシミュレートしてみましょう。

　ユーザーがウェブでなんらかの目的（情報の閲覧や、商品の購入など）を持って行動しようとしたとき、そこにはユーザーの行動を妨げるハードルがいくつか存在します。具体的には、以下のものです。

①見込みユーザーが使う（と想定している）検索キーワードで、自社サイトがヒットしない
②検索結果に、不親切な紹介文が表示されている。
③ランディングページにユーザーの知りたい情報、興味を喚起する情報が掲載されていない。または検索キーワードとずれた内容が記載されている。
④他のウェブページへの移動がスムーズに行えない。
⑤ウェブページの不備でユーザーがアクションを起こせない。

ユーザー行動を妨げる5つのハードル

ユーザーの行動	ハードル
検索する	サイトがヒットしない
検索結果を見る	紹介文が不親切
サイトへ訪問	ランディングページに知りたい情報が掲載されていない
サイト内の移動	他ページの移動がスムーズでない
購買・申込アクション	ページの不備でアクションを起こせない

これらは、ネットユーザーが検索をして行動に至るまでに出会うハードルです。ご自身のユーザーとしての経験に照らし合わせても、思い当たる節があるのではないでしょうか？　実際、これらのハードルの存在が、競合サイトへユーザーが流れるなどのチャンスロスを招いているケースが驚くほど多いのです。そして、これらのハードルを解消するのが、SEOの本質なのです。

☐ SEOの作業フロー

では、前述のハードルを踏まえた上で、SEOの作業フローを確認しておきましょう。簡単なフローは下記の通りです。

①キーワードを選定する
②選定したキーワードを含んだウェブページを適切なhtmlのタグを使いつつ制作
③制作後は告知活動を行う
④効果測定し、調整を加えていく

これらの作業を行うことで、先ほどの5つのハードルを解消することができます。それでは、各ステップではどんなことを行い、その結果どのようにハードルが解消されるのか、次節より見ていきましょう。

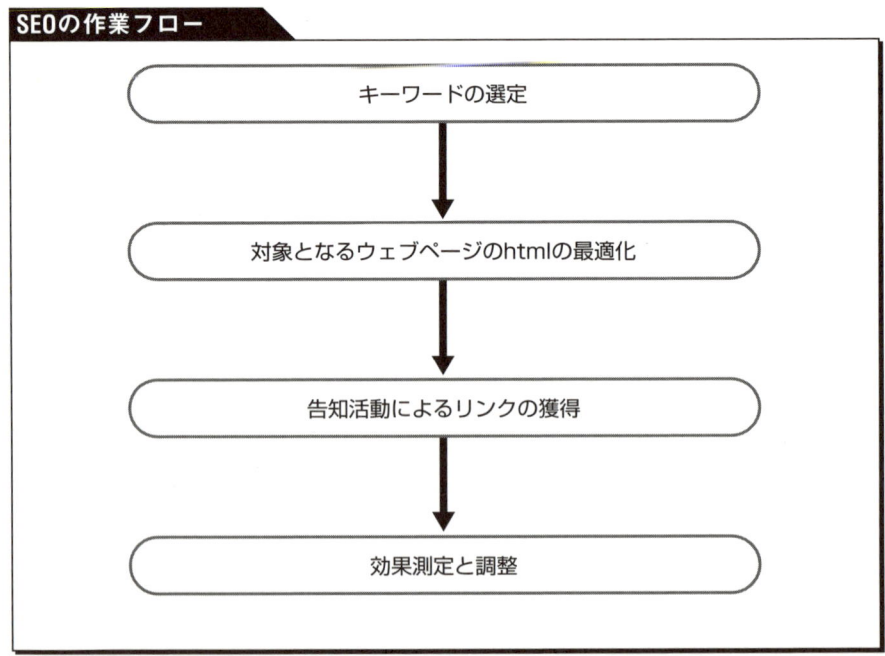

SEOの作業フロー

3-1 キーワードの重要性

◻ キーワードの争奪戦が始まっている

　SEOは、まずどのキーワードの検索結果ページで自分のサイトを上位表示させたいのかを確認するところから始めます。

　現在、SEOが浸透してきたことで、キーワードは争奪合戦になっています。Google Adwordsなどのリスティング広告の出稿トレンドを見ると、1社における出稿量は桁違いに多くなりました。3桁は当たり前、4桁の数の検索キーワードに出稿している企業も少なくありません。

　『1億円稼ぐ検索キーワードの見つけ方』(滝井秀則著、PHP出版刊)では「キーワード検索結果に1位表示していることを前提として、クリック率は10％前後、そこからアクションに至る率(コンバージョンレート)は1％前後」と経験則から想定される数字が挙げられています。検索回数が1,000回あれば、リスティング広告をクリックしてくれる人が100人、さらにそこからアクション(資料請求や購買)を起こしてくれる人が1人いる、ということです。

　1,000回の検索回数で1人のアクションを促すことができるのであれば、10人のアクションを起こさせたいときには、10,000回の検索回数を確保しなくてはなりません。ということはキーワードを相当数ピックアップしなくてはならない、ということになります。4桁の数の検索キーワードに出稿する企業が出現したのも、頷ける話です。

　このような状況の中で、自分のビジネスに関するキーワードでSEOをしていないサイトが、ユーザーに選ばれるはずがありません。

◻ ユーザーニーズにフィットしたキーワードを探そう

　では、どのような視点で、キーワードを決めればいいのでしょうか？

　ここで大切なのが、ユーザーの立場に立ち、想起しやすいキーワードを探すことです。ここを間違うと、先ほどの5つのハードルのうち、「①見込みユーザーが使った検索キーワードの検索結果に表示されない」という事態になってしまいます。

　ところが、自分が考えているキーワードと、ユーザーの検索キーワードは意外と一致しないものです。サイト運営側は、取り扱う商品や商材・競合から市場まで豊富な商品知識を持っているのに対し、実際に商品を購入するユーザーは、あなたが取り扱う商品やサービスに精通しているわけではないなど、意識や知識の違い起因します。

　したがって、キーワードは自分の思い込みだけで決めるのではなく、「実際にユー

ザーが使っている検索キーワードは何なのか」ということを調査して決めるべきです。そのための方法は、第2章で解説します。

◻ ページ内容とキーワードは一致させなければ意味がない

　また、ある検索キーワードで検索結果に表示されたとしても、そのキーワードとリンク先ページの内容が一致していないと、「③ランディングページにユーザーの知りたい情報、興味を喚起する情報が掲載されていない。またはキーワードとずれた内容が記載されている」というハードルが発生することになります。

　「どんなキーワードでも、とにかく検索結果に引っかかりさえすればOK」というのは、SEOではないのです。

　せっかくユーザーがあなたのウェブサイトにアクセスしても、「そのページに知りたい情報がない」と判断すると、ユーザーは即座にブラウザーの「戻る」ボタンを押して、検索結果ページへと帰ってしまいます。そこで、最近では、検索結果とウェブページの内容のギャップをなくそうとするLPO（Landing Page Optimization：ランディングページ最適化）という考え方も出てきています。

　これについても、詳しくは第2章でお話ししましょう。

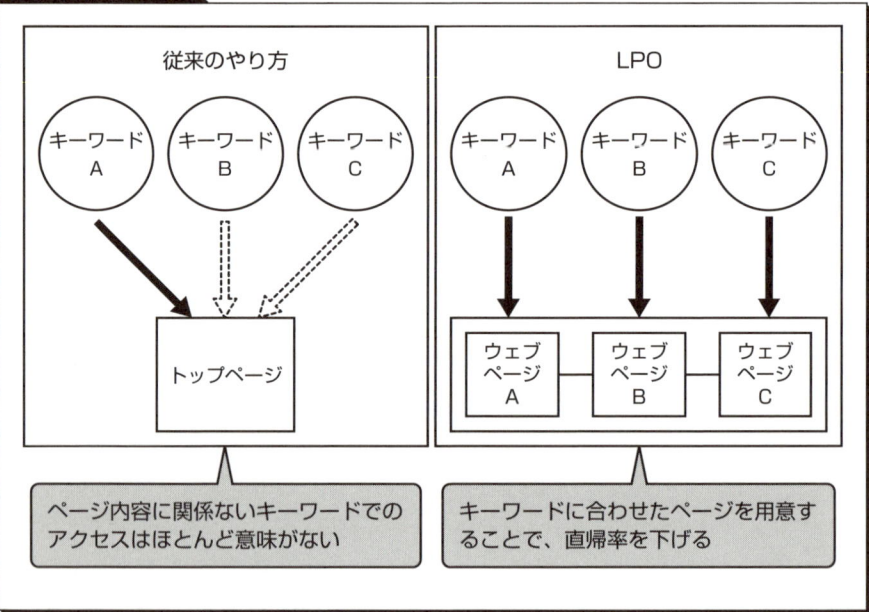

LPOの考え方

1-4 内部要素と外部要素

☐ SEOを構成する2つの要素

　キーワードを選定したら、そのキーワードで検索したときに検索結果上位に来るように、ウェブページにSEOを施しますが、その際、内的要素と外的要素の2要素の改善を目指します。

　内部要素は、htmlを検索エンジンに好まれるように調整することです。P24で挙げたSEOの手順の「②選定したキーワードを含んだページを適切なhtmlのタグを使いつつ制作」にあたります。

　一方、外部要素は、主に外部リンク対策を指し、外部の有力なサイトにリンクを貼ってもらうことやソーシャルブックマークに登録してもらうことを狙います。これはSEOの手順の「③制作後は告知活動を行う」にあたります。

　順に、詳しく説明しましょう。

☐ htmlを調整する内部要素対策

　内部要素のSEOでは、htmlタグを調整して、検索エンジンが読みやすいページを作成しますが、これがうまくいっていないと、P23で紹介した5つのハードルのうち「①見込みユーザーが使った検索キーワードの検索結果に表示されない」や、「②検索結果に、不適切な紹介文が記載されている」が起こります。

　SEOにおいては、こちらが想定したキーワードで検索したときに、ウェブサイトが上位に表示されることはもちろんですが、その検索結果にどのような紹介文が記載されるかも重要なポイントです。

　ユーザーは、検索結果に表示された多くのウェブサイトの中から、タイトルや紹介文を見て、訪れる価値があると判断したウェブサイトにアクセスします。

　したがって、いかに検索エンジンに適切な紹介文を表示させるか、言い換えると「そのページでのテーマは何なのか」をいかに検索エンジンに上手に伝えるかが大切になってきます。

　もっとも、実際のhtmlタグの調整は、一定の手順に従うだけですので、取り立てて難しいものではありません。<meta>タグ、<title>タグ、<hx>タグなど、これだけ押さえていれば大丈夫という厳選したタグの最適化方法を第3章で解説しますので、それに添って実施すれば問題ありません。

被リンクを確保する外部要素対策

　一方、「外的要素」は、端的にいえば「被リンクを確保する」ことです。Google・Yahoo!を始め、多くの検索エンジンは、被リンクの質と量でそのサイトを価値を計りますので、被リンクを獲得することは、検索順位を上げるために非常に重要になります。

　検索していると、取り立ててSEO対策を取っていないように見えないサイトが検索結果上位に来ることがありますが、このようなサイトは良質な情報を提供し、多くのユーザーの支持されている（リンクを貼られている）サイトなのです。被リンクの力がいかに大きいか分かるでしょう。

　被リンクを得ることをは、当然、外部の協力が必要なため、つい「コントロール不能な他力本願的なもの」と考えてしまいますが、実は自分でできることも少なからずあります。リスティング広告などのSEMの活用法も含めて、詳しくは第4章で説明していきますので、参考にしてください。

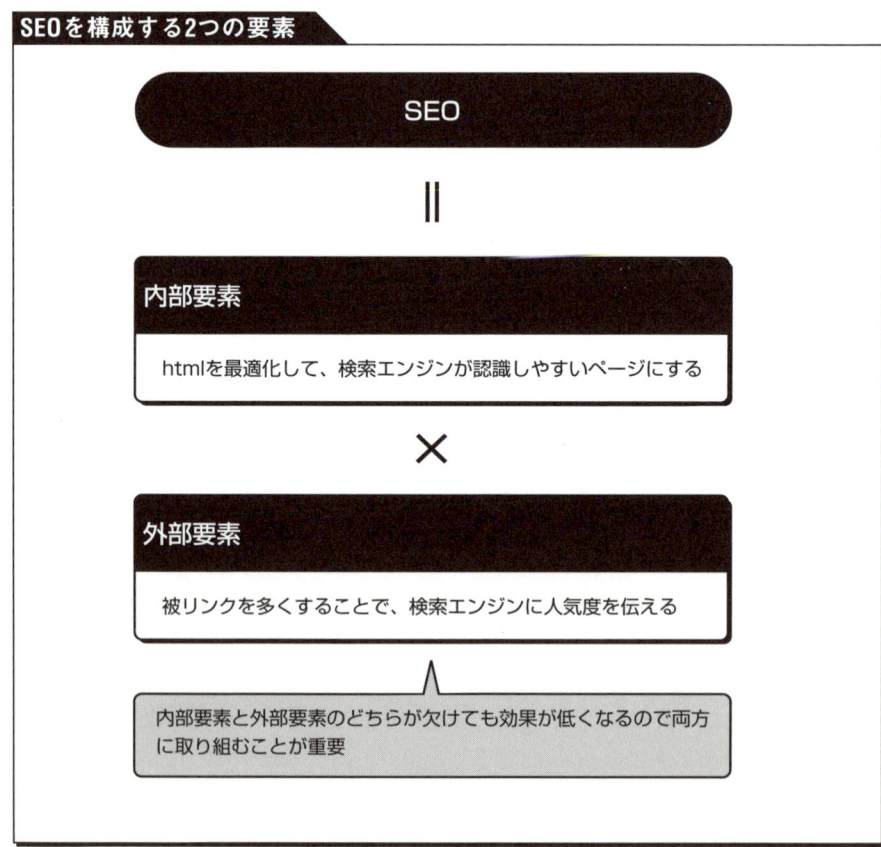

SEOを構成する2つの要素

1-5 SEOの効果測定

❏検索エンジンスパムには気を付けよう

　内部要素と外部要素のSEOが終わったら、最後に「④効果測定し、調整を加えていく」作業を行います。

　ここで一番気を付けなければならないのは、ここまでの作業で施したSEOが、検索エンジンに検索エンジンスパムと判定されていないかという点です。検索エンジンスパムと判定されると、最悪の場合、検索結果から外されてしまうことになります。過剰なSEOは、そのままリスクになり得るのです。

　実際に、2006年3月、サイバーエージェント運営のサイト群が不適切なリンクを貼っていたとして、Googleのデータベースから一時抹消されました。サイバーエージェントのサイトが一切、検索結果に引っかからなくなったのです。同様の事件は海外でも起きていて、2006年2月、独BMWサイトと独RICOHサイトが、JavaScriptのリダイレクト機能を悪用したとして、Googleのデータベースから抹消されました。

　Google検索にヒットしないのは、ウェブサイトの存在がなくなるほどのダメージを意味します。数日後、全サイトとも問題箇所を修正したため、Google検索に復活を果たしましたが、Google八分で受けたブランドダメージやチャンスロスは看過し得ないもの甚大なものだったでしょう。

　また、検索エンジンスパムと判定されないまでも、サイトの作りによっては検索エンジンからやってきたユーザーが「④他のウェブページへの移動がスムーズに行えない」「⑤ウェブページの不備でユーザーがアクションを起こせない」というハードルを生み出してしまうこともあります。

　どんなことが検索エンジンスパムと判断されるのか、あるいはユーザビリティに問題を生じてしまうのかは、第5章で詳しく説明しますので、くれぐれも注意してください。

❏目先の数字に一喜一憂しない

　また、ウェブサイトで成果を挙げようとするならば、定期的なサイト情報の分析は欠かせません。SEO施工後の結果分析や、成果に繋げられているか否かをアクセスログを分析しながら検証し、その検証データを元にウェブサイトを改善していく必要があるのです。

SEOは、手順の①（キーワード選定）から④（効果測定）を順に行っていったら終わり、という短期的な施策ではありません。④での効果測定の結果を元に、さらに①のキーワード選定に戻り、このサイクルを常に回していく、長期的なウェブ戦略なのです。

　ただし、効果測定では目先の数字に一喜一憂しがちになり、対処療法を繰り返してしまうという罠に陥りがちです。PVやユニークユーザー数の増減は気になるところですが、最終的なゴールはサイトで成果を出すことであり、表面的な数値の増減にばかり目を奪われては大局的なサイト運営はできません。

　アクセス分析でも、PVやユニークユーザー数よりもチェックしておかなくてはならないデータもありますし、そもそもSEOを施したページの意図を検索エンジンはちゃんと読み取っているか、ということも重要な分析対象です。

　SEMに出稿していればその効果測定は当然やっておかなくてはなりませんが、ここでも広告の表示回数や売上だけに捕らわれると先に進めません。リスティング広告の飛び先（ランディングページ）の違いによる成果は変わるのか、というトライ＆エラーを繰り返しながら、検証していきます。

　数字の落とし穴にはまらないように、的確に状況を掴み、多角的にデータを分析・検証していくことが重要です。

　目先の数字に捕らわれないための分析手法については、第6章で触れていきます

SEOのサイクル

- キーワード選定
- 効果測定
- htmlの最適化
- 被リンクの獲得

SEOは1回やったら終わりではなく常に効果を測定して改良を続けていかなければ、効果は維持できない

1.6 ブログとSEOの関係

☐ もともと相性が良いブログもSEO対策が必要

さて、ここまで、一般的なウェブサイトのSEOについて説明してきましたが、最後にブログについても考えてみましょう。

以前から、ブログと検索エンジンの相性がいいことは、ご存じの方も多いでしょう。ブログツールが生成するhtmlソースは、CSSと分離されているなどの理由で、検索エンジンと相性が良いのです。

また、ブログのエントリーは通常、トラックバックやコメントなどのテキスト情報が他のブロガーによって書き加えられますが、トラックバックによる相互リンクの獲得とコメントによるページ強化は、SEOを強力にバックアップしてくれます。

このため、ブログツールをウェブ日記を書くだけのツールとしてではなく、CMS（Contents Management System：コンテンツ管理システム）として活用しているウェブサイトは数多くあります。企業ブログとしてだけではなく、企業のプレス配信ページや新着情報発信ページをブログツールで更新しているのです。

しかし、もともとこれらのツールが生成するhtmlソースが検索エンジンと相性が良いとはいえ、SEOを十分に意識されているとは限りません。さらに検索エンジン好みのhtmlソースを生成させるために、その設定をチューニングする必要があります。

また、ブログはコンテンツ更新時に、RSSフィードという更新情報などを記したコードも生成します。最近次々とリリースされているブログ検索エンジンは、このRSSフィードの情報をインデックスしますので、RSSフィードもまたブログ検索エンジン向けに最適化しなくてはなりません。

ブログのSEOについては、第7章を参照してください。

☐ ウェブ2.0の変化に対応するために

なお、こうしたSEOの変化は、今後、さらに大きくなっていくでしょう。なぜなら、ウェブ自体が、現在、大きく変化しているからです。

ウェブ2.0という言葉を聞く機会が多くなってきました。ブログも、ウェブ2.0的なサービスのひとつです。

IT系書籍としては異例のベストセラーとなった梅田望夫氏の『ウェブ進化論』では、「（ウェブ2.0とは）ネット上の不特定多数の人々を（中略）積極的に巻き込んでいくための技術やサービス開発姿勢」と説明しています。言葉にすれば難しいことのよう

に感じてしまいますが、「ウェブがコミュケーションツールとして、さらなる進化を遂げようとしている」と言い換えてもいいでしょう。ウェブが情報の流通をスムーズにすることを期待されながら、一方通行でしかなかったのが、ここにきてやっとインタラクティブ性を帯びてきたということです。

そして、この変化の流れは、SEOとも強く関係しています。

ウェブ2.0の定義のひとつが「情報の共有化」です。情報量の爆発的な増加に伴い、検索エンジンのインデックスが追いつかないケースが増えてきたために、ユーザーは有益な情報を効率よく収集する手段として様々なツールを駆使し始めました。

このため、従来であればYahoo!ディレクトリに登録されることなどが外部要素の強化に繋がったわけですが、被リンクの確保において「ソーシャルブックマーク」と呼ばれる共有ブックマークサービスに登録されたり、RSSを通じて被リンクを確保したりなど、ウェブ2.0的な手法を取り入れることが求められつつあります。

既に、朝日新聞のニュースサイト「asahi.com」の一部の記事では、SBM国内最大手サービスのはてなブックマーク登録ボタンが付加されました。産経新聞社系列のニュースサイト「iza!」は記事に対するトラックバックを受け付けています。誰でも一度は目にしたことがあるYahoo!ニュースもトラックバック機能が付き、ソーシャルニュースとしてリニューアルされました。

既存のメディアであっても、一方的な情報配信からの脱却を図り、ユーザーとのネットワークを構築することを模索しているのです。

こうした動きに対応する方法についても、第7章で説明していますが、まだまだ変化はあるでしょう。

そういったとき、その変化に対応できるかどうかは、基礎が分かっているかどうかに掛かっています。基礎が分かっていれば、新しいサービスが出てきても、それがどのようにSEOに応用できるのかを自分で思いつくことができるでしょう。次章より、SEOの基礎を学んで、ぜひそのような応用力を身に付けてください。

それでは、始めましょう。

6 ● ブログとSEOの関係

はてなブックマークの登録ボタンが付いた「asahi.com」

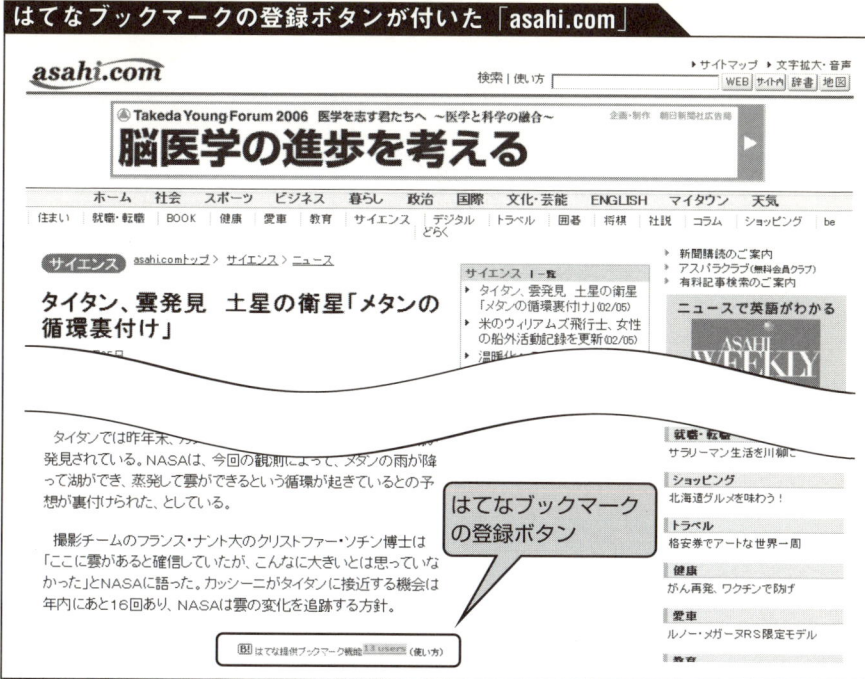

トラックバックを受け付ける「iza！」

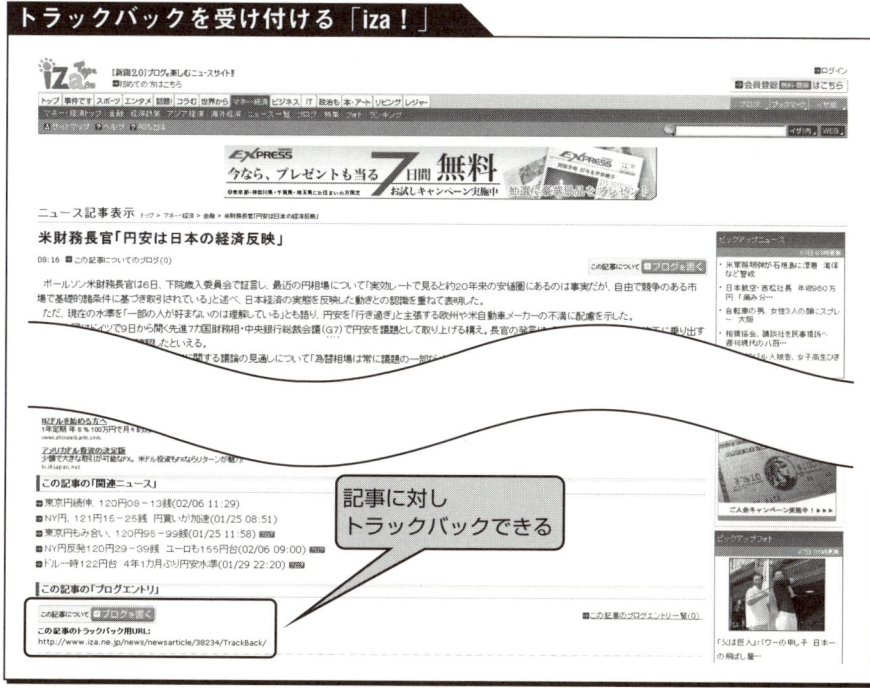

SEO「検索エンジン最適化」の教科書

第 2 章

キーワード選定

ガンガン集客できるキーワードを見つける方法とは

2.1 キーワード選定

□「どんなキーワードでも上位表示」を目指しては成果は出ない

　SEOのファースト・ステップは、「ユーザーにどういうキーワードで検索されたいか？」「あなたのビジネスのターゲットユーザーはどのようなキーワードを使うか？」を確定するところから始まります。

　キーワード選定は、その後のSEOを左右する大事な作業になります。サイトのコンセプトに沿った絶妙なキーワードを設定できれば、大きな成果が見込めます。

　あるミリタリーショップは、「ミリタリー」以外に「自衛隊」というキーワードにも最適化しています。これは「自衛隊」で検索するユーザーは、ミリタリーと嗜好性が近いだろうという予測の元に選ばれましたが、実際にその読みがあたって着実に成果を挙げているようです。キーワード選びで勝利した好例でしょう。

　一方で、ロングテールを誤解して「サイトに関係があろうがなかろうが、ひとつでも多くのキーワードで上位表示させればいいんだろう」と考えている人は要注意です。それでは一昔前の検索エンジンスパムとなんら変わりがありません。

　いかに適切なキーワードを見つけるかが、SEOの成否を決める鍵となるのです。

□適切なキーワードを選定するための5つの方法

　とはいえ、ゼロからやみくもに考えても、なかなか適切なキーワードの選定はできないものです。そこで、本章では、以下の方法を紹介していきます。

- アクセスログを解析する
- 競合サイトを参考にする
- ツールを使う
- 複合キーワードを狙う

　既にサイトが存在している方は、アクセスログ解析から入っていくのが常道です。その上で競合サイトを分析することで、効果的なキーワードを分析します。まさに、「敵を知り己を知れば百戦危うからず」の言葉通りです。

　また、これからサイトを立ち上げるというときは、競合サイトの分析やツールを使うことから始めるといいでしょう。

2.2 アクセスログから ユーザーニーズを探る

◻ 検索窓にはユーザーのニーズが反映される

　お客さんの心を開かせることは、ベテランの販売員でも困難を伴います。北風と太陽の寓話にもあるように、営業トークを一方的にまくし立てるだけでは、お客さんの心を開かせることはできません。お客さんが進んで心を開いてくれるために、工夫をしなければならないのです。

　ところが、お客さんが100％心を開いてくれる場があります。欲求や願望、期待に満ち溢れた言葉を、お客さん自らが語る場があるのです。それが検索窓です。ユーザーは、検索窓を通して「今一番何がしたいか」「何が欲しいのか」「何が知りたいのか」を語りかけてくれます。

　したがって、「どういった検索キーワードで、自分のサイトに訪問したのか」が分かるアクセスログ解析は、キーワードを選定する上で必須といえます。

◻ アクセスログ解析の3つの種類

　アクセスログ解析には、htmlにアクセス解析用のタグを埋め込む「ウェブビーコン型」、サーバーログを分析する「サーバーログ分析型」、ネットワーク上のデータ（パケット）を監視する「パケットキャプチャ型」の3種類があります。

　どのタイプも一長一短ありますが、導入のハードルや効果を総合的に判断すると、ウェブビーコン型がベストといえるでしょう。もしアクセスログ解析ツールを導入していないならば、「Google Analytics」など無料で使えるツールも提供されていますので、一刻も早く導入されることを強くお勧めします。

　ただし、ウェブビーコン型は、対象となるウェブページすべてにタグを埋め込まなくてはいけません。タグの貼り忘れがあれば、正確なアクセス解析を行うことができません。何百ページもあるサイトともなれば、その手間だけで膨大です。

　ブログであれば、テンプレートにタグを書き足して再構築するだけですので、かなり楽ですが、もしブログツールやCMSなどのサイト更新ツールを使っていない場合は、weavecode（http://www.gesource.jp/soft/weavecode/）などhtmlを対象とした一括置換ツールを使って、該当箇所を一括置換することをお勧めします。

　なお、収集したログデータをサイトに反映させていくための手法は、P122で詳しく説明していますので、ご覧ください。

weavecodeでの一括置換のやり方

①インストールする

②設定する

- Google Analyticsのコードを織り込む対象となるファイルが置いてあるフォルダを指定する
- 対象となるファイルの拡張子を指定する。通常は、htm、html、xhtml、shtml
- ファイルの文字コードを指定する
- 織り込むコードに別途取得したGoogle Analyticsのコードをコピー&ペーストする

③対象の確認を押し、そのファイル群で間違いがないことを確認

④「実行」を押す

⑤コードが織り込まれたファイルをアップロードする

2-3 競合サイト調査からキーワードを選ぶ

◪ 競合サイトのキーワードを調査する

　競合サイトや同業他社サイトのキーワードの傾向を参考にすると、スムーズにキーワードを選定することができます。個人サイトであれば、目標としているサイトやコンセプトが似通っているサイトを分析してみましょう。

　まずは競合サイトで使われているキーワードをピックアップします。競合サイトの<title>タグ、<hX>タグ、アンカーテキストを抜き出して、どのようなキーワードが使われているのかをリサーチすればOKです。そして、その中で、自分のサイトに欠けているキーワードがあれば、それを取り込んだコンテンツを用意します。

　なぜ競合サイトのキーワードを取り込む必要があるのかといえば、アクセスログからは見えてこないユーザーの取りこぼしを防ぎたいからです。

　自分のサイトに存在しないキーワードで検索されると、検索にすらヒットしないのですから、そこからのユーザーの誘導もなく、結果的にアクセスログに何の痕跡も残りません。自分達が知らない間に、成果に結び付きやすいキーワードでどんどん検索されて、競合サイトに流れているかもしれないのです。そういった事態を避けるためにも、競合サイトで使われているキーワードには常に注意を払っておきたいものです。

競合サイトのキーワード調査の方法

- 競合サイトの〈title〉タグ、〈hx〉タグ、アンカーテキストを抜き出す
    ↓
- 抜き出したキーワードの中で、自分のサイトに欠けているキーワードを探す
    ↓
- 欠けているキーワードがあれば、それを取り込んだコンテンツを用意する

2-4 ツールを使ってみよう

❏ 代表的な無料ツールは？

　ネット上には、キーワード選択を助けてくれる便利な無料ツールがあります。せっかくタダで使えるのですから、これを利用しない手はありません。ここでは、以下の3つのツールを紹介したいと思います。

- オーバーチュアのキーワードアドバイスツール
- Google Trend
- Google ウェブマスターツール

　それでは、それぞれについて詳しく説明しましょう。

❏ オーバーチュアのキーワードアドバイスツールを使う

　オーバーチュアのキーワードアドバイスツールは、SEOをする上で定番ともいうべきサービスです。キーワードを入れると、ユーザーがどのようなキーワードと一緒にそのキーワードを使ったのかということが分かります。後述の複合キーワードを選び出すときにも効果的ですが、ここでは検索回数に注目してみましょう。

　たくさんある複合キーワードの中のどれに注力していけばいいのか、狙い目の複合キーワードはどれなのか、KEI（Keyword Effectiveness Index：キーワード有効性指数）を使って判断します。KEIは、検索回数を検索結果数で割ったものです。

- KEI ＝ 検索回数 ÷ 検索結果数

　ここで、検索回数はオーバーチュアの「キーワードアドバイスツール」、検索結果数はGoogleで検索したときに画面右上に表示される件数を用いて、KEIを計算します。検索回数はいわばユーザーの需要で、検索結果数はウェブでの情報の供給具合を表しています。

　KEIが高いということは、検索回数の割りに検索結果数がそれほど表示されないということです。つまり、需要があるのに供給が追いついていない状態ということですから、KEIが高いキーワードは、狙い目のキーワードになります。

なお、KEIを「検索結果の2乗÷検索結果数」としているところもあります。同じ計算式を使って比較・計算すればいいだけの話ですので、どちらでも構いません。同じ土俵で比較すれば、それでいいのです。

KEIの計算の仕方

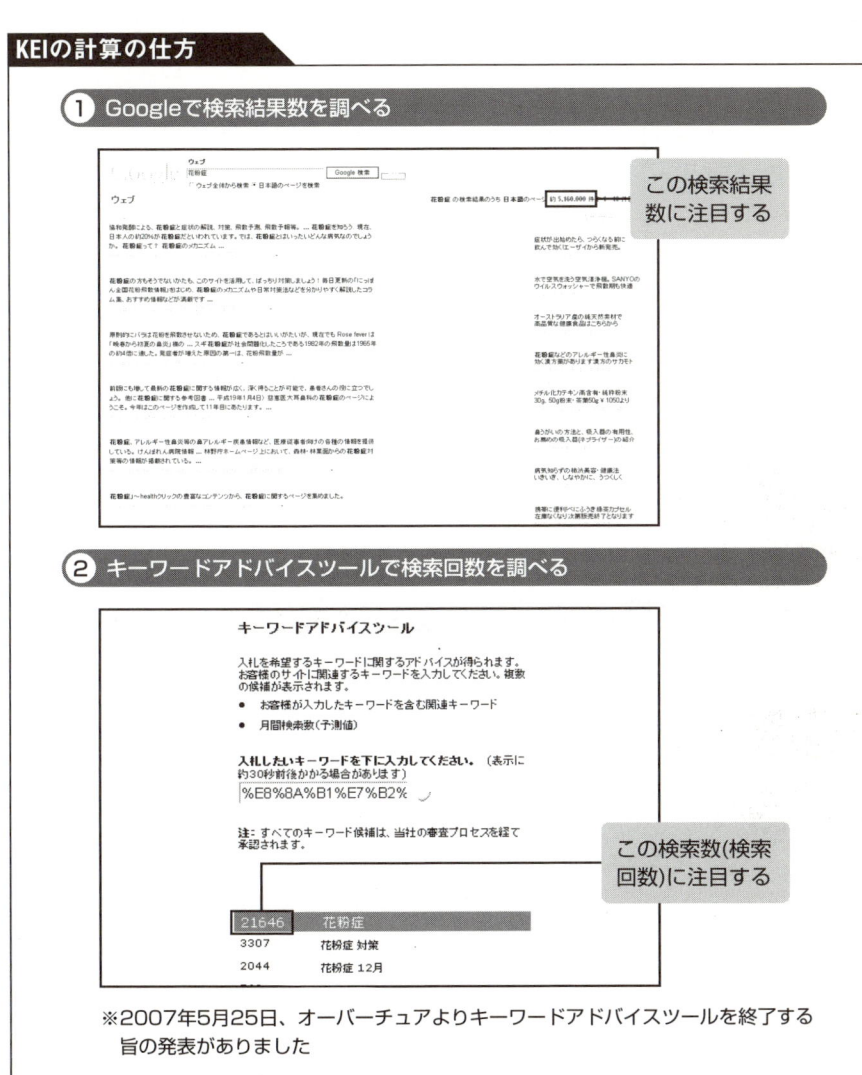

① Googleで検索結果数を調べる

② キーワードアドバイスツールで検索回数を調べる

※2007年5月25日、オーバーチュアよりキーワードアドバイスツールを終了する旨の発表がありました

③ KEI＝検索回数÷検索結果数

☐ Google Trendを使う

　一方、Google Trends（http://www.google.com/trends）は、「トレンド」と銘打たれているように、検索キーワードのトレンドを知ることができるサービスです。気になるキーワードを入力するだけで、過去2年間の検索数の推移や、急激に増加したときのニュースを表示してくれます。さらに、その検索をしたユーザーの国、地域なども示してくれます。

　また、複数のキーワードを同一画面で比較することもできます。例えば、2006年末から2007年初頭に掛けては次世代ゲーム機が話題になりました。任天堂の「Wii」、ソニー「PS3」、マイクロソフト「Xbox360」などのゲーム機が相次いで登場しましたが、これらのゲーム機の注目度は検索ニーズに表れてくることは明白ですので、Google Trendsで調べてみましょう。

　複数のサービスや商品を扱っているとして、そのどれに注力するべきかは悩ましいところです。下手すると、1ページの中にとにかくキーワードを詰め込んで、結局何のことだかよく分からないページになってしまいます。

　そのようなときには、今どの商品やサービスが勢いがあって、狙っていくべきかを天秤に掛けて判断するために、このサービスを使うといいでしょう。

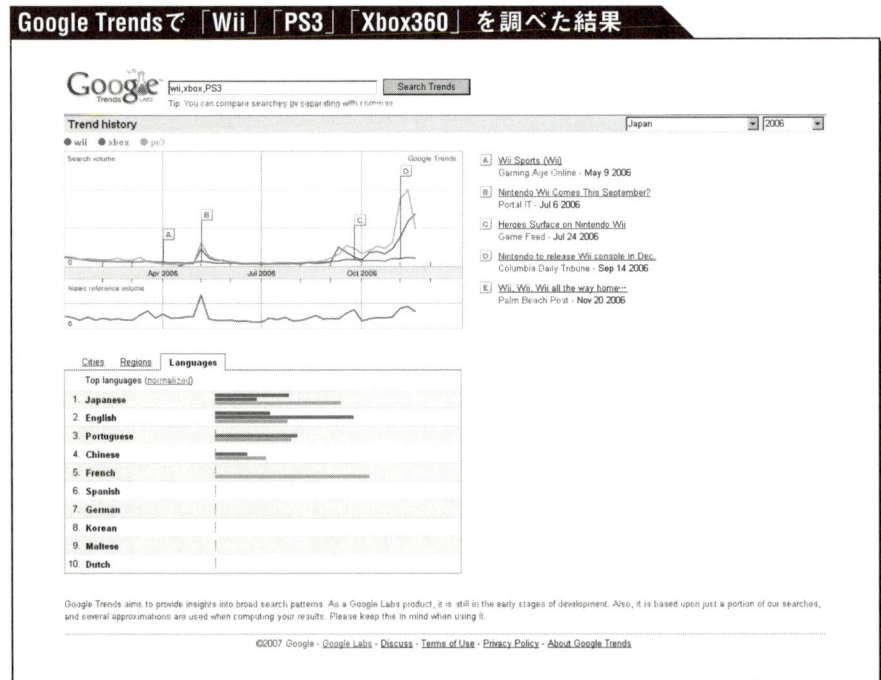

Google Trendsで「Wii」「PS3」「Xbox360」を調べた結果

■Googleウェブマスターツールを使う

　Googleウェブマスターツールは、本来は、サイト構成情報を正しくGoogleに伝えることで、より正確にクロールしてもらうことを目的としたサービスです。ただ、その付帯サービスのひとつに、「上位の検索クエリ」「上位の検索クエリのクリック数」閲覧機能があり、これが適切なキーワード選定の武器になります。

　「上位検索クエリ」はそのサイトがより多く検索されたキーワードの上位一覧、「上位の検索クエリのクリック数」は実際にサイトの訪問に至ったキーワード一覧です。

　つまり、上位検索クエリのランキングには入っているのに、上位の検索クエリのクリック数ランキングには入っていないキーワードがあれば、それは「検索結果ページには表示されるものの、サイトへの誘導力が足りないキーワード」ということになります。おそらく検索結果ページに表示されている説明文やタイトルが、その検索をしている人の興味をそそるものではない、ということが考えられますので、この場合には<description>の見直しなどで少しでも興味を喚起させるようにします。

　また反対に「上位検索クエリ」のランキングには入ってないのに、「上位の検索クエリのクリック数」にランクインしているキーワードがあれば、検索回数がもっと上がればかなり効果が見込めることを示していますので、そのキーワードに特化したコンテンツを作って検索回数の底上げを図るなどの対策が取れます。

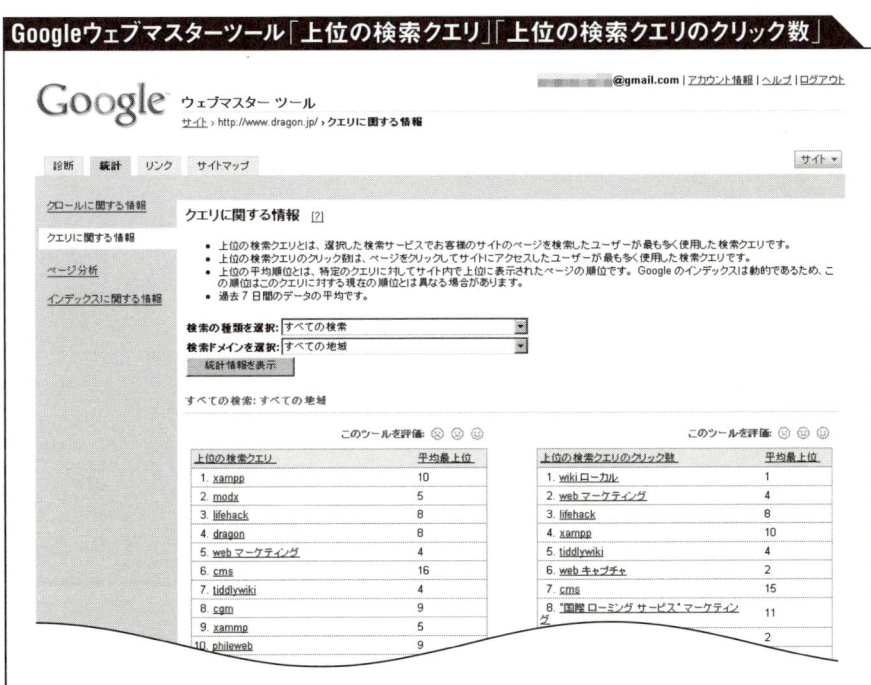

◻BIGLOBEの指標からキーワードの激戦度を探る

　BIGLOBEの検索サービスを使うことで、そのキーワードが激戦区かどうか判別することができます。BIGLOBEで検索すると、それぞれのサイトタイトルの横にバーが表示されるのですが、10本並んだバーのうち、赤いバーが何本があるかで、そのキーワードにおけるそのサイトの重要性を推測できるのです。

　たいていの場合、検索結果1位は赤棒が10本立っています。そして2位、3位と順位が落ちるに従って、赤棒の数が減っていくのですが、減り方はキーワードによって異なります。2位が9本、3位が8本ということもありますし、2位が3本、3位以降は1本ということもあります。

　棒の数がそのままサイトの価値を相対的に表しているので、僅差でひしめいているということは激戦区であり、上位サイトと逆転しやすいということでもあり、同時に下位から逆転される可能性も高いと言うことになります。常に研鑽していく必要があるということです。

　検索結果で自分のサイトよりすぐ上のサイトと棒の数が5,6本開いているときには、そのキーワードにおいてはそのサイトよりも上位になることは難しいということです。逆に、検索結果ですぐ下のサイトとかなり差が開いている場合は、安泰ということですので、別のキーワードでのSEOに注力をすることになります。

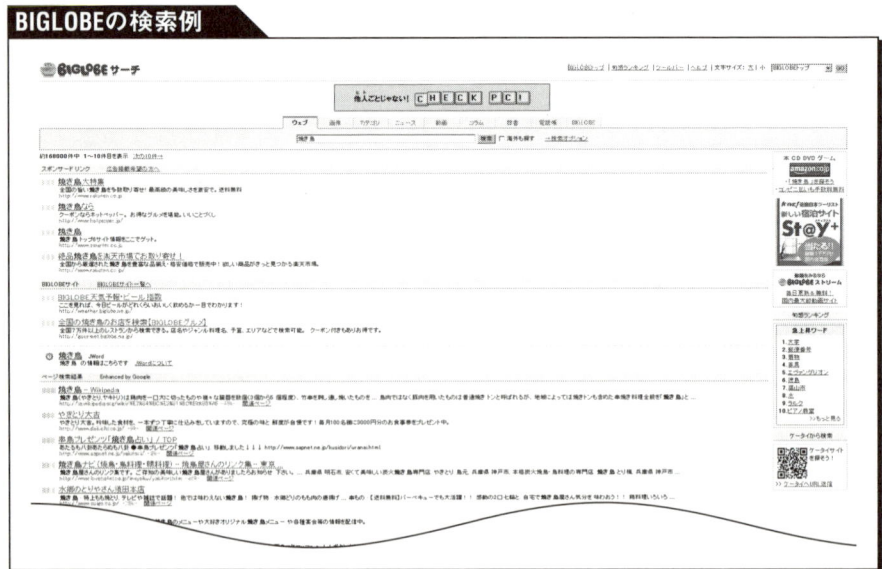

BIGLOBEの検索例

2-5 複合キーワードを狙う

□ 90％のユーザーは複合キーワードを使っている

　ここまでで、狙うべきメインのキーワードは固まってきたと思います。
　しかし、競争が激しい現在のSEOでは、キーワードは単体で考えるべきものではありません。検索キーワードは「複合キーワード」を前提として選定します。
　これは、「旅行」という単体キーワードで上位を目指すよりも、「旅行　北海道」「旅行北海道　宿泊」のような複数キーワードでどれだけのロングテールを拾って全体への流入数を上げられるかを考えた方が、よほど効果が高いためです。
　ここで、「旅行」など検索頻度が高い一般名詞をビッグキーワードといい、地名や人名・商品名などの検索頻度が低い固有名詞をスモールキーワードといいます。キーワード選定の際には、「ビッグ」＋「スモール」の複合キーワードで、検索結果上位を目指した方が効率的です。
　オランダのOneStat.comが2006年7月に実施した調査によると、「検索エンジンに1語だけ入力するネットユーザーは11.43％」という結果が出ました。つまり、約90％のユーザーは2語以上のキーワードで検索をするということです。
　そして、その割合は増加し、一方1語で検索するユーザーは減少の一途を辿っているのです！
　SEOを希望するクライアントの中には、いまだに一般名詞1語での上位ポジショニングを切望するところがありますが、1語検索は「検索キーワード訴求型広告（"○○で検索してください"とアピールしている広告）」や「誰が聞いてもその名称でそのブランドしか想起しないだろうというようなナショナルブランド（商品、サービス、会社）」「人名などの固有名詞」を調べるときくらいにしか用いません。「1語SEOの効率・効果はいちじるしく低い」ということを、認識しておきましょう。
　特に、B2C業界、とりわけサービス業は総じてSEOを含めウェブ活動に熱心なため、そういった激戦業界では、複合キーワードが威力を発揮します。「旅行」というキーワードで検索結果1位になるのは困難でも、「旅行」＋「北海道」の複合キーワードならば1位になれる、というように、自分の強みを活かしたキーワードでSEOを行うことが重要です。
　「旅行」あるいは「北海道」の単一キーワードで検索された場合、その人がどういうニーズを持って検索したかを判別することは困難です。ところが、「旅行」＋「北海道」で検索した人ならば高い確率で、北海道旅行について考えているはずなのです。

このように複合キーワードにはユーザーニーズが如実に反映しますので、その後の成果に繋がる可能性が高いのです。

□ツールを使って複合キーワードを探す

では、効果的な複合キーワードを選定するには、どうすればいいのでしょうか？

手軽で効果が高いのが、Googleの「関連検索」を参考にする方法です。関連検索は、何かの検索キーワードに対して、その第2キーワードを教えてくれるサービスです。

あるキーワードで検索をすると、検索結果ページの最下部にその検索キーワードと関連度が高い複合キーワードがいくつか表示されます。実際にこれらの複合キーワードはユーザーが使ったものですので、これらの複合キーワードを取り込んでウェブページを制作するか、あるいはこの複合キーワードでリスティング広告を出稿するとより効果が期待できます。

また、関連語を探すツールとして、レリパッドのReleKeyも有力です。キーワードを入力するだけで、そのキーワードに対する関連性の高いキーワードが表示されます。オーバーチュアのキーワードアドバイスツールと似ていますがこちらは実際に検索された回数ではなく、別のアルゴリズムから弾き出された関連語ですので、ニッチなキーワードが表示されることも少なくありません。

もちろんSEOとしてこれらのキーワードを反映させることは重要ですが、同時にリスティング広告でも活躍が期待できるサービスです。リスティング広告では見込みがありそうなキーワードのとにかくひとつでも多く出稿する必要がありますので、その際の力強い味方になってくれるはずです。

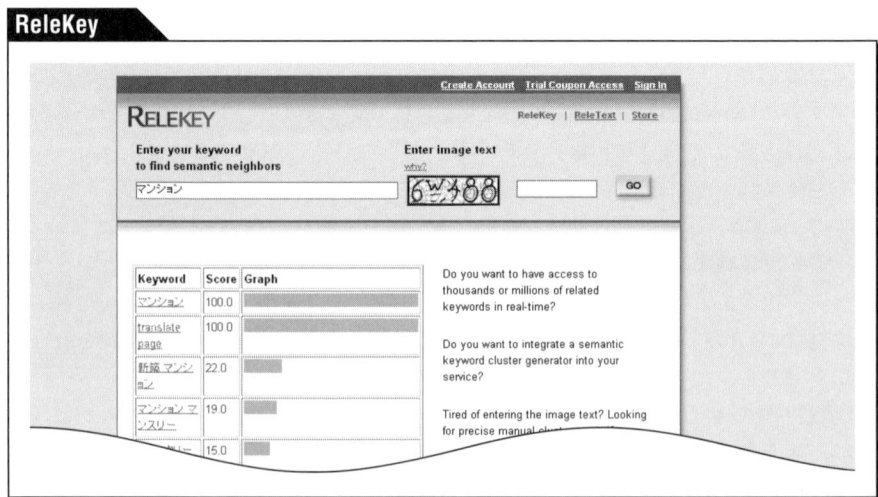
ReleKey

2-6 キーワードに対応するランディングページを用意する

□LPO（ランディングページ最適化）とは何か

　狙いたいキーワードが決まったら、最後にそのキーワードでSEOを施す「ランディングページ」を決めておきましょう。

　ランディングページとは、検索エンジンの検索結果から、ユーザーが最初にやって来る受け皿となるページを指します。このページを次章から説明する各種SEOテクニックによって、検索エンジンに最適化することになります。

　誤解している方も多いのですが、SEOは必ずしもウェブサイトのトップページを検索結果上位に表示させることを目指すのではありません。むしろ、狙ったキーワードごとにランディングページを用意して、そこを起点にサイトを回遊してもらおうとするのが、現在のSEOの主流となっています。いわば、大きな玄関をひとつ用意してそこに誰も彼もを誘導するのではなく、検索ユーザーのニーズに応じて小さくても複数の入口をたくさん用意しておくというイメージです。

　ユーザーニーズに合った受け皿ページをきちんと用意して、成果に繋げようとする考え方を、「LPO（Landing Page Optimization：ランディングページ最適化）」と呼びます。

□ランディングページの有無で成果は大きく変わる

　LPOの考え方を理解していないと、SEOは十分な効果を発揮しません。

　例えば、ある食品メーカーでは懸賞キャンペーンを行っていました。そのキャンペーン名で検索すると、Google Adwords枠に「○○キャンペーンページはこちら」と誘導を促すリスティング広告が表示されるというものです。ここまでは問題ないのですが、そのリスティング広告の飛び先は、キャンペーンページではなくその食品メーカーのトップページだったのです。そして、トップページからキャンペーンページに誘導しようと考えていたようなのです。

　サイト運営者の心情を察すれば、キャンペーンページに来て、そのまま直帰されるのが嫌だったのかもしれません。「もっと他のページを知ってもらいたい」という意識も働いたかもしれません。

　しかし、その思いが逆効果になっているのです。

　たしかに、トップページはサイトの顔であり、個々の商品ページやサービスページ

への入口です。しかし、キャンペーン名で検索して訪れたユーザーにとっては、どうでしょうか？　せっかくそのキャンペーンに興味を持ってやってきたのに、その食品メーカーのトップページから、あらためてそのキャンペーンページへのリンクを探すことを強いられるわけです。ユーザーによっては、「なんだ、キャンペーンのページじゃないんだ」と直帰する可能性もあります。

　SEOを駆使して検索結果上位に表示されても、ユーザーの直帰率が高ければ何の意味もありません。

　ユーザーが検索エンジンを使うのは、何かしらの課題やニーズを抱えているからです。したがって、検索結果に表示されたページがトップページかどうかということは大した問題ではありません。自分のニーズを満たすものがない、あるいはなさそうだと感じ取れば、すぐに検索結果画面に帰ってしまいます。

　情報ニーズを満たしてくれそうだと感じたときに、はじめてそのサイトに興味を持ってくれるのです。そういった意味でも、検索エンジンからやってきたユーザーに対して受け皿となるページを用意しておくことは重要なのです。

□検索キーワードにユーザーニーズは宿る

　では、どのようなキーワードにどのようなランディングページを用意すればいいのでしょうか？

　検索エンジンユーザーと一口にいっても、そのニーズは様々です。既にあなたのサイトを知っており「再度訪問したい」と考えているユーザーもいれば、サービスや商品の情報を比較検討するために検索しているユーザーもいるでしょう。このような多種多様なユーザーニーズに適格に応えるには、検索キーワードを元にユーザーを分類し、それぞれにふさわしいページを用意する必要があります。

　例えば、検索エンジン登録代行サービス「さぶみっと！JAPAN」であれば、ユーザーが使う検索キーワードは以下の3タイプに分類できます。

```
①会社名、製品名、サービス名、キャラクター名など
　　例）「さぶみっと！JAPAN」「イー三六五」
②複合キーワード
　　例）「検索エンジン登録 代行」「登録代行 料金」
③一般名称
　　例）「検索エンジン」
```

　①は、会社名やサービス名で検索していることから、もっとも関心が高い層といえます。当然、その際のリンク先は「会社情報ページ」「サービスのトップページ」に

設定し、商品の購入やサービスの成約に向けての導線を確保します。関心の高さは緊急度が高いことも考えられます。検索エンジンからの誘導がもっとも効くユーザーですので、会社名だったら会社情報、サービス名だとサービス情報を情報ニーズに対してダイレクトに答えが出ているコンテンツに誘導します。

②は、サービス・商品の購入を比較検討しているユーザーです。複数キーワードを使っていることで、何を重要視しているのか分かります。「登録代行 料金」では料金が気になっていることが分かりますし、「検索エンジン登録 代行」では代行業者を探していることが伝わってきます。それらの悩みを解決するページを用意して、誘導することが重要です。

③は、漠然と情報を集めているユーザーです。どのような目的で情報を探しているのかは、この段階では分かりませんので、サービスの詳細ページに飛ばしてしまうとユーザーニーズとずれている場合もあります。しかし、自社サービスと無縁とはいえないキーワードで検索しているので、この先お客さんになる可能性を秘めています。この場合だと「検索エンジン」についての用語辞典やコラムなどを用意しておき、まずはサービスや会社を覚えてもらい、できればリピーターにまで育てていきたいところです。

なお、検索エンジンユーザーは、何かの問題を解決するために検索エンジンを使うのですが、特定の何かについて知識を深めたいときには、「○○とは」というように「とは」を付けて検索します。ということは、「とは」を付けたユーザーは、ほぼ100%の確率で知識ニーズを満たしたいと考えていると推測できます。

このように、キーワードに応じてユーザーのニーズを考え、適切なランディングページを用意しておけば、SEOは単にサイトのアクセスを増やすだけでなく、その先にあるビジネスの成約率向上などに、大きな力を発揮するでしょう。

SEO・SEMの言葉が独り歩きして、検索結果上位に来ればいいだろうとするウェブマスター、あるいはSEO業者がまだまだ存在するのも事実です。しかし、検索結果上位に来るのはあくまでも手段であって、それが目的ではないことを今一度確認しておきましょう。

❏ デザインやナビゲーションも重要

なお、ランディングページはサイトの入口ですので、そのウェブサイトの他のページへの移動が簡易であることも重要です。ランディングページを見て「ここには自分の求めている情報がある」と思えば、ユーザーはさらに詳しい情報を求めて、サイト内の他のページも見ようと思います。そんなとき、他のページへのリンクが存在しなかったら、大きな機会損失となってしまいます。

「他ページへのリンクがないなんて、そんな変なことはするわけがない」と思う方もいるかもしれません。しかし、残念ながら現実問題として、そのようなページが存

在するのです。

　あなたのウェブサイトは、どのページに直接来訪されても、他のページに移動できるようになっているでしょうか？　そして、自分がいるページがウェブサイトのどこに位置しているのかが、すぐに分かるようになっているでしょうか？

　これは、サイトデザインやナビゲーションの問題でもありますので、詳しくはP108で説明しましょう。

SEO「検索エンジン最適化」の教科書

第 **3** 章

htmlの最適化

検索エンジンが理解しやすいウェブページ作成の
テクニック

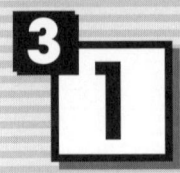
内部要素のSEO

❏検索エンジンが理解しやすいhtmlを書こう

　キーワードを選定したら、そのキーワードを軸に据えたウェブサイトを制作していきます。

　いくら良質のコンテンツを作ったとしても、それが検索エンジンに表示されなければ、それはウェブに存在しないも同然です。そこで、少しでも検索エンジンに拾われるように、htmlに工夫を凝らします。これが内部要素のSEOです。

　いうなれば、検索エンジンが理解しやすいようにhtmlソースを書くのが、本章での目的となります。

❏SEOに関係するタグは？

　ご存じの通り、htmlは<head>要素と<body>要素の、2つの要素から成り立っています。<head>部分には、文字コードやページの概要など主にhtml自体の情報が書かれています。一方、<body>要素はブラウザーに表示され、ユーザーの目に触れる部分です。このそれぞれの要素にSEOを施していきます。

　<head>要素のSEOに関係してくるのは、以下の2つのタグです。

- <title>タグ
- <meta>タグ

　<title>タグはそのページのタイトルになり、<meta>タグはそのページの概要や含まれるキーワードなどを検索エンジンに伝えます。

　<body>要素のSEOの対象となってくるのは、以下の、主にテキスト情報に影響を与えるタグです。

- <hX>タグ
- <a>タグ
- <strong>タグ、<em>タグ
- <img>タグの<alt>属性
- <acronym>タグ、<abbr>タグ

また、内部要素のSEOには、ページに書かれた文章全体や、ページレイアウトも関係してきます。具体的には、以下の工夫が挙げられます。

- キーワード出現頻度の最適化
- サイドメニューの配置
- JavaScriptやCSSの外部化
- サブドメイン
- サイトマップ

これらを適切に使うことで、内部要素のSEOは完了します。本章では、これらのテクニックについて説明していきます。

SEOに関係するhtmlのタグ

\<head\>要素内

- \<title\>タグ
- \<meta\>タグ

\<body\>要素内

- \<hx\>タグ
- \<a\>タグ
- \<strong\>タグ、\<em\>タグ
- \<ing\>タグの\<alt\>属性
- \<acronym\>タグ、\<abbr\>タグ

さらに「キーワードの出現頻度」「サイドメニューの配置」「CSSやJavascriptの外部化」「サブドメインの活用」「サイトマップ」など、コンテンツなどの改良も内部要素に含まれる

3.2 <title>要素におけるSEO

■検索エンジンにもユーザーにも最重要な<title>タグ

　<title>タグは、数あるhtmlタグの中でユーザーの目に触れる機会が多いタグのひとつで、その名の通りページタイトルを表します。
　<title>タグに書かれたページタイトルは、メニューバーやお気に入りの登録名、あるいは検索結果に表示され、そのページの内容を端的に表すことになります。
　検索結果には「ページタイトル」「スニペット」「URL」という数少ない情報しか表示されませんので、ページタイトルはユーザーの価値判断にも重大な影響を与えます。当然、検索エンジンも<title>タグを重要視しますので、<title>タグにはユーザー並びに検索エンジンを意識したページタイトルを付けるのは当たり前といえるでしょう。

■タイトルは30字以内で付けよう！

　では、SEO的には、どのようなタイトル付けが望ましいのでしょうか？
　検索エンジンユーザーは何かしらの課題を解決したいがために検索するわけですから、その課題への答えがあるような文言を<title>タグに忍ばせておくことで、サイトへの誘導率がアップします。

タイトル付けの考え方

ユーザーの課題	→	タイトル
○○とは？		○○の基礎知識 ○○について

ユーザーがそのキーワードをどんな気持ちで使ったのかを考えて、それに応えるようなタイトルを付けよう

例えば、前述の「○○とは」検索（→P49参照）を想定したページならば、「○○の基礎知識」や「○○について」というタイトルが効果的であることはお分かりいただけるでしょう。つまり「ユーザーがどのようなシチュエーションや気持ちでその検索キーワードを使ったのか」ということを想定して、ページタイトルを付けていくことが大事です。

なお、検索結果に表示されるページタイトルの文字数は、Googleでは全角30文字程度、Yahoo!は全角40文字（半角80文字）程度ですので、全角30文字を目処にタイトルを付けます。それ以上だと、せっかく工夫したタイトルの一部分しか検索結果に表示されず、ユーザーにサイトの概要を正しく伝えることができないかもしれません。

❑ <title>タグで気を付けるその他のこと

また、<title>タグは、SEOに重要なだけに取り扱いには注意を要します。

例えば、<title>タグがSEOで重要だからとはいえ、無闇に多数のキーワードを埋め込んでしまうと検索エンジンスパム（→P100参照）と判断されてしまう可能性があります。検索エンジンスパムと捉えられるリスクを考えると、小手先のテクニックに走るよりは、<title>タグはシンプルにまとめることをお勧めします。ページタイトルに含むキーワードはひとつにとどめます。これは1ページに1テーマと言うこと鉄則に従うなら当然の結果です。逆にいくつもキーワードを含めると、検索ユーザーは何について書かれているページか検索結果から読み取ることができません。

<title>タグに、長い社名や一般的ではない正式名称・略称を入れるのも避けましょう。ユーザーの立場に立ち、商品名やサービス名を想定すれば、おのずと<title>タグに盛り込むキーワードが浮かび上がってきます。大手SNSのmixiの運営会社は、今でこそ「株式会社ミクシィ」ですが、以前は「イー・マーキュリー」という社名でした。そのときに、mixiのトップページタイトルに「mixi - イー・マーキュリー」と付いてあったらどうでしょうか。どこまでがサービス名なのか、軽く戸惑うでしょう。トップページタイトルには、色々な情報を詰め込みたいのが人情ですが、ユーザーに戸惑いを与えないように配慮すべきです。

逆に、社名に商品名やサービス名がまったく入っていない場合や、同じ商品を他社も扱っている、サービス名が混同しやすい場合には、「商品名－社名」あるいは「商品名－キャッチコピー」のようにページタイトルから会社名と商品名・サービス名が繋がるように、情報を補ってあげることも必要です。

また、<title>タグのページタイトルと、<body>内の内容がかけ離れていることもマイナスに働きます。検索ロボットは、<title>タグと<body>内のテキストを総合的に分析し、そのページ内容を理解しますので、その2つがまったくリンクしないものだとしたら、検索エンジンスパムと判断されないまでも、ページの評価は落ちてしまうの

です。例えば、ページコンテンツはヤクルトスワローズの戦力分析なのに、ページタイトルには「セ・リーグの戦力分析」では、ページコンテンツとページタイトルの関連性は薄いと判断されてしまいます。この場合は「ヤクルトスワローズ編 - セ・リーグ戦力分析」とすべきでしょう。

表記も同様です。ページ内のコンテンツでは、SEOについて書かれているのに、ページタイトルには「検索エンジン最適化について」とあれば、やはり関連性は薄いと判断されてしまいます。

さらに、<title>タグに「★」「●」などの記号を入れることも、検索ロボットにマイナスに働くことはあっても、プラスに働くことはありませんので、避けた方が無難です。

<title>タグの注意点

- タイトルは全角の30文字以内

- タイトルに含むキーワードは1つ

- 長い社名や一般的でない名称は入れない

- <body>内のテキストとかけ離れたタイトルにしない

- <body>内のテキストと表記を統一する

- 「★」「●」などの記号は使わない

<title>タグはSEOでもっとも重要な存在。簡潔に、かつユーザーにわかりやすいタイトルを心掛けよう!

3 <meta>タグのSEO

☐ 検索エンジンにだけ働きかける特殊なタグ

　<meta>タグは、ユーザーではなくて検索エンジンにだけ働きかけるタグです。

　ただし、「<meta>タグにまったく関係ないキーワードを埋め込む」「同じキーワードを繰り返し使う」などの不正使用が多かったため、その影響度は徐々に低下しています。Yahoo!など検索エンジンによっては、<meta>タグの内容が検索結果に反映されることがあるものの、現在<meta>タグの重要度はほとんどありません。

　したがって、SEO的な効果はそれほど期待せずに、やれる範囲でやっておけば十分というスタンスで構いません。

☐ 本当に必要な<meta>タグは4つだけ

　<meta>タグには様々な種類がありますが、SEO的に必要な<meta>タグは、以下の4つだけです。

- <charset>
- <description>
- <keywords>
- <robots>

　それ以外の<meta>タグは、意味がない上に、シンプルなhtmlソース記述を心がけるというSEOの原則にも反しますので必要ありません。

　特に、ホームページビルダーのように、勝手に<meta>タグを追加してしまうホームページ作成ソフトもありますので、ファイルをアップする前にその箇所は削除しておきましょう。<head>はシンプルにすることが鉄則です。

☐ <charset>で文字コードを指定する

　<charset>タグは、そのページの文字コードを伝えるタグで、検索エンジンがそれを読み込むことで、その下のテキストを適切な文字コードで読み取ってくれます。

```
<meta http-equiv="Content-Type" content="text/html";charset="XXXX">
```

XXXXの部分には「utf-8」「Shift_JIS」など、そのページで使われている文字コードが入ります。

検索した際、まれに文字化けしているページを検索結果で見かけることはないでしょうか？ これは言語指定が正確に行われなかったため、検索エンジンが正しい文字コードを判別しなかったためです。

文字化けすれば、検索エンジンも当然キーワードを認識してくれないので、htmlファイルの先頭では必ず言語指定を行うよう心がけましょう。

❏ <description>で説明文を伝える

<description>タグは、そのページの説明文（スニペット）を伝えるタグです。

```
<meta name="description" content="XXXX">
```

XXXXの部分に、説明文を記載します。

検索エンジンによっては、ここに書かれた説明文が検索結果に表示されますので、検索エンジンユーザーの目に触れる可能性があります。大手の検索エンジンは大体120文字くらいまで表示されるので、ユーザーを呼び込むためのライティング技術の見せどころです。

また、この説明文には、そのページのキーワードを含めることを忘れないようにしましょう。

❏ <keywords>でキーワードを明示する

<keywords>では、そのページ内で使われているキーワードを列挙します。

```
<meta name="keyword" content="X,X,X">
```

上のタグ例だと、「X」の箇所にキーワードを埋めていきます。キーワード間は「,」で繋いでいきます。

無関係のキーワード（大企業名や芸能人名など）や、膨大な量のキーワードを埋め込んで、検索にヒットされやすくするというテクニックがあったため、現在ではこの<keyword>は検索表示順位にそれほど影響を与えませんが、この情報を見る検索エンジンもありますので、きちんと書いておいた方が無難です。

しかし、キーワードを何十個、何百個も埋め込んだり、同一キーワードの多用や連続記載すると、検索エンジンスパムとしてペナルティを課せられるか、後半部分は無視されます。

適正なキーワード数は、3～10程度、しかもページ内容に関係したキーワードを書く必要があります。

<robots>で検索エンジンの振る舞いを指示する

<robots>は、SEOとは直接関係しないものの、検索エンジンに対して何からのアクションを促すことができるタグです。

例えば、検索エンジンへの登録の可否を指示できます。

```
<meta name="robots" content="noindex,nofollow">
```

<meta name="robots" content="noindex,nofollow">と記述すれば、検索エンジンに対して、「登録しない（noindex）」「ここからリンクされている他のページも登録しない（nofollow）」と拒否の意思を伝えることになります。

<meta name="robots" content="noindex,follow">ならば、「このページは登録しないが、リンクされているページは登録する」ということになります。

「検索エンジンに登録されたくないページがあるのか？」と思われた方もいると思いますが、むしろ登録させない方が好ましいケースというのもありますので（→P140参照）、ページの用途に合わせて使い分けます。

また、<robots>には、別の使い方もあります。

```
<meta name="robots" content="noodp">
```

検索結果ページには、ページタイトル、URL、スニペット（説明文）が表示されますが、このスニペットはいくつかのパターンがあります。

①<meta>タグの<description>がそのまま表示される。
②検索キーワードと一致した<body>内の該当箇所がキーワードの前後の文章と共に表示される。
③ディレクトリ型検索エンジンに登録されているスニペットが表示される。

この中で問題になってくるのが③です。①②はある程度こちら側でコントロールできるものの、Yahoo!ディレクトリあるいはDMOZ（Directory Mozilla）やODP（Open Directory Project）と呼ばれるディレクトリ型検索エンジンに登録されたサイ

トの説明文は、自分でアップデートすることができません。修正を依頼することはできますが、それが反映されるには時間が掛かります。スニペットに古い情報が表示されてしまえば、ユーザーの誘引力は激減です。

そこで、ページ自体の情報は刷新されて、<description>やコンテンツの内容が表示される方が望ましい場合には、<meta name="robots" content="noodp">と<meta>タグに明記することで、検索結果にディレクトリ型検索エンジンに登録されているスニペットを表示させないようにできるのです。歴史が古いウェブサイトならば、このタグを導入する価値はあるでしょう。

<meta>タグの表記例

文字コードを指定する

`<meta http-equiv="Content-Type"content="text/html;charset="XXXX">`

文字コードとしてEUP-JP, shift_JIS, ISO_2022-JP, utf-8 などを指定

説明文を伝える

`<meta name="description"content="XXXX">`

検索結果に表示させたい説明文を120文字程度で書く

キーワードを明示する

`<meta name="keyword"content="X,X,X">`

そのページのキーワードをカンマで区切って列挙する(3~10個)

検索エンジンへの登録の可否を伝える

`<metaa name="robots"content="noindex, nofollow">`

noindexなら検索エンジンに登録しない、indexなら登録する意志を表す

nofollowならリンク先ページを登録しない、followなら登録する意志を表す

検索エンジンにディレクトリ型検索サイトの説明文を表示しない

`<meta name="robots"content="noodp">`

3-4 <hX>タグのSEO

□ タイトルと並んで重要な見出しタグ

　たいていのWebページは、タイトル、大見出し、小見出し、本文ごとに文字の大きさや太さ、色を変えてアクセントが付けられています。

　そして、多くの場合、大見出しはページの内容を、小見出しはそのページの小センテンスの内容を端的に表していますが、これらの見出しは、<hX>タグを使って表現します。<hX>のXの部分には、1～6までの数字が入り、<h1>がタイトル、<h2>は大見出し、<h3>は中見出し……という風に使い分けられています。

　そこで検索エンジンは、<title>タグと同様に、<hX>タグもまたページの内容を表していると判断します。数字が小さくなるほど、その注目度は高くなり、<h1>に至っては<title>と同等の重要性を持っているのです。

□ <h1>には<title>と近似の内容を入れよう

　このように<hX>タグは<title>タグと並んでSEOで重要なタグといえますので、<hX>タグの中には、サイトテーマに沿ったキーワードをしっかり入れておきましょう。

　逆説的にいえば、そのページのキーワードを<h1>に反映させれば、おのずと<title>と近似の内容になるはずです。

　例えば、会社概要のページならば、当然ページタイトルは「会社概要 - ドラゴンフィールド株式会社」となり、<h1>も「会社概要」となるはずなのです。

　ここで<h1>に「採用情報」としてしまうと、このページの主題となっているものは何なのか、検索エンジンはおろか、そのページを見たユーザーですら分からなくなってしまいます。

□ 文章構造に見合った見出しタグを使おう

　ただし、<h1>が重要視されるからといって、文章すべてを<h1>で挟めばいいのかといえば、答えは当然Noです。

　一般的な文章の流れとして「タイトル→大見出し→小見出し→段落→小見出し→段落→……」のようになっているはずです。ですから、見出しタグの流れもそのように

なっていなければ不自然なのです。

　<h1>が頻繁に現れたり、<h3>の後に<h2>が続けて出てきたり、文章が<h2>から始まっていたりなど明らかに文章構造に問題があると判別された場合、検索ロボットはそのページを検索エンジンスパムと判断します。セオリーとしては、<body>の直下に<h1>タグを使って、そのページのキーワードを入れた形で表示されるようにすることが一般的です。

　また<h1>が効果的だからといって乱発することやめましょう。1ページに使える<h1>タグは1回だけです。<h2>タグは2～3回程度、<h3>タグは4～5回程度が目安となります。これは、表題、大見出し、小見出し、という通常の文章構造から見れば当然の帰結といえます。もし表題や大見出しが目安よりも増えるのであれば、内容が詰め込み過ぎなのでページを分割して別コンテンツにすべきだと言うことになります。

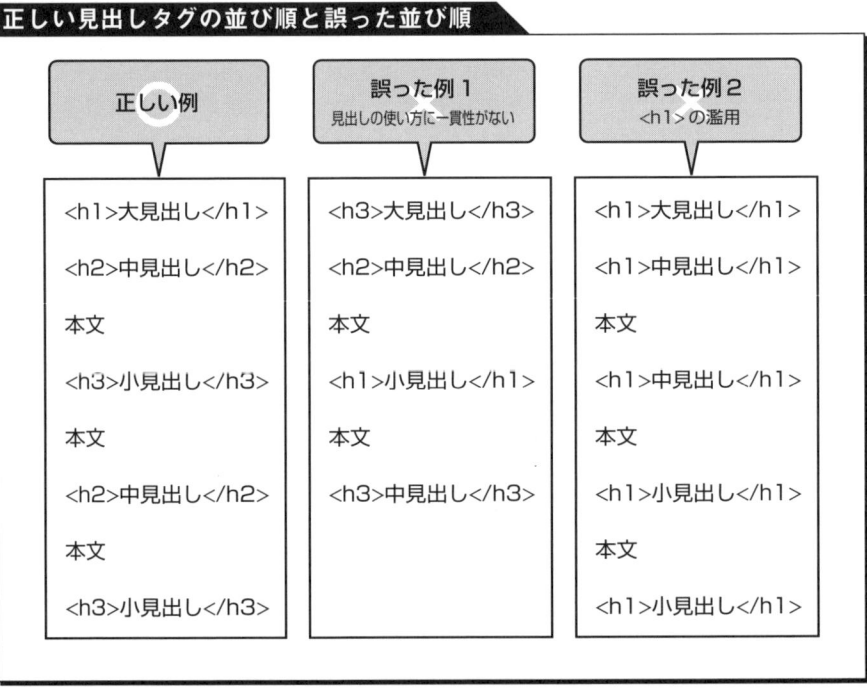

3-5 <a>タグのSEO

□アンカーテキストとリンク先の内容を一致させよう

　<a>タグは「アンカータグ」ともいい、他ページや画像へのリンクを貼るときに使われるタグです。

　SEOを考えた場合、内部リンクを適切なアンカーテキストで密接に繋いでいくことを忘れてはいけません。それはナビゲーションであっても同様で、「トップページ」だけでは不十分で、「サイト名トップページ」が望ましいのです。

　検索エンジンは、<a>タグ内で使われている文言は、リンク先のコンテンツ内容を端的に表しているキーワードが使われているであろうと判断します。したがって、リンクを設定する際に「こちらへ」や「クリック」といった抽象的な表現は避けましょう。<a>タグにはリンク先の説明を入れておかなくてはなりません。

　例えば、リンク先が「液晶テレビ」について書かれたページだとします。SEOとして正解なのは、以下の2つのうち、どちらのリンクでしょうか?

①<a href="（URL）">クリック!!</a>
②<a href="（URL）">液晶テレビ</a>

　答えは、アンカーテキストとリンク先の内容が一致している②です。

□相互リンクの書式を徹底させよう

　これは、外部からのリンクについても同様です。外部リンクを貼ってもらうときには、適切なアンカーテキストとして貼ってもらうことが重要です。

　もちろん、相互リンクを獲得することは、それだけでも歓迎すべきことといえるでしょう。検索エンジンは外部リンクの量と質で、そのサイトの価値を計るからです。またSEOとして機能する他に、他のサイトからユーザーを誘導することができるというメリットもあります。

　ただし、せっかく外部リンクを貼ってくれるということであれば、少しでも効果的に貼ってもらうように働きかけましょう。

　相互リンク用のバナーを用意しているWebサイトは多いのですが、バナーでリンクを貼ってもらうよりも、テキストリンクを貼ってもらった方が効果は期待できます。

そのためには　ソースコードを示して、「このソースをお使いください」と促しましょう。

□ リンクスパムを防止するための<nofollow>属性

また、<meta>タグで、rel="nofollow"という属性が付けると、検索エンジンに登録されないことはP59で紹介しましたが、これと同様のことを<a>タグでも実現できます。<a href="XXXX" rel="nofollow">とすることで、「リンク自体は有効なもののリンク先のページランクには何の影響を及ぼさない」という姿勢を検索エンジンに伝えられます。

ブログなどで、コメントスパム、トラックバックスパムと呼ばれる手法があります。これは、見境なしに他ブログへコメントやトラックバックを打ち、自分のサイトへのリンクを貼ることで、大量の被リンクを確保して、自サイトのページランクを上げようとする行為です。

これらのスパム行為を牽制するために採用されたのが、この<nofollow>属性なのです。Googleはもちろん、YST、MSN Searchでも同様に、<nofollow>属性を採用しています。また多くのブログサービスで、コメントをトラックバックを貼ると、多くの場合自動的に<nofollow>属性が付記されます。

相互バナーの提示例

	（例）
× （どのようなリンクの貼られ方をするのか明示されていない）	「Dragon.jp｜Webマーケティング情報サイト」←このバナー画像を使ってください。
△ （バナー画像によるリンクだが、貼り方まできちんと指示されている）	「Dragon.jp｜Webマーケティング情報サイト」←このバナー画像を使ってください。その際のソースは、<a href="http://dragon.jp"><img src="dragon.gif" alt="Webマーケティング Dragon.jp"></a>としてください
○ （アンカーテキストによるリンクを提示している）	トップページへのリンクを貼られる場合のソースは、<a href="http://dragon.jp"><img src="dragon.gif" alt="Webマーケティング Dragon.jp"></a>をお使いください。

3.6 \<strong\>タグと\<em\>タグ

□ 論理タグと視覚タグ

　\<strong\>タグと\<em\>タグは強調タグと呼ばれますが、これらも\<a\>タグや\<hX\>タグ同様、検索エンジンがチェックするタグのひとつです。

　本文中で強調したいキーワードがあるときは、\<strong\>タグや\<em\>タグを使います。なお、\<strong\>タグの方が\<em\>タグより強い強調の意味を持ちます。

　ここで、強調といえば\<B\>タグや\<I\>タグも同じではないか、と思われる人もいるかと思います。たしかに、\<B\>タグは「挟んだ文字を太字にする」、\<I\>タグは「斜体にする」という働きを持つタグで、\<B\>タグと\<strong\>タグ、\<I\>タグと\<em\>タグの見え方は同じです（なお、\<strong\>タグ、\<em\>タグは、何の設定もしていない場合はそれぞれ太字と斜体で表示されますが、CSSで見え方を設定してあげることで、デザインを自由に変更することができます）。

　しかし、その意味合いは違います。

　\<strong\>タグや\<em\>タグは、本文中で強調したい箇所という意味を持っていますので、強調タグの中でも特に「論理的強調タグ」と呼ばれています。

　一方、\<B\>は挟んだ文字をただ太字にする以上の意味を持っていないため、「視覚的強調タグ」と呼ばれます。

　検索エンジンが重視するのは、論理的強調タグの方です。視覚的強調タグについては、検索エンジンは無視します。

　したがって、強調したいキーワードをマークアップするときは、\<strong\>タグや\<em\>タグを使うべきなのです。

□ 強調したいキーワードだけに適用する

　なお、注意していただきたいのですが、強調タグは、他の文章との差別化のために使われるタグです。

　したがって、文章すべてを強調タグで囲んでしまうと、どこが重要かということを検索ロボットに伝えることができず、結果的に強調タグがまったく無効化してしまいます。最悪の場合、強調タグの多用は検索エンジンスパム行為と認識されますので、文中のキーワード1種類に対して使うのが目安です。

　また勘違いしやすいのが、強調するのはあくまでもキーワードだけということです。

文脈で強調したい箇所があって、その箇所にキーワードを含んでいないのであれば、<B>タグで囲んだ方がいいかもしれません。

論理的強調タグと物理的強調タグ

論理的強調タグ

- <strong>タグ
- <em>タグ

強調して伝えたい単語をマーキングするタグ。検索エンジンがページの内容を判断する際に利用する

物理的強調タグ

- <B>タグ（太字にする）
- <I>タグ（斜体にする）

単に見た目を変えるタグ。検索エンジンには考慮されない

どちらも見た目は同じように表示されるが、SEO的には意味がまったく異なるので注意する！

3-7 画像に<alt>属性を付ける

□ <alt>属性で検索エンジンに画像情報を伝える

　画像をアップロードするときには、その画像が何であるかを<alt>属性を付けて、検索エンジンに画像情報として伝えます。この<alt>属性はイメージ検索に反映されますので、確実に付けておきます。

　ただし、この<alt>属性はSEOとして以外にも、アクセシビリティ的側面も持っています。具体的には、画像が表示されなかった場合に表示される代替テキストや、音声読み上げブラウザーで読み上げられるテキスト情報としても使われます。

　したがって、多数のキーワードを埋め込んだりすることはその働きを阻害してしまい、ユーザーの利便性を欠くばかりか、検索エンジンスパムと判断されることもありますので、注意が必要です。ひとつの画像に対しては、キーワードを2～3個程度埋め込むのが妥当です。

<alt>属性の使い方

	（例）
× <alt属性>にキーワードが過剰（10個以上）に盛り込まれている。検索エンジンスパム対象となる。	<img src="dragon.gif" alt="Webマーケティング Dragon.jp SEO SEM アクセス解析 Webサービス Web2.0 Google Yahoo! MSN 検索エンジン最適化 LPO ロングテール" >
△ <alt>属性に何もつけられていない	<img src="dragon.gif">
○ <alt>属性に適切な数（2～3）のキーワードが含まれている	<img src="dragon.gif" alt="Webマーケティング Dragon.jp" >

3-8 <acronym>タグと<abbr>タグ

略称を定義できるタグ

　SEOは、ご存じの通り「Search Engine Optimization」の略称です。
　このように正式名称と略称のように複数の表記が存在するような場合で、そのどちらの名称でも検索エンジンにヒットさせたいのならば、html内に双方を記述する必要があります。本文中に、「SEO（Search Engine Optimizationの略称）」と書けば、とりあえず「SEO」と「Search Engine Optimization」のどちらでも検索エンジンにヒットします。しかし、複数ページに渡るコンテンツがあったとして、文中に出てきた「SEO」に対して、「SEO（Search Engine Optimizationの略称）」と書くのが果たしてスマートといえるでしょうか？
　そのような場合には、htmlタグには正式名称と略称を同一のものだと認識させる役割を持った<acronym>タグを使います。<acronym>タグは、Aという単語がBという単語の略称であることを宣言するタグです。
　例えばこのタグを使って「SEO」が「Search Engine Optimization」の略称であることを定義付けておくと、html内にわざわざ双方を記述することなしに「SEO」と「Search Engine Optimization」のどちらで検索されても、そのページがヒットするようになります。またP2P（Peer to Peer）やblog（weblog）など頭文字ではない略称は、<abbr>タグで定義付けをします。
　文章の1番目に出てきた略称だけは、テキストで略称と正式名称（ここでは、「SEO（Search Engine Optimizationの略称）」）を記述して、その後の略称は<acronym>タグで正式名称を指定しましょう。

<acronym>タグと<abbr>タグの見本

<acronym>タグ

<acronym title=" Search Engine Optimization">SEO</acronym>は検索エンジン最適化を意味します。
<acronym title=" Search Engine Marketing">SEM</acronym>は検索エンジンマーケティングを意味します。SEOは検索エンジン最適化を意味し、SEMは検索エンジンマーケティングを意味します。

<abbr>タグ

<abbr title=" HyperText Markup Language ">HTML</acronym>はウェブページを記述するときに用いる言語で、<abbr title=" Extensible HyperText Markup Language ">XHTML</abbr>のベースとなりました。HTMLはウェブページを記述するときに用いる言語で、XHTMLのベースとなりました。

3-9 キーワードの出現頻度

◻ キーワードの出現頻度と近接度

　ここまでは、タグの使い方についてのテクニックを紹介してきました。しかし、内部要素のSEOは、タグの使い方に限りません。ページ内のテキスト自体も、SEOに関係してきます。

　特に重要なのが、ページ内テキストに占めるメインキーワードの出現頻度率です。1ページ中に、メインキーワードの出現頻度率が5％前後含まれていることがとりあえずの目安になります。つまり、SEOについて書かれたページ内で、「SEO」という語句が全体の総単語量の5％程度になっていれば、検索エンジンはこのページがSEOについて書かれたものであると判断する、ということです。

　5％という数字はあくまでも目標値ですが、別に難しく捉えることはありません。ためしに何かキーワードをひとつ決めて、それについて文章を書いてみてください。そのキーワードは全単語数の5％程度の出現率に収まっているはずです。

　これが10％以上含まれていればそれは明らかに不自然ですし、逆に2、3％しか含まれていなければ、そのキーワードはテーマとみなされませんので、出現数を増やす必要があります。

　また、複数キーワードを設定している場合は、そのキーワード同士が近接するように記述することも重要です。「リンゴ」と「ダイエット」なら、「リンゴを使ったダイエット」よりも「リンゴのダイエット」の方が、検索エンジンは「リンゴ」と「ダイエット」に関する内容なのだと判断するのです。

◻ 表記は統一させよう

　また、日本語は4種の文字（漢字・ひらがな・カタカナ・アルファベット）を併用する、世界でも類を見ない言語体系を持っていますので、同じ単語をひらがな・カタカナで使い分けたり、漢字をあえてひらがなで表記することで微妙なニュアンスを伝えたりすることがあります。

　しかし、こうした表記の揺れは、SEO的にはマイナスに働きます。検索エンジンはカタカナとひらがなで区別を付けますので、もしキーワードがカタカナ・ひらがな両表記がある場合、ページの中に両表記が混在していると、キーワードの出現頻度が半減することになります。

したがって、こういった場合は、カタカナ表記かひらがな表記か、いずれかに統一すべきなのです。

ここで、どちらの表記を選ぶかは、色んな判断指標がありますが、オーバーチュアのキーワードアドバイスツールで調べて、より多くの回数で検索されているキーワードを選択するのもひとつの手です。

キーワード表記のポイント

- メインキーワードの出現頻度率は5％前後にする

- 複数キーワードを狙う場合は、それらのキーワードがなるべく近接するように記述する

- 漢字・ひらがな・カタカナ・アルファベットの表記は統一する

> 複数の表記のどれに統一すればいいのか迷ったら、オーバーチェアのキーワードアドバイスツールで調べて、より多く使われている表記を使うといい。

3-10 サイドメニューの配置

□検索エンジンは<body>直後のテキストを重要視する

　サイドメニューがあるレイアウトがありますが、右側と左側、あるいは両側、どちらにサイドメニューを置いた方がいいのでしょうか？
　ユーザビリティ的にはサイトのコンセプトに合わせてどちらでも構いません。
　しかし、検索エンジンは<body>直後のテキスト100文字を特に重要視するともいわれていますので、メニューの位置がどこにあろうとも、センター部のコンテンツ本文が<body>の直後に来ることが最優先です。
　ところが、htmlはページの右から左、上から下の順に記述されていきますので、例えばヘッダーと左右メニュー、一番重要なセンター部、そしてフッターという一般的なサイトのレイアウトの場合、通常のhtmlソースだと<body>の下にはヘッダー部、右サイトメニュー、センター部、左サイドメニュー、フッター部の順に並ぶことになります。この場合は、肝心のキーワードを含む主要コンテンツ部分が出てくるのが<body>の中頃ということになり、SEO的には不利になってしまいます。
　したがって、サイドメニューは左側もしくはフッター部分に置くのが、正解となります。

□CSSで、<body>直下にメインコンテンツを持ってくる

　ただ、左側やフッターにしかメニューを置けないとなると、デザインがかなり制限されてしまいます。そのため、一昔前は、右側にサイドメニューを置きながらも、SEO的に不利にならないようにhtmlソースの<body>直下にセンター部を持ってくるために、かなり複雑なテーブルレイアウトを駆使しているケースも多く見られました。
　しかし現在は、CSSレイアウトを使うことで、<body>直下にセンター部のコンテンツが来る2段組、3段組のレイアウトを簡単に実現できます。
　つまり、CSSを使うことで、左右のサイドメニューがありながら、<body>直下にセンター部のコンテンツを配置することができるのです。CSSを使った2段組と3段組のソースコードを記しますので、参考にしてください。

<body>直後にメインコンテンツが来る2段組記述

CSS

```
div.main {
       float: right;
       width: 80%;
       }

div.left {
       width: 20%;
       }
```

html

```
<body>
<div class="main">
メインのコンテンツの内容
</div>
<div class="left">
左メニューの内容
</div>
```

> 左メニューよりも上にメインコンテンツの内容が来る

<body>直後にメインコンテンツが来る3段組記述

CSS

```
div.main  {potision: relative;
      width: 100%;
      }

div.center  {margin-left: 100px;
      margin-right: 200px;
}

div.left  {position: absolute;
      top: 0;
      left: 0;
      width: 100px;
      }

div.right  {position: absolute;
      top: 0;
      right: 0;
      width: 200px;
      }
```

html

```
<body>
<div class="main">
<div class="center">
メインのコンテンツの内容
</div>
<div class="left">
左メニューの内容
</div>
<div class="right">
右メニューの内容
</div>
</div>
```

> 左右のメニューよりも上にメインコンテンツの内容が来る

3-11 CSSとJavaScriptの外部化

☐ 外部化することの2つのメリット

　前節でも触れたように、SEOを考えるにあたって、CSSの使用は必須の条件といえます。また、SEO的には好ましくないのですが、サイトを制作するにあたってJavaScriptを使わなければならないことも多いでしょう。

　こうしたCSSやJavaScriptなど、htmlではない部分に関しては、htmlソースに含めるのではなくて、外部ファイルとするのが原則です。

　これらファイルの外部化のメリットは、2つあります。

　ひとつめは、htmlのファイルサイズをコンパクトにできること。Googleは100KB以上のhtmlはうまく読み込めませんので、htmlの<head>部分に膨大な量のCSSやJavaScriptの記述があれば、html全体をうまく読みきれない可能性も出てきます。CSSやJavaScriptを外部化することで、<head>部分の肥大化が避けられ、html自体のファイルサイズを20～30％の減少させることができます。

　ふたつめのメリットとして、CSSの分離はアクセシビリティの向上に寄与することが挙げられます。レイアウトやフォントの修飾など見栄え的な要素をCSSに渡して、htmlソース自体をテキスト情報だけにすることで、ユーザーにとっても見やすいサイトになるとともに、検索エンジンにとって分かりやすい構造になります。CSSとJavaScriptを外部化することで、より検索エンジン好みのWebサイトを作ることができるということです。

CSSとJavaScriptの外部化

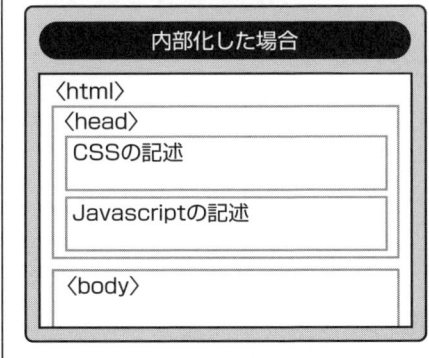

3-12 サブドメインの活用

□サブドメインを使う3つのメリット

　企業サイトの一般的なURLアドレスは「http://www.XXXXX.co.jp/」ですが、この「www」にあたる部分をサブドメインと呼びます。

　サブドメインを使うにあたって新たにドメインを取得する必要はなく、サーバーの設定を変更するだけで済みますので、簡単に独立サイトを立ち上げることができる利点があります。サブドメインを複数使い分けることで、複数の独立サイトを所有することができます。

　一部の企業では、サブドメインに商品名やサービス名、あるいは取り扱っているジャンル名を付けて、それぞれのサイトを差別化させています。例えば、Yahoo!の場合、各コンテンツページをサブドメインで使い分けています。

　これは、実は、このサブドメインでコンテンツを分散させることに、SEO的な効果があるからなのです。具体的には、以下の3つの効果が期待できます。

- サブドメイン間のリンクは外部リンクとして扱われる
- 検索結果にすべて表示される
- エイジングフィルタ対策になる

それぞれ詳しく見ていきましょう。

□サブドメイン間のリンクは外部リンクとして扱われる

　サブドメインを使うSEO上のメリットのひとつめは「検索エンジンは、サブドメインが異なるサイト群を、同一サイトではなく、外部サイトと認識する」ということです。つまり、同じグループのサイトであっても、サブドメインが異なれば、それぞれ独立したサイトであると判断されるということです。

　そうすると、サブドメインごとに独立したサイトだと認識されるわけですから、他のサブドメインサイトからのリンクは内部リンクではなく、外部リンクだと認識されることになります。これは、SEO的に大きなメリットです。

　ご存じの通り、Googleの検索順位は、外部リンクの質と量に左右されます。多くの人気サイトからリンクを貼られるほど、Google内におけるサイトの価値は上がっ

ていきます。つまり、複数のサブドメインサイトの相互リンクにより、リンクポピュラリティを稼ぐことができるのです。

外部リンク、特に有力サイトからリンクを増やすことは一朝一夕でできるものではありませんが、サブドメインを使えば、内部リンク並みの平易さで外部リンクを増やすことができるのです。

検索結果にすべて表示される

ふたつめのメリットは、検索結果にたくさん表示されやすいということです。

Googleの検索結果では、同一ドメインのサイトは2つまでしか表示されません。しかし、サブドメインサイトは異なっているサイトと認識されているため、検索条件に合致すれば、すべて検索結果に表示されます。

ためしに、「yahoo!」でGoogle検索してみると、Yahoo!本体の下にサブドメインサイトがずらりと表示されます。

エイジングフィルタ対策になる

さらに、サブドメインサイトを立ち上げることは、Googleエイジングフィルタ対策としても機能します。これが3つめのメリットとなります。

新規ドメインによるサイト立ち上げは、立ち上げから半年〜1年程度、Googleの結果上位表示されません（これを「エイジングフィルタ」といいます）。しかしサブドメインで立ち上げることで、それを回避することができるのです。

したがって、立ち上げ後、すぐに検索結果に反映してほしいキャンペーンサイトや新商品サイトは、サブドメインで立ち上げることをお勧めします。

Yahoo!のサブドメイン活用例

コンテンツ名	URL（太字がサブドメイン）
Yahoo!テレビ	http://**tv**.yahoo.co.jp/
Yahoo!スポーツ	http://**sports**.yahoo.co.jp/
Yahoo!路線情報	http://**transit**.yahoo.co.jp/
Yahoo!ショッピング	http://**shopping**.yahoo.co.jp/

サブドメインを活用することで検索結果に表示されやすくしている

❏ サブドメインを使う注意点

　このように、サブドメインサイトを使ったSEO対策は効果的ですが、悪用すると検索エンジンスパム行為と判断されます。

　例えば、サブドメインが異なるだけのダミーサイトを多く立ち上げ、リンクポピュラリティを稼ぐという手法もありましたが、検索エンジンスパム行為とみなされペナルティを課せられました。

　また、際限なくサブドメインサイトを立ち上げると、個々のサイトの影響力が分散されてしまう危険性もあります。

　テーマごとにサブドメインサイトを立ち上げれば、たしかにSEOとして効果的です。しかし、テーマをあまりに細分化してしまったために、ひとつひとつのサイトが数ページ程度になってしまえば何の影響力も持ちません。多くの弱小サイトが寄り集まってリンクを貼りあっても、何の相乗効果は期待できないのです。

　したがって、サブドメインサイトは、ある程度のボリュームのコンテンツを持つことが条件となります。

❏ サブドメイン対応のブログサービス

　なお、「livedoor blog」「FC2ブログ」など、各社ブログサービスを提供していますが、これらのブログサービスのURLは「下位ディレクトリ型」「サブドメイン型」の2タイプに分かれます。下位ディレクトリ型は、「http://www.XXXX.jp/ユーザーID」といったURLが与えられます。一方、サブドメイン型は「http://ユーザーID.XXXX.jp/」というURLを割り当てられることが多いです。

　一例を挙げると、livedoor blogは、下位ディレクトリ型ですので、「http://blog.livedoor.jp/ユーザーID/」というURLになります（ただし、有償のlivedoor blog Proはサブドメイン型のブログサービスを提供しています）。

　一方、サブドメイン型であるFC2ブログは、「http://ユーザーID.blogXX.fc2.com/」というURLでブログが提供されます。

　検索結果ページには同一ドメインでは2サイトまでしか表示されませんので、ある検索キーワードで検索した場合に、下位ディレクトリ型のlivedoor blogは2つのブログしか表示されませんが、サブドメイン型のFC2ブログではすべてのブログが検索結果に表示されます。

　検索結果に表示されるか分からない下位ディレクトリ型に比べて、すべてのブログが検索結果に表示されるサブドメイン型のブログサービスが圧倒的に有利なことがお分かりいただけるでしょう。

サブドメイン型のレンタルサーバーサービスの例

サービス名	初期費用	月額費用
ステップサーバー	600円	250円〜
ロリポップ	3150円	263円〜
マックスサーバ	3000円	900円〜
さくらインターネット	1000円	125円〜
ハッスルサーバー	1000円	208円〜

サブドメイン型のブログサービス/ディレクトリ型ブログサービスの例

サブドメイン型		ディレクトリ型	
FC2ブログ	http://アカウント.blog(数字).fc2.com/	gooブログ	http://blog.goo.ne.jp/アカウント名/
livedoor Blog Pro(有料)	http://blog.livedoor.jp/アカウント名/ http://アカウント名.livedoor.biz/	livedoor Blog	http://blog.livedoor.jp/アカウント名/
ココログ	http://任意の文字列.cocolog-nifty.com/	Yahoo!ブログ	http://blogs.yahoo.co.jp/アカウント名/
エキサイトブログ	http://アカウント名.exblog.jp/	アメーバブログ	http://ameblo.jp/アカウント名/
Seesaaブログ	http://アカウント名.seesaa.net/	はてなダイアリー	http://d.hatena.ne.jp/アカウント名/
JUGEM	http://アカウント名.jugem.jp/	楽天ブログ	http://plaza.rakuten.co.jp/アカウント名/

3-13 サイトマップの役割

□ユーザーだけでなく検索エンジンも利用する案内板

　サイトマップは、サイトの案内板や目次というべき存在で、多くの場合、サイトの構造と全コンテンツを階層構造と共に表しています。どのサイトでも普通に見かけるコンテンツのひとつです。

　このサイトマップも、SEOとして、大きな意味を持ちます。サイトマップは、ユーザーにとっての案内板であると同時に、検索エンジンに対しての案内板としても機能します。

　特に、FlashやJavaScriptを使ったナビゲーションを採用しているサイトでは、必須のコンテンツといえるでしょう。

　FlashやJavaScriptを検索ロボットは苦手にしています。グローバルナビゲーションにこれらの技術が使われていると、検索ロボットはウェブサイトを不完全にしか理解できません。したがって、そもそもFlashやJavaScriptを使ったナビゲーションをウェブサイトで使うべきではありませんが、使わざるを得ない場合であっても、アンカーテキストだけでシンプルにデザインされたサイトマップがあれば、検索エンジンは、サイトマップのリンク情報を辿ってサイト内を移動し、リンク元のアンカーテキストとリンク先のコンテンツを比較して、リンク先の情報を判断します。

　現在はGoogleサイトマップというサービスが始まり、検索エンジン専用のサイトマップをxmlファイルで作成して検索エンジンに読み込ませることで、確実にウェブ情報を拾ってくれるように促すことができるようになりましたので（→P84参照）、今までの形でのサイトマップの重要度は低くなりましたが、ユーザーのことを考えれば今までのような形でのサイトマップも用意しておきましょう。

□内部リンクの充実にも効果的

　また、内部リンクの充実という面から見ても、サイトマップはSEOに効果的なコンテンツといえます。

　いくらリンクの充実度がGoogleの検索順位に反映されるからといって、普通のウェブページでは、アンカーテキストだけで埋め尽くすことはデザイン上、実現不可能です。しかし、サイトマップだけは、アンカーテキストで埋め尽くされていても不自然ではありません。作っておかない手はないのです。

12 ● サブドメインの活用

サイトマップの例

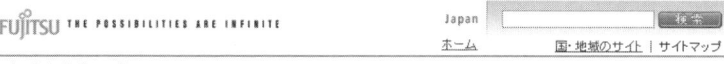

※富士通サイトより引用

SEO「検索エンジン最適化」の教科書

第4章

制作後の告知活動

サイトの存在を知らしめて被リンクを獲得する
テクニック

4.1 外部要素のSEO

□ 内部要素だけではSEO効果は8割減

　ウェブサイトの内部要素の最適化が終わったら、次に外部要素の最適化に着手しましょう。

　外部要素のSEOとは、すなわち被リンク（バックリンク）の確保と同義です。サイトの存在を知らしめて、積極的にリンクを貼ってもらい、外部リンクを確保していくこともSEOでは重要なことです。欲をいえば、有名サイトからのリンクを多数得ることができればいうことなしです。もちろん検索エンジンにインデックスされると言うことも、被リンクの獲得のひとつといえるでしょう。

　内部要素対策としてやれることには、限りがあります。逆にいえば、どのサイトでもある程度のレベルのSEOは施すことができると言うことです。となると、サイトの価値の優劣を決める要素は「どれくらい外部から支持されているか」になってきます。実際、ほとんど外部要素によってサイト価値が判断されているといわれています（もちろん、しっかりとした内部要素のSEOの裏付けがなければ意味はありませんので、内部要素対策・外部要素対策はSEOの両輪であることを忘れないでください）。

　筆者はプライベートサイトをひとつ持っています。簡易的なものとはいえ、公開できるくらいのコンテンツ量を持っていますが、あえて検索エンジンへの告知もせず、外部リンクも一切貼られていない状態にしているため、半年経った今でも検索エンジンにはヒットしません。

　つまり、どこからもリンクが貼られていない状態では、検索エンジンにインデックスされる確率はゼロに等しいことが分かります。

　いくら内部要素をチューニングして、検索エンジンに好まれるページを作ったとしても、そもそも検索エンジンが来てくれないのでは何の意味もありません。だからこそ、外部要素のSEO対策は疎かにしてはいけません。ユーザーと検索エンジンを自分のサイトに誘導するために重要なのです。

□ 自力で被リンクを獲得しよう

　外部要素のSEO、つまり「外部からの被リンク」を充実させるのは、一朝一夕ではいきません。基本的に誰かがサイトを見つけてリンクを貼ってくれるのを待つ、受け身の姿勢にならざるを得ないからです。

しかしながら、そもそも被リンクが少ない状態では、なかなか人目に触れることもなく、したがっていつまで経っても被リンクを得られない、という負のループに陥りがちです。

ですので、最初の一歩として、なんとかして自力でどこかに接点を設ける必要があり、そのためにできる施策は2つに分かれます。

- 検索サイトからのリンクを獲得する
- 検索サイト以外からのリンクを獲得する

本章では、以上の2つの方法について、詳しく解説していきます。

特に、検索サイトからのリンクを獲得（検索エンジンのデータベースに登録されることと同義）するには、ある程度自分から働きかけなくてはいけません。また全ページの情報を漏れなく、検索エンジンに拾ってもらうには、それなりの手段を講じなくてはなりません。本章で解説することを、しっかりと実践してください。

被リンクの2つの獲得方法

検索サイトからのリンク

- Google, Yahoo！などの検索サイトへの登録
- SEMの併用　　　　など

検索サイト以外からのリンク

- プレスリリース
- メールマガジン
- wikipedia
- ソーシャルブックマーク　　　など

どんなにhtmlを最適化しても、外部からのリンクのないサイトは検索エンジンに認識されない！

4.2 検索エンジンへのサイト登録

❏Googleウェブマスターツールを使ってみよう

「サイトができました」と検索エンジンに伝えなくては、データを収集しに来てはくれません。もちろん、外部リンクから辿っていつかはサイトに来てくれることはあるかもしれませんが、その可能性は極めて低く不確実です。ですから、サイト立ち上げと同時に、自分自身で検索エンジンに登録しておくことが大切です。

Googleにサイト情報を告知する手段はいくつかありますが、ここではGoogleウェブマスターツール（旧：Googleサイトマップ）を使います。

このツールは、Googleのクローラーにサイト情報やページURL、サイト構成を告知するためのサービスで、具体的には検索エンジン専用のサイトマップを用意してクローラーに読み込ませます。このサービスを使うことでサイト更新情報を告知できると共に、Googleクローラーが実際にそのサイトから収集したデータの一部も確認できるという一石二鳥のメリットがあります。

また、Googleウェブマスターツールで読み込むxmlファイルのフォーマットは、Yahoo!とMSNとも共通ですので、SEOとしてもぜひ取り入れていきたいところです。

利用の手順としては、以下の通りとなります。

---
①Googleウェブマスターツールのアカウント（無料）を取得して、サイトのURLを登録
②認証作業で、登録したサイトの持ち主であることを証明する
③サイト構造を記したxmlファイルをアップロードする

順に、詳しく説明してきましょう。

❏アカウントを取得してURLを登録する

まずGoogle アカウントを取得します（https://www.google.com/accounts/NewAccount）。

このアカウントは、Googleウェブマスターツールのアカウントと共通ですので、このアカウントを使ってGoogleウェブマスターツール管理画面にログインします。

ログインすると、「サイトを追加」という入力フォームがありますので、ここに自

分のサイトのURLを入力します。

□認証作業で、登録したサイトの持ち主であることを証明する

　サイトのURLを入力しただけでは、まだGoogleウェブマスターツールへの登録は完了していませんので、続いてあなたが登録したサイトの本当のオーナーであることを証明しなくてはなりません。そのためには、以下の2つの方法があります。

> ①Googleウェブマスターツールの管理画面に表示されたhtmlファイルをサイト内にアップロードする
> ②トップページのhtmlの<head>部分に指示された<meta>タグを埋め込む

　①と②、どちらを選んでも、機能や効果が変わるわけではありませんので、どちらを選択していただいても構わないのですが、通常、FTPでファイルをアップロードできる場合は①、ブログサービスのように自由にFTPでアクセスできない環境では②を選びます。

　①では、テキストエディタで新規ファイルを開いた上で、指定されたファイル名で保存し、指定されたディレクトリにアップします。

　②は、ブログサービスでは、テンプレートのindexページの<head>部に指定の<meta>タグを埋めるだけです。

□サイト構造を記したxmlファイルをアップロードする

　認証が終了すると次は、Googleウェブマスターツールに更新情報を伝えるための、xmlファイルやテキストファイルなどをサイト内にアップします。

　詳細な形式はGoogleウェブマスターツールのヘルプに書かれてありますのでご確認いただくとして、簡単にいえばURLリストを列挙しただけのテキストファイルでも大丈夫です。クロールしてもらいたい全URLを1行ごとに列挙していき、そのテキストファイルをGoogleウェブマスターツールに読み込ませるだけで、Googleの巡回リストに追加されます。

　また、ブログサービスの中にも、FC2やSeesaaブログのようにGoogleウェブマスターツールに対応しているものもあります。

　ブログツールのMovable TypeやWordPressをお使いの方は、簡単にGoogleウェブマスターツール用のxmlファイルを生成する方法（→P148参照）をご覧ください。また一般のウェブサイトを運営している方はや、ウェブで提供されている様々なツールを活用するといいでしょう。

　「Create your Google Sitemap Online」（http://www.xml-sitemaps.com/）では、サ

イトのURLを入力するだけで、Googleウェブマスターツール用のxmlファイルを生成してくれます。手順は下記の通りです。

①URLを入力して、Create Mapボタンを押す。
②しばらく待つと、xmlファイルが生成される。
③xmlファイルの生成が終了したらxml SiteMapを押す。
④出てきたファイルをテキストファイルに保存
⑤保存したxmlファイルをサイトにアップロード

これでxml形式のサイトマップファイルの作成が完了します。このファイルのURLを検索エンジンに伝えることで完了です。

注意すべき設定

なお、Googleウェブマスターツールでは、「使用するドメイン」という設定項目があります。
「www」が付くドメインと付かないドメインを区別することができるのです。
お恥ずかしい話ですが、弊社サイト「Dragon.jp」はその設定で失敗を犯してしまいました。Googleウェブマスターツールで、登録するときに「URLをwww.dragon.jpと表示する」と設定してしまったのです。すると、今まで検索結果には「http://dragon.jp」と表示されていたのが、「http://www.dragon.jp」と表示されるようになりました。その結果、「www.dragon.jp」という新サイトが立ち上がったと判断されたのでしょうか、以前6あったページランクが0になってしまいました。

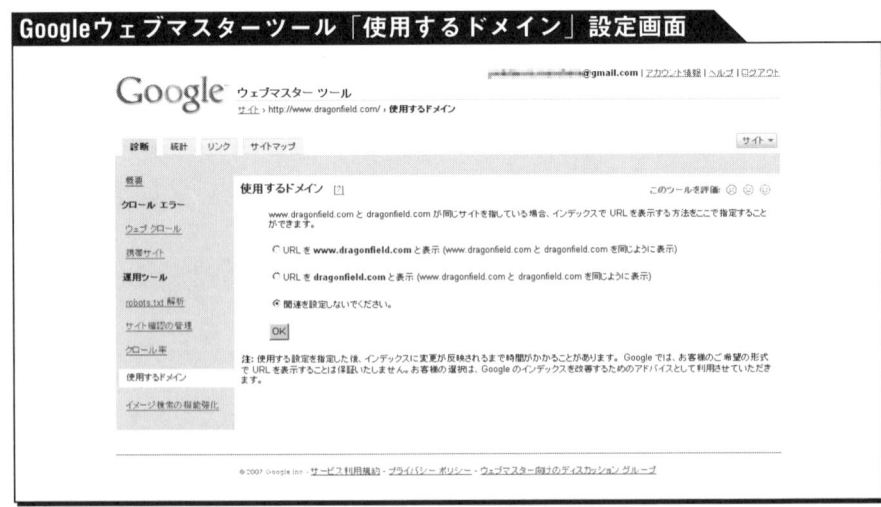
Googleウェブマスターツール「使用するドメイン」設定画面

その設定ミスに気づいて「URLをdragon.jpと表示する」と修正したのですが、時既に遅し。たしかに検索結果こそ「http://dragon.jp」と表示されるようになりましたが、ページランクは0のままで回復していません（2007年2月8日現在）。

「www」を付けないURLを持ったサイトは多いと思いますが、Gooleウェブマスターツールを使うときにはくれぐれも設定を間違わないように気を付けましょう。

❏Yahoo! Site Explorerへの登録

Googleに、Googleウェブマスターツールがあるように、Yahoo!にもサイトの告知手段が用意されています。それがYahoo! Site Explorerです。米Yahoo!が提供しているサービスですが、日本のサイトも登録できます。手順は以下の通りで、基本的にGoogleウェブマスターツールを使ったときとほとんど一緒です。

> ①Yahoo!IDを取得する
> ②登録したサイトの持ち主であることを証明する
> ③xmlファイルのURLを登録する

すべて英語ですので敷居が高く感じられるかもしれませんが、米Yahoo!のインデックス情報は、Yahoo!JAPANにも反映されますので、挑戦する価値は大です。やり方を詳しく説明しましょう。

①Yahoo！IDを取得する

Yahoo!JAPANのIDは使えませんので、新規取得する必要があります。登録画面は当然英語ですが、それほど難しい単語が並んでいるわけではありませんので、心配要りません。Yahoo！IDの登録が終わると、次はそのアカウントでYahoo! Site Explorerの管理画面（https://siteexplorer.search.yahoo.com/mysites）からログインします。

②認証作業

Yahoo! Site Explorerにも、Googleウェブマスターツール同様に認証作業があります。やはり、指定されたhtmlファイルをサイトにアップするか、指定された<meta>タグをウェブページに埋め込むかの方法を取ります。もちろんどちらでも構いませんので、対応可能な方で認証をしてください。通常24時間以内に認証が終わります。

③Feedを登録する

認証を待っている間、Feed（xmlファイル）を登録します。これはYahoo!が読み込むxmlファイルのURLを登録するですが、Googleウェブマスターツールで制作した、sitemap.xmlのURLをそのまま登録して問題ありません。

> Googleウェブマスターツールで製作したxmlファイルを使って、Yahoo！にもサイトを告知することができる

☐ディレクトリ型検索エンジンに登録される

　なお、従来は外部リンクを増やす手段として、「Yahoo!ディレクトリに登録される」というSEO手法がありました。Yahoo!の検索結果に、Yahoo!ディレクトリに登録されているサイトが優先的に表示されていたからですが、Yahoo!の検索結果がYST中心になってしまったこともあり、その重要性は薄らいでしまいました。

　しかし、Yahoo!ディレクトリに登録されていることは今でもYST対策として少なくともマイナスには働きませんので、少しでも検索結果上位を目指すのであれば有料審査サービス「Yahoo!ビジネスエクスプレス」を活用することをお勧めします。

　他にも、エキサイトが提供するディレクトリ型検索エンジンサービス「モンキーポッド（MonkeyPod）」への有料登録審査サービス「Xrecommend（クロスレコメンド）」の活用もディレクトリ型検索エンジン対策として有効に機能します。

　ただし、CGIを使って自分のサイトにディレクトリ型検索エンジンを設置して相互リンクを獲得する手法は、検索エンジンスパムと認定される可能性があるので（→P105参照）避けましょう。

4-3 エイジングフィルタ対策

□ 立ち上げから半年は検索エンジンに表示されない!?

　前節で、Googleへのサイト登録の方法を解説しましたが、それだけでは十分とはいえません。

　実は、新規ドメインで新たにウェブサイトを立ち上げても、最初の一定期間（半年程度）はGoogleの検索結果上位には表示されないのです。きちんとSEOを施しても、です。これは「Google エイジングフィルタ」と呼ばれている現象で、検索エンジンスパム対策の一種だと考えられています。

　通常、サイトが立ち上げと共に、大量の被リンクを獲得して、数日や数週間で大人気サイトに成長するなんてことはまずありません。もしそういうことがあるのならば、意図的に仕組まれた可能性が大きく、そのようなサイトを検索上位に表示するのはリスクが高いとGoogleは判断しているのでしょう。

　もちろん半年を過ぎれば、SEOの効果が反映された検索結果になりますが、それではビジネスチャンスを逃してしまうかもしれません。期間限定のキャンペーンサイトなどはその最たる例で、キャンペーンサイトが検索結果に反映する前に、キャンペーン自体が終了を迎えるなんてことも起こり得ます。

　前出のGoogleウェブマスターツールに登録したとしても、やはりエイジングフィルタを回避することはできません。

□ 情報を小出しにして更新頻度を高めよう

　では、どうすればいいのでしょうか？

　一気に完成形を目指さないで、コンテンツを小出しにしていくということもSEOとしては一考の価値があります。

　新規サイト立ち上げの半年前から、例えば「×月×日オープン」と書かれたページ1枚だけをプレサイトとして立ち上げておいて、徐々にコンテンツを追加しながら盛り上げつつ、半年経った頃に正式オープンするのです。米MicrosoftがAppleのiPodとiTunesに対抗する音楽製品「Zune」のティーザー広告サイトを立ち上げましたが、まさしく情報を小出しにしていく手法を取っていました。

　こうすることで、エイジングフィルタ対策になるだけでなく、ユーザーの好奇心も高められますし、コンスタンスに更新頻度を保つこともできます。更新頻度が高いと、

それだけ頻繁にクローラーが巡回することになり、その結果、検索結果には新しい情報が掲載されることになります。

また、企業ではサイト構築において段階的に予算が下りるということも少なくありませんので、今期の予算内で完成形を目指すのではなく、来期の予算も見据えた上でフェーズを切り、徐々にコンテンツを追加していくこともウェブサイト戦略としてよくあります。あくまでもウェブサイトは育てていく媒体であることを忘れてはいけません。

□ SEMやサブドメインを併用することでチャンスロスを抑える

ただし、ティーザー広告は綿密な計画性が要求されるプロモーション手法です。タイミングや仕掛け方にはそこまで凝ったことはやれないものの、しかしながら半年間のチャンスロスを最低限に抑えたい場合も出てきます。

そういうときには、リスティング広告を併用することでチャンスロスは最小限に抑えます。詳しくは次節で説明しますが、SEOとリスティング広告を併用することで、短期間でサイトの認知度を上げることができますので、とにかくスピード勝負という場合には有効な手段です。

また、P74でも説明しましたが、既にサイトを持っていてそれが検索エンジンに登録されているのであれば、新規サイトはそのサブドメインで立ち上げる方法もあります。

エイジングフィルタを回避する方法

- 段階的に情報を公開していく
- サブドメインを使う
- リスティング広告を併用する

新規ドメインは半年程度はGoogleの検索結果に反映されないので、即時性が求められる場合は対策をとっておこう

4-4 SEMの併用

□ SEOとの使い分けがますます重要になったSEM

　先に述べた通り、新サイトはオープンから少なくとも半年は、Googleの検索結果上位に表示されません。これはGoogleの仕様なので、テクニックで挽回することができません。

　米Enquiroは、検索結果1位～3位は100％クリックされるが、10位になると20％しかクリックされない、という調査結果を発表しました。検索結果3位までに入ることがいかに重要なことか分かるデータです。

　ただ現実問題として、一朝一夕で検索結果上位3位以内入りすることが困難なことも事実です。そこで、即効性が高いリスティング広告と組み合わせて検索エンジン対策をする必要があります。リスティング広告は、あらかじめ登録しておいた検索キーワードでユーザーが検索したときに結果結果の横、あるいは筆頭に広告文とリンクを表示させる広告で、こうした検索エンジンの検索結果画面を使ったプロモーション手法を、SEM（Search Engine Marketing）といいます。

　先の調査では、リスティング広告のクリック率にも言及されていて、それによると、1位が50％、2位40％、3位30％、4位20％、5～8位10％ということです。検索結果で10位ならば、リスティング広告で3位以内に表示される方がクリック率が高いということです。

順位によるクリック率の違い

表示順位	検索結果のクリック率	リスティング広告のクリック
1	100%	50%
2	100%	40%
3	100%	30%
4	85%	24%
5	60%	10%
6	50%	10%
7	50%	10%
8	30%	10%

◻SEMなら検索結果順位をコントロールできる

　SEOとSEMは相互補完する関係にあります。SEOとSEMは検索エンジンを使ったプロモーション活動という点では一致していますが、その特性はまったく異なりますので、その違いをよく理解しておきましょう。

　SEOは、その検索結果に対して働きかけることはできません。あくまでも、検索エンジンの検索結果算出アルゴリズムで弾き出された結果に従うしかないのです。完璧なSEOを施したとしても、検索結果最上位に表示される確約は得られませんし、どのような検索キーワードで検索されたときにヒットするかも、サイト運営者側ではコントロールできません。

　一方、リスティング広告はほぼ入札額によって表示順位が決まるので、「どうしてもこの検索キーワードで上位表示させたい」と思えば、ある程度コントロール可能です（もっとも相応の料金が必要になってきますが）。Google Adwordsには、掲載順位を指定できる「掲載順位設定」機能もあります。

　ここで、検索キーワードを指定できるというのは、実は重要なポイントです。

　例えば、あるSEO案件で、トイレの芳香剤メーカーが、「トイレ」を想定キーワードとして挙げてきたことがありました。

　たしかに、「トイレ」と検索するユーザーの中には、トイレの掃除や芳香剤などの情報を探している人もいます。しかし、実際に調べると、「トイレ」というキーワードはアダルトコンテンツ絡みで検索されていることが多いと言うことが分かりました。

リスティング広告の表示例

このように、同じ検索キーワードであっても、まったくユーザー層もニーズも異なる場合があります。その場合、単なるSEOではどうしようもありませんが、Google Adwordsなら複合キーワードで除外キーワードを設定できます。

この例では、「トイレ」そのものを除外するわけにはいきませんが、複合キーワードからユーザーニーズを汲み取り、明らかにユーザー層が異なるキーワードを除外できます。例えば「トイレ 盗撮」で検索しているユーザーが、芳香剤に興味があるとは思えませんので、「盗撮」を除外キーワードに設定するわけです。

このように、リスティング広告は表示させたい検索キーワード、表示させたくない検索キーワードをあらかじめ設定できるので、ターゲットユーザーが使うと想定している検索キーワードを登録しておけば、効率的にターゲットユーザーを誘導することができます。

□キーワード単位で効果測定ができるのもメリット

さらに、効果測定がしやすいのもSEMの特徴です。

SEOだと想定しているキーワードがどれだけ検索されて、そこからどれくらいのユーザーが流入してきたかが重要になってきます。そしてどのキーワードで検索してきたユーザーがどれくらいのコンバージョンに繋がったか、ということを分析して、コンテンツの最適化に繋げていきます。

それに対して、リスティング広告は、検索キーワードに対して出稿しますので、キーワード単位でコンバージョンを計っていくことができます。キーワード単位の費用対効果を割り出すことができるのです。

この効果測定については、後ほどP124で詳しく説明します。

SEOとSEMの違い

	SEO	SEM
コントロール	不可能	可能
ターゲットへのアプローチ	投網	一本釣り的
成果基準	検索エンジンからの流入数と流入者のコンバージョンレート	キーワード単位のコンバージョンレート

重要性を増していくSEM

SEOは「人事を尽くして天命を待つ」的な受動的なプロモーションですが、SEMは広告を出稿する能動的なプロモーション活動です。個人サイトやIRサイト、会社情報ページなど特にビジネス的な成果を求められているわけではないサイトならばともかく、サイトになんらかのビジネスゴールが設けられているのであれば、SEOとSEMはセットで使い分けていかなくてはいけません。

特に今後は、よりSEMの重要性が高まっていくでしょう。

日本におけるリスティング広告の双璧は、Yahoo!やMSNに出稿しているオーバーチュアと、Googleの検索結果に表示されるGoogle Adwordsですが、検索連動型広告は従来型のバナー広告に代わってネット広告の主流になるほど急成長を遂げていることを受け、各社虎視眈々と参入機会を狙っています。

今までは、Google Adwordsとオーバーチュアのスポンサードサーチがら SEM の双璧でしたが、米MSNも広告プラットフォーム「AdCenter」を開設し、自前で検索連動型広告（P4P）分野に名乗りを上げました。執筆時点では、日本版のAdCenterは開設されていませんが、検索連動型広告も3強時代に突入するものと予想されます。

また、他にもリスティング広告を提供しているところがあります。

Jリスティングの「Jアドリスティング」や、クロスリスティングの「REMORA Listing（レモーラ リスティング）は、これらでしか扱っていない媒体や、独自の出稿形態の存在などに違いがあります。大手ポータルサイトで、これらのリスティング広告だけに出稿しているところはないのですが、中小のメディアサイトではこれらのリスティング広告しか扱っていないところは数多くあります。かなりニッチな分野のサイトが多いので、ニッチなターゲットにアプローチしたいときには、Googleやオーバーチュアではなくあえてこれらのサービスを利用します。

JアドリスティングとREMORA Listingの掲載先

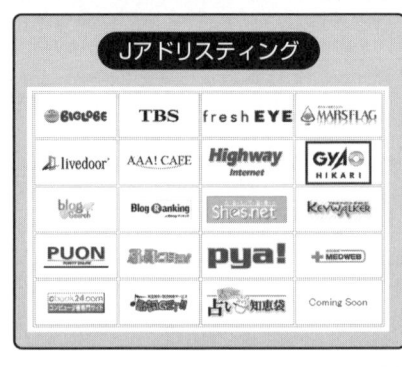
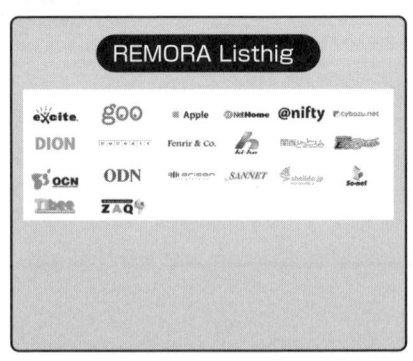

4-5 検索エンジン以外の外部リンクを確保する

❏ 外部リンクを確実に獲得する3つの方法

　ここまでは検索エンジンからの被リンク獲得方法を考えてきましたが、最後に検索サイト以外のサイトからの被リンクを獲得する方法を考えてみましょう。

　一般には、他サイトからの被リンクの確保は、一般ネットユーザーからリンクを貼ってもらうことになるため他力本願の色合いが濃くなっていますが、それでも積極的に被リンクを確保する手段はあります。具体的には、以下の手段が考えられます。

- プレスリリース
- メールマガジン
- Wikipedia
- ソーシャルブックマーク

　こちら側が働きかけることでリンクを貼ることができる貴重な手段です。必ずしも高い効果を望めるとは限りませんが、ひとつでも多くの導線を確保することは重要ですので、やれることはしっかりと確実に押さえておきましょう。

　それでは、それぞれの方法について説明します。

❏ プレスリリースを流す

　サイトがリニューアルした、あるいは新商品のマーケティングサイトが新しく立ち上がったなど、ニュース事項があれば、積極的にプレスリリースを流しましょう。うまくいけば、ニュースサイトから自分のサイトにリンクを貼ってもらえます。

　なお、個人的な経験則ですが、毎月中旬は比較的ニュースが少ないようです（時期によっても変わってきますが）。したがって、ニュースバリューが低いニュースでも、中旬辺りで流してみると、取り上げられる確率が多少上がるかもしれません。

　自分でプレスリリースを流す場合は、各ニュース媒体が持っている連絡先メールアドレスに対してプレスリリース文を書いたメールを送るか、プレスリリースを書いたドキュメントファイルを添付して送付します。

　現実問題として、各メディアの連絡先メールアドレスの収集も労力が掛かりますので、プレスリリース配信代行会社に配信委託する選択肢もあります。

プレスリリースの書き方にもコツがあるのですが、大事なことは受け皿となるページをきちんと設けることです。新サービスや新商品の発表しても、それを紹介するページがなければ、記事として取り上げにくいのです。よくあるのが、プレスリリースの配信時にそのページがまだ完成していないということです。これでは各メディアからの被リンクを得ることはできませんので、プレスリリースを出すときはきちんと受け皿ページを用意すべきです。

□メールマガジンを発行する

メールマガジンを発行すると、告知媒体を入手できる上、大手メールマガジン配信スタンドから被リンクを得られます。Yahoo!もメルマガ配信サービスを開始しましたので、ぜひ利用しましょう。漏れなく、Yahoo!からの被リンクを獲得することができます。

さらに、メルマガを発行するとバックナンバーが残りますので、ロングテール効果が期待できます。ちなみに、メルマガ配信スタンドのバックナンバーページは文中のリンクが無効化されているか、<nofollow>属性が加えられていることがほとんどですので、できればナックナンバーは自分のサイトでも公開するといいでしょう。

□Wikipediaに会社情報を登録する

Wikipediaというユーザーの手によって編纂されている百科事典サイトがあります。誰でも執筆・編集に参加できるというもので、集合知を活かした、まさにウェブ2.0的なコンテンツの代表といえるでしょう。

Wikipediaは回遊率の高いサイトとして知られており、芋づる式に情報が読まれています。企業情報を入れておけば、それだけユーザーの目に留まる機会も多いということです。誰でも執筆可能なのですから、会社の沿革や歴史などの企業情報を書き込んでおくといいでしょう。

もちろん、あくまでも百科事典サイトですから、あからさまな宣伝活動は逆効果です。しかし宣伝行為ではなく、事実関係のみであれば掲載は可能です。

なお、Wikipediaからのリンクは、<rel="nofollow">の属性が付けられるので、被リンク確保には繋がりません。あくまで認知度アップと導線確保の手段と割り切りましょう。

□ソーシャルブックマークに登録する

P32で、既存ニュースメディア各社が、ユーザーに対して記事をソーシャルブックマークしてもらうように働きかけていることを説明しました。自分自身でソーシャル

ブックマークに登録することも可能です。はてなブックマークであれば、はてなでアカウントを開き、自分のソーシャルブックマークに登録するだけです。他のソーシャルブックマークサービスも同様で、簡単に自分のサイトをソーシャルブックマークに登録することができます。

　それが他のブックマークユーザーの目に留まり、立て続けに被ブックマークを獲得することになれば、はてなの注目エントリーに表示され、さらに注目度を集めることとなります。ただし、多くのユーザーアカウントを使って同時にブックマークし、作為的に注目のエントリーに登録されるという手法も一時期流行りましたが、不自然なブックマークのされ方はすぐに露見してしまいますので、注意が必要です。

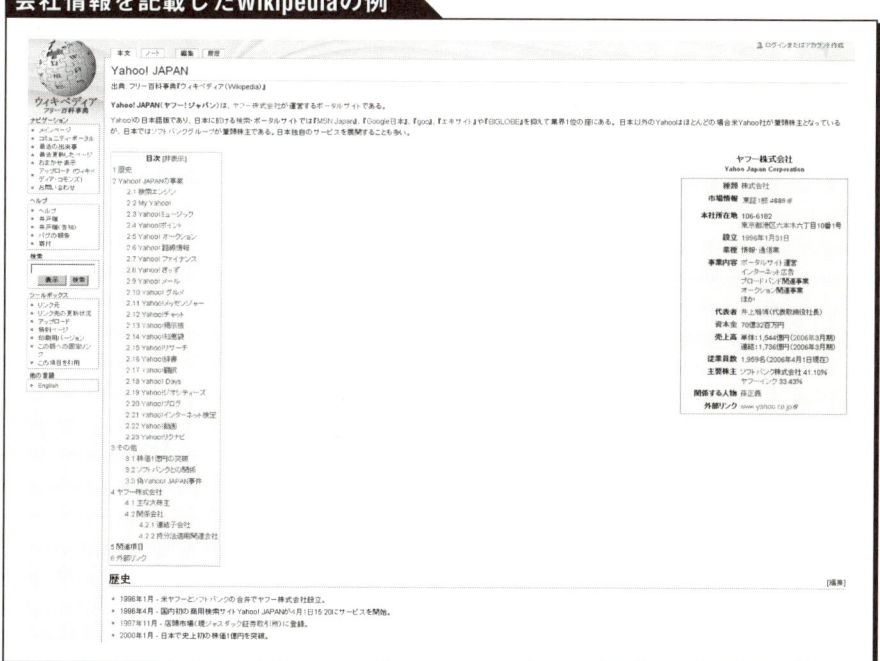

会社情報を記載したWikipediaの例

SEO「検索エンジン最適化」の教科書

第5章

検索エンジンスパム

行き過ぎたSEOテクニックにはペナルティが待っている

5.1 検索エンジンスパムとはなにか？

◻過度のSEOにはペナルティがある

ここまで、SEOの様々なテクニックを紹介してきました。その解説の中でも、折に触れ言及してきましたが、実は、SEOを進める上で、やってはいけない禁じ手がいくつかあります。

それが、検索エンジンの仕組みを逆手にとって、イレギュラーな手法や過度のSEOを施し検索結果上位を目指す「検索エンジンスパム」と呼ばれる行為です。

検索エンジンスパムとは、ユーザーの閲覧ではなく、専ら検索エンジンへの働きかけを目的としている手法と定義することができます。

検索エンジンスパムと判断されると、悪質の度合いによって「検索順位が下がる」「検索結果から除外される」「Googleのデータベースから完全削除される」のいずれかのペナルティが課せられます。

検索結果除外やデータベースから完全削除となってしまった場合、復活する可能性は限りなくゼロに近く、新たにサイトを立ち上げてまた1から再出発しなくてはなりません。当然、訪問者数の激減や企業ブランドの失墜を招くことは明らかです。

P29でも触れましたが、独BMW、独RICOHリコー、サイバーエージェントが検索エンジンスパムと判断されてデータベースから一時期削除されてしまいました。大手企業サイトであっても検索エンジンスパムは許さないという強い意思を感じますし、今後も似たような事件が見せしめ的に起きると予想されます。

そのような結果を招かないよう、スパム行為についての知識を深め、対策を打ちましょう。

◻検索エンジンスパムの種類

なお、検索エンジンスパムは、コンテンツスパムとリンクスパムの2つに別れます。

検索エンジンは内部要素と外部要素の両軸により検索結果を判定しますが、内部要素のスパム行為として「コンテンツスパム」、外部要素には「リンクスパム」と、それぞれが対応します。

また、検索エンジンスパムではありませんが、検索エンジンの仕組みやアルゴリズム上、不利になる手法もあります。

それぞれ、詳しくは次節より説明していきます。

ただし、検索エンジンスパムの手法は日々進化しており、それに対応する形で、常に検索エンジン側の判断基準も変化しています。常にいたちごっこは続いているわけで、今日まで大丈夫だった手法が明日からNGになることも十分起こり得ます。そうなってから、「今まではOKだったじゃないか！」「検索エンジンは横暴だ！」といっても通用しません。検索エンジンの使命は、ユーザーが望む情報を提供することにあり、検索品質は検索エンジンの生命線です。品質を保つために、検索エンジンは強権を振るうことも厭わないのです。

したがって、本書で紹介していないからといって、「これは判断基準に引っかからないから大丈夫」と検索エンジンスパムまがいのテクニックを駆使するのはやめておきましょう。

あくまで「ユーザーにも検索エンジンにも優しい」サイト作りが、SEOの本来の姿なのです。検索順位を意識し過ぎるあまり、検索エンジンを騙すような行為にまで発展すると、かえって逆効果です。

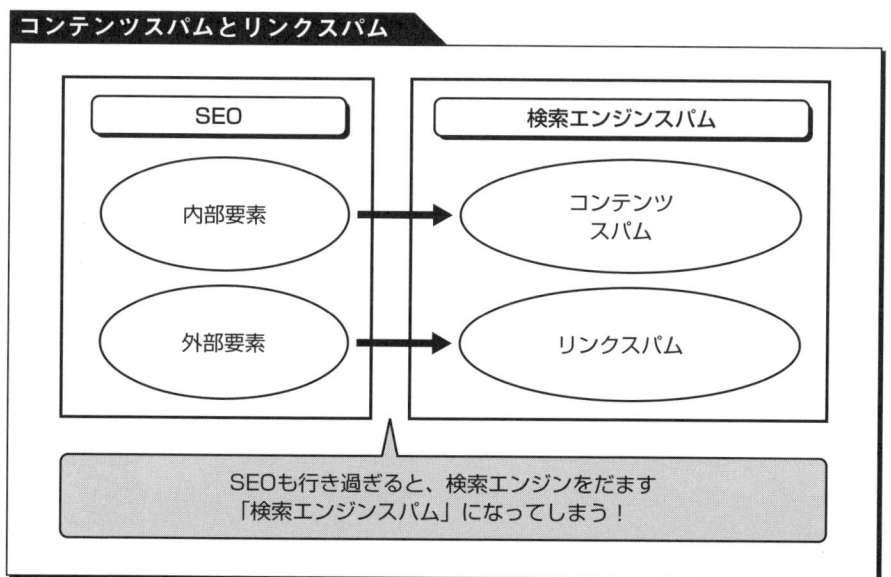

コンテンツスパムとリンクスパム

5.2 コンテンツスパムの手法

◻ 代表的な3つの手法

それでは、まずはコンテンツスパムから確認していきましょう。

コンテンツスパムとは、内部要素のスパム行為です。代表的な手法としては、以下のものがあります。

- 見えない文字を使う
- キーワードの詰め込み
- ＜noflames＞タグや＜noscript＞タグの濫用

これらは、場合によっては、ついうっかり使ってしまうケースもありえますので、気を付けたいところです。

では、それぞれ詳細を説明しましょう。

◻ 見えない文字を使う

普通に表示すると、人間の目には見えない（または見えにくい）文字を記述するのは、検索エンジンスパムとみなされます。

例えば、背景色と同じ色や、限りなく背景色に近い色で文字を表示するのは、NGです。また、人が読み取れないほど小さいサイズで文字を表示するのも同様です。スタイルシートを用いて、ブラウザーの表示からはみ出た部分や、非表示部分にテキストを記述するのも、検索エンジンスパムとみなされます。

人間の目に触れない部分に大量のテキストを埋め込んで、検索エンジンの目を欺こうとするこういった行為には、厳しいペナルティが下ります。

うっかりこういった手法を選択しないためにも、出来上がったページを、テキストベースのブラウザーである「Lynx」で逐次確認しましょう。Lynxでのページ閲覧が不自然ならば、それは検索エンジンスパムと判断される可能性があります。

◻ キーワードの詰め込み

SEO初心者がついやってしまいがちなのが、ページ内のキーワードの詰め込みです。

たしかにSEOにおいて、html内にキーワードをきちんと入れ込んでいくことは重要なのですが、これが行き過ぎると検索エンジンスパムと判断されることがあります。

<meta>タグの箇所でも触れましたが（→P57参照）、<keywords>の部分にキーワードを詰め込んだり、同一キーワードを多用したりすると、検索エンジンスパムと判断されます。また、画像の<alt>属性にキーワードを詰め込む行為もスパムとみなされます。あからさまな例だと、1×1ピクセルという人が見ることができないような極小画像の<img>タグの<alt>属性にキーワードをぎっしりと詰め込んだり、画像にまったく関係ないキーワードを羅列したりという手法もありますが、これらも当然スパム行為と判断されます。

また、上記の例に限らず、htmlソースの<body>内にキーワードを過剰に詰め込む行為も、検索エンジンスパムとみなされます。全体の単語数に占めるキーワード数の割合が20%を超えてくると、検索エンジンスパムと判断されるといわれていますので、その比率は常に気に掛けておきましょう。

◻ <noflames>タグや<noscript>タグにキーワードやアンカーテキストを埋める

<noscript>タグは、JavaScriptが動作しないブラウザーのために代替文を表示させるタグです。JavaScriptに対応していない、あるいはJavaScriptを実行しない設定にしているブラウザーで表示されます。一方、<noframes>タグは、フレームに対応していないブラウザーに代替テキストを表示させるタグです。

もちろん、これらのタグを通常の使い方で用いる分には問題ありませんので、<noscript>タグや<noflames>タグを使ったら即検索エンジンスパムと判断されるわけではありません。

しかし、<noscript>タグや<noflames>タグにキーワードやアンカーテキストを詰め込むことは「隠し文字」と判断されて、検索エンジンスパムとされる可能性がありますので注意してください。

コンテンツスパムの種類

見えない文字
背景色と近い色の文字、極小の文字、表示領域外に表示される文字など

キーワードの詰め込み
1ページ内にキーワードをたくさん入れたり、文章中に同じキーワードがひんぱんに現れ過ぎるなど

<neflames>タグ<noscript>タグの悪用
<neflames>タグや<noscript>タグにキーワードやアンカーテキストを詰め込むなど

5 検索エンジンスパム―行き過ぎたSEOテクニックにはペナルティが待っている

5.3 リンクスパムの手法

代表的な6つの手法

次に、リンクスパムについて説明しましょう。リンクスパムは外部要素のスパム行為で、被リンクを稼ぐために不当な手段でリンクを増やす行為を指します。具体的には、以下のような手法が挙げられます。

- 隠しリンク
- リダイレクト
- ドアウェイページ
- リンクファーム
- トラックバックスパム・コメントスパム
- リファラースパム

特にサイトを立ち上げた直後は、サイトの存在を知ってもらいたい気持ちが先行して、これらのリンクスパム行為に手を染めてしまうことがあります。しかし、現在ではこのようなリンクファームを用いたスパム行為はほとんど無効となっています。やるだけ損、ということです。

そもそも、サイトのテーマからかけ離れた被リンクを獲得したところで、検索エンジンのサイト価値判断に寄与しませんので、十分に注意したいところです。

それでは、それぞれの詳細を見ていきましょう。

隠しリンク

隠しリンクとは、サイト内に背景と同色の文字で設置されたリンクです。同色でなく、近似色であったとしても検索エンジンスパムとしてペナルティを与えられます。

コンテンツスパムの一種で、見えない文字を使ってキーワードを入れ込むスパム行為がありましたが、それのリンク版というところでしょうか。当然、検索エンジンスパムと判断されてしまいます。

これは、内部リンク・外部リンクを密接にしていくことは重要なことではあるので、ページ内に大量のリンクを埋め込むことでリンクポピュラリティを稼ごうという狙いで行われます。たくさんのリンクがあると不自然なので、同色にしてユーザーの目か

ら隠すのです。

■リダイレクト

あるページに来たユーザーを別のページに自動的に移動させてしまうのが、リダイレクトです。通常はサイトを移転したときやコンテンツを移動したときなどに、旧ページから新ページへの転送目的で使われます。

これを悪用して、検索エンジンに読ませることを目的としたページを作る一方で、自サイトにやって来たユーザーにはユーザー向けのページへ転送させてしまうことができますが、Googleを始め検索エンジンの多くは、この手法に大変厳しいペナルティを与えています。特に、0秒で別サイトに転送するよう設定すると、スパム行為としてみなされる可能性が高くなります。

現に独BMWサイトがGoogle八分になったときは、JavaScriptを使ったリダイレクトが原因といわれています。リダイレクトを新しいサイトへの転送などで使う場合には、検索エンジンスパムと判断されないように配慮する必要があります。

■ドアウェイページ

リダイレクトの悪用と共によく用いられるのがドアウェイページです。これはサイトのトップページを別のドメインでいくつも作り、同一サイトの入口を増やす行為です。

ドアウェイページを悪用すると、検索結果に異なるドメインのサイトがずらりと表示されたとしても、実は飛び先はすべて同じ、と言うことになります。つまり検索結果ページからライバルサイトを弾き出してしまうのです。したがって、もちろん検索エンジンスパムとされています。

■リンクファーム

通常の被リンクの獲得は、相互リンクやトラックバックで成立しますが、もっと大規模に何百、何千というサイトが集まり、それぞれリンクを貼りまくり一大リンクネットワークを構築するのがリンクファームです。リンクのためだけに存在する集団行為といってもいいでしょう。

しかし、被リンク獲得のためだけに無理矢理作った無意味なリンク群は、検索ユーザーにとっては何の存在意義もありません。ですから当然、検索エンジンスパムと判断されます。

サイバーエージェントが、Google八分に陥る事件が起きましたが、これも自社サイト群でリンクを貼りまくっていた行為がリンクファームと判断されたからです。こ

のときは、自社サイトのいくつかのトップページ隅のユーザーの目に付かないような小さなスペースに自社サイトへのリンク集を設けていました。

また、yomiサーチと言うCGIがあります。自サイト内にディレクトリ型検索エンジンを設置できるCGIなのですが、これを濫用し大量の被リンク獲得の手段として使っているSEO業者もいました。これらのサイトは2007年1月に行われたGoogleのアルゴリズム変更ではほスパム行為と断定されてしまい、ウェブページの影響度を表すといわれているページランクも軒並み下落してしまいました。

そもそも機械的に被リンクを大量獲得していた時点で、SEOとしてグレーゾーンだったわけですが、Googleはそれをはっきりと「黒」と認定したわけです。

今後は今まで以上に、被リンクの質と量に気を付けなくてはなりません。ウェブ上にはこうした機械的に被リンクを獲得するためのツールや手法が公開されていたり高額販売されていたりしますが、こういった被リンク獲得に対して、今後も厳しいペナルティが加えられるのは必至です。

☐ トラックバックスパム・コメントスパム

トラックバックは、ブログにおいて簡単に相互リンクを生成することができる機能です。コメントもその記事に対する意見を書き込めると共に、自サイトへのリンクを書き込むことができます。本来ならば、情報交流のための手段である、有用な機能といえます。これらの機能を悪用したのが、トラックバックスパムやコメントスパムです。とにかく無作為に多数のブログに対して、トラックバックとコメントを書き込んでいきます。結果的に大量の相互リンクを獲得することができ、サイトの価値を上げることを期待します。

本来の「情報交流」を邪魔するやっかいなノイズであるこれらのスパムですが、実は、どこまでやれば検索エンジンスパムなのかという線引きはまだはっきり定まっていません。

ただし対策として、多くのブログサービスで、トラックバックやコメントに書かれた外部リンクには<nofollow>属性（→P64参照）が付与されるようになりました。これにより、トラックバックスパムやコメントスパムの実効性はなくなっています。

なおブログサービスによっては、<nofollow>属性を付けない対象の指定もできますので、友人からのトラックバックに対しては<nofollow>属性を取る、ということもできます。

☐ リファラースパム

トラックバックスパムやコメントスパムの実効性が低くなったことで、代わりに最近出てきているのがリファラースパムです。

ブログサービスの中には、アクセスしてきたアクセス元のURLを一覧表示できる機能を提供しているところがあります（サイドメニューあたりに「本日のリンク元一覧」などと表示されています）。そこに表示させるために、無作為にアクセスしてきて、もしそのサイドメニューに自分のサイトへのリンクが貼られれば、被リンクが得られるというわけです。

　mixiでも、足あとを大量に残してアクセスを稼ぐという手法がありましたが、それと似ています。これは、被リンク獲得によるSEO効果、導線確保を狙っているわけですが、明らかにスパム行為に該当します。もっと悪質になると、アクセス元のURLを偽装しているケースもあります。

　普通にアクセスしていくだけですので、お手軽なスパム行為なのですが、決してやってはいけません。

リンクスパムの種類

隠しリンク
背景色と近い色で配置されたリンク

リダイレクト
極端に短い時間で他のページに転送されるページ

ドアウェイページ
同一サイトに対して意味もなく複数の入り口となるページを作る

リンクファーム
内容に関係なく相互リンクされたサイト群

トラックベックスパム・コメントスパム
ブログで記事内容に関係なく付けられたトラックバックやコメント

リファラースペム
アクセス元のサイトの一覧からのリンクを期待した過剰なアクセス

5-4 ユーザビリティ的に避けるべき行為

❒ 代表的な4つのNG手法と回避策

　検索エンジンスパムではありませんが、検索エンジンの仕組みやアルゴリズム上、不利になる手法もあります。代表的なものを以下に挙げます。

- 文字を画像にしてあるページ
- Flash、JavaScriptをページ移動用の手段にする
- フレームを使ったページ
- 動的ページ生成

　これらの手法は、検索エンジンが情報を拾いにくくなるため検索結果などに影響を与えます。
　また、検索エンジンが情報を拾いにくいサイトは、ユーザーにとっても使いづらかったり、分かりにくいサイトとなりがちです。したがって、ユーザビリティの観点からも改善が必要になってきます。それでは、それぞれを詳しく説明しましょう。

❒ 文字を画像にしてあるページ

　検索エンジンは、テキストデータを取得して、そのページにどんな情報があるのかを判断します。画像の場合も、<img>タグの<alt>属性に書かれているテキストによってその内容を判断していますので、画像そのものは判断材料になりません。
　ところが、文章をすべて画像にしているページを見かけます。デザインによほどこだわりがあるか、あるいは既存の印刷物をそのまま取り込んだのでしょうか?
　こういったページは、画像が置いてあるだけのページと判断され、画像上にどんな文章が書かれてあったとしても、検索結果にはまったく反映しません。
　文字情報は基本的にテキストデータで記すべきなのですが、画像で表現したい場合には、少なくとも<alt>属性には、その画像を示すキーワードを含んだ説明文を加えるべきです。もし文章を画像にしている場合には、<alt>属性にその文章をまるごと加えましょう。

SEO上不利になる手法

- **文字を画像にしてあるページ**
  画像になった文字は検索エンジンは読めない

- **Flash、JavaScriptをページ移動の手段にする**
  検索エンジンはFlashやJavaScriptは苦手

- **フレームを使ったページ**
  フレーム内のページに直接アクセスされると混乱が生じる

- **動的ページ生成**
  検索エンジンは動的ページを低く評価する

❏ Flash、JavaScriptをページ移動用の手段にする

　約70%のユーザーはトップページ以外のページにやって来ます。検索技術の進化で、どのページであっても入口になってしまうのです。

　したがって、どのページに来ても、「そのページがウェブサイトのどこに位置するのか」を示すパンくずリストと、FlashやJavaScriptを使用しないグローバルメニューを完備するべきです。

　検索エンジンはリンクを辿ってサイトの各ページの情報を拾っていきますが、JavaScriptやFlashでメニューやナビゲーションを作っていると、検索エンジンが下位のページに移動できません。

　例えば、最近ではあまり見かけなくなりましたが、JavaScriptの「javascript:history.back()」を使って「前に戻る」機能を付けているウェブページは、SEO的にはありえないといえるでしょう。

　こういったページに、検索エンジン経由で直接移動してきた場合、履歴を辿れば直前の検索結果ページに戻ってしまうだけです。JavaScriptやFlashは、検索エンジンにも人にも優しくないのです。

　しかも、アンカーテキストによる内部リンクを増やすことにも寄与できていません。すべてのリンクをきちんとパーマリンク（固定リンク）で指定しておくのは、SEOの鉄則です。

　もし、グローバルメニューにFlashやJavaScriptを使用せざるを得ないときは、アンカーテキストを充実させたサイトマップや、html版のサイトを用意するなどの代替手

段を用意しておくか、あるいはフッター部分に、アンカーテキストによる予備的なメニューを置いておきましょう。

　また、通常だと、Flashコンテンツ内でページ遷移してもURLは同じということがほとんどですが、Nikeのサイトは基本的にフルFlashで構成されているにも関わらず、ページ遷移するとそれがURLに反映するようにJavaScriptに工夫が凝らしてあり、擬似的にパーマリンクを表示させています。

　このようにフルFlashサイトや、ページのナビゲーションにFlashを使っていても（擬似的にとはいえ）十分にパーマリンク化することができますので、ぜひそうすべきです。

　なお、Nikeサイトのように、Flashにパーマリンクを付けたいときには、「SWFAddress」（http://www.asual.com/swfaddress/）というFlash埋め込み用JavaScriptライブラリを使います。同梱されているサンプルを見ていただければお分かりいただけると思いますが、ActionScript内でアクションに紐付いたページタイトルを埋め込んでいくことで、擬似的にページタイトルを表示させています。

Nikeのサイト

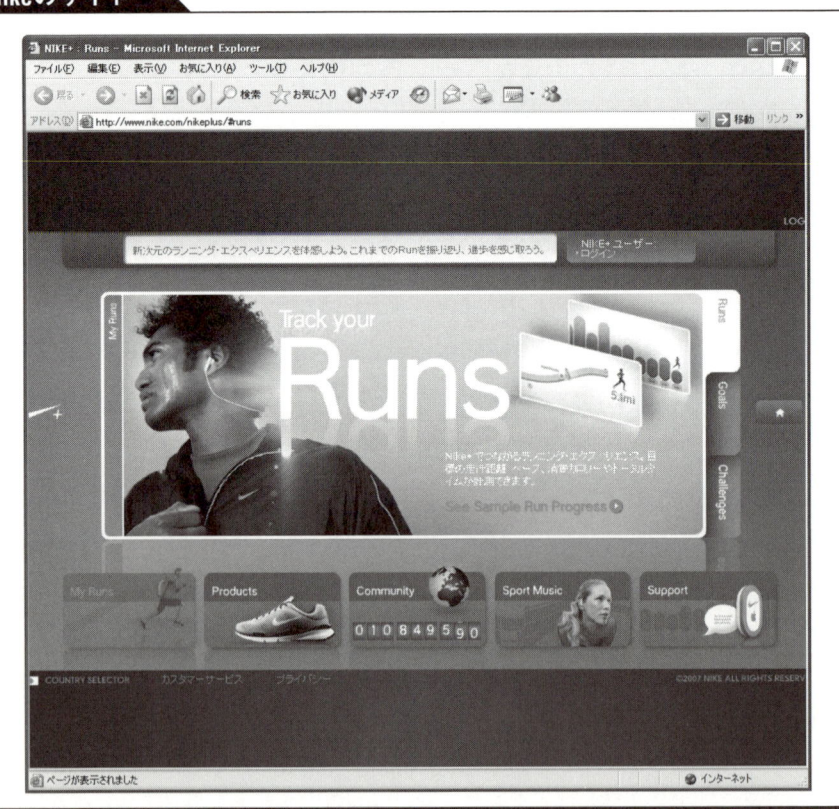

◻フレームを使ったページ

　フレームとは、1枚のページの中に複数のページを表示させる手法です。衰退しつつある手法ですが、今でも有名企業サイトの中に根強く残っていたりします。

　以前は、ウェブサイト制作において、フレームは効率的な手法でした。ナビゲーション部分とコンテンツ部分を別々に管理できるため、ウェブサイトのメンテナンス面でも最低限の労力で済んだのです。

　しかし、フレームを使ったページでは、もっとも重要な「index.html」ページが、フレームの配置を示す情報だけで他には何のテキスト情報も記載されていないため、検索ロボットはそのサイトを低く評価してしまいます。

　また、ほとんどの場合、フレームのメインとなるページにはグローバルメニューが配されていて、フレーム内ページには情報だけが記されています。つまり、フレーム内ページ自体には、他のページへのリンクが存在しないことが多いのです。そういうページに、検索結果から直接アクセスしてきたユーザーは、もっと他の情報が知りたいと思っても、別ページに移動する手段がないため、結局そのサイトから帰らざるを得ません。

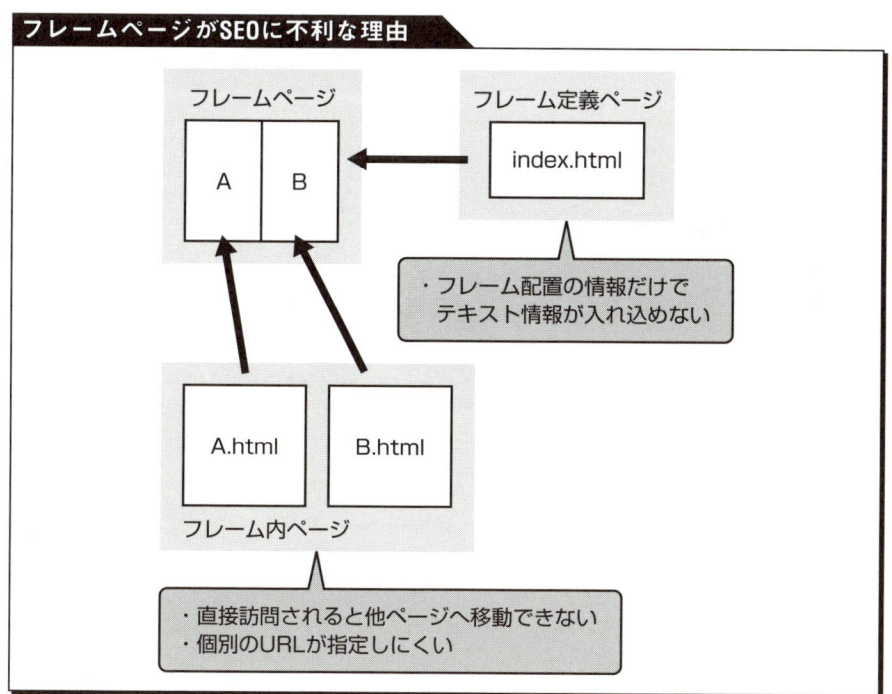

フレームページがSEOに不利な理由

さらに、フレームを使うと、個々のウェブページのURLアドレスが分かりづらいということも大きなマイナスポイントです。アドレスが分かりづらいということは、ユーザーは、各コンテンツに対してリンクを指定しづらいということです（URLアドレスを指定することは不可能ではないのですが）。各コンテンツに対してリンクが貼れない（あるいは貼りづらい）ということは、被リンクを重要視するGoogleなどに対しては大きな不利が発生することを意味します。

つまり、SEO的に見るならば、フレームを使っているだけで大きなハンデを抱えているといえるでしょう。

フレームを極力使うことなく、各ウェブページにグローバルメニューを付け、独立したページとして完結するようなアクセスしてくることを前提にしなくてはなりません。少なくとも、どのページからでもトップページ、あるいは上位階層のページに戻れるようなウェブサイトを心がけるべきでしょう。

□ 動的ページ生成

CGIなどで、ユーザーの操作に応じて動的に生成されるウェブページ（動的ページ）は、検索エンジンが不得手とされています。改善されてはきていますが、URLの中に「&」「？」「＝」が含まれている動的ページは、検索エンジンにインデックスされにくいのです。

Amazonの例

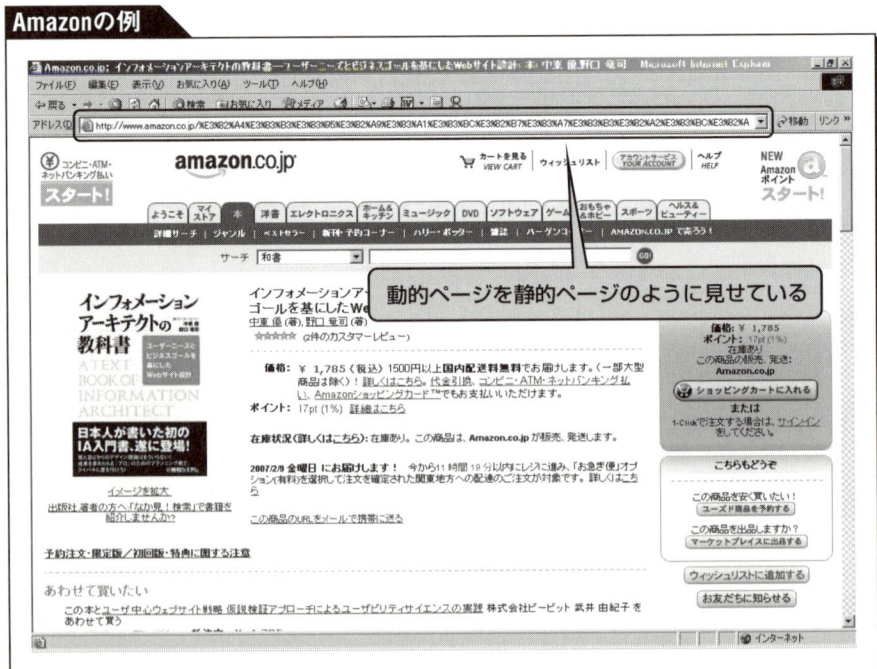

動的ページを静的ページのように見せている

Amazonは、ページのほとんどを動的に生成していますが、検索結果によく出てきます。これはすなわち、動的ページを静的ページのように見せているからです。ページのURLに「&」「？」「＝」が含まれていないことからもそれは分かります。

　したがって、もし動的ページを生成するのであれば、「mod_rewrite」を使って、動的ページのURLを静的ページのURLに見せかけましょう。「mod_rewrite」はApacheサーバー側で要求されたURLを書き換えたり、リダイレクトしたりしてくれるモジュールのことで、具体的には、「.htaccess」ファイルを書き換えることで発動します。

SEO「検索エンジン最適化」の教科書

第 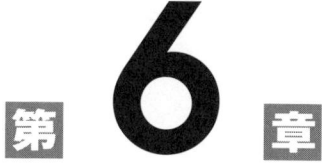 章

効果測定と調整

PDCAサイクルを回して効果を維持するには

6.1 効果測定の必要性

□PDCAサイクルを回そう

　SEOというのは、一度施してしまえば、それでOKという性質のものではありません。サイトの立ち上げ当初は内部要素・外部要素共にほぼ理想的なSEOが実施できていたとしても、時間が経つにつれてその効果は薄れてきます。

　アクセスログだけを定期的に見てPVやユニークユーザー数の増減に気を付けていればそれで十分、と考えているのであればその認識を改めましょう。

　例えば、「SEO」で検索するユーザーよりも「検索エンジン最適化」で検索するユーザーが多いとします。それなのに、あなたのウェブサイトに「検索エンジン最適化」というキーワードが使われていなければ、知らないうちに多くのユーザーを取りこぼしているということになります。

　このようにキーワードの方向性やトレンドがユーザーニーズとずれていると、ユーザーに背を向けて走っているかのように、SEOが進めば進むほど集客力が落ちていくことになります。

　そうならないために、効果測定やデータ分析を通じて、サイトがユーザーの方を正しく向いているかを常に確認しましょう。

　例えば、AmazonはP125で紹介しているA/Bスプリットテストを常に実施して、よりユーザーに支持されるデザインやコンテンツを模索しています。大手サイトといえども、常にユーザーの方を向くための努力をしているのです。それよりも規模が小さいサイトならなおさら、Amazon以上の努力なしにユーザーの心を掴むことができないでしょう。

　マーケティングでは、PDSA（Plan-Do-See-Act）のサイクルを回さなくてはいけない、といわれます。計画（Plan）を立て、実行（Do）し、確認（See）、改善（Act）に繋げる、というサイクルですが、ウェブに限っていえば、最後のAはAnalyse（分析）ではないかと思います。

　ウェブは様々な効果測定を行うことができるメディアです。その特性を活かさない手はありません。

■効果測定の4つの手法

では、効果測定とは、一体何をすればいいのでしょうか？

アクセスログの結果分析や、出稿しているリスティング広告のコンバージョンレートの確認など、確認しなくてはいけない事柄は数多くあります。本章では、具体的には以下の方法について説明します。

---

①SEO TOOLSを使う
②Google AdSenseを使う
③アクセスログを分析する（Google Analytics）
④SEMの効果測定をする

これらの方法を使うことで、検索エンジンの視点（①と②）と、ユーザー視点（③と④）の両方の視点で、効果を分析することができます。

それでは、次節より詳しい説明を始めましょう。

効果測定の4つの手法

- 検索エンジンの視点
  - SEO TOOLS
  - Google AdSense
- ユーザーの視点
  - アクセスログを分析（Google Analytics）
  - SEMの効果測定

これらの方法を利用して、常に検索エンジンやユーザーの反応をチェックすることが重要！

6.2 SEO TOOLSで効果を測定する

◻ 複数の検索エンジンを横断的にチェックするツール群

　まずは今現在、サイトにSEO効果がきちんと現れているかを確認します。

　そのために提供されているのが「SEO TOOLS」(http://www.seotools.jp/)です。SEOの効果が出ているかどうかを、複数の検索エンジンを横断的にデータ収集して、一覧表示してくれる利便性の高いサービスです。

　このサイトでは、以下の3種類のツールが公開されています。

- SEOアクセス解析ツール
- SEOアクセス解析履歴
- 順位チェックツール

　どれもSEOの効果測定の心強い味方になってくれるツールばかりです。では、3種類のツールを順に説明していきます。

◻ SEOアクセス解析ツール

　SEOアクセス解析ツールは、サイトのURLを入れるだけで、SEOの実施状況を自動分析してくれます。URLを入れるだけですので自分のサイトはもちろん、競合他社サイトのSEO状況も確認することができます。

　分析項目は、Googleのページランク、Alexaを使ったトラフィックランキング（トラフィック世界ランク、世界100万人あたりのサイト来訪者数、サイト来訪者の平均ページビュー）、そのサイトがどのようなキーワードで表すことができるかというキーワード分析、検索エンジンへのインデックス数、被リンク数、はてなブックマークを使った注目度、そしてそれらの指標を合算した総合指数、と多岐に渡ります。

　これほどのサービスが無料で提供されていることに驚きますが、一番役に立つのは各項目に添えられたコメントでしょう。SEOをやっていく上で案外気になるのが、「SEOをやってみたはいいがページランクはどれくらいあればいいのか？」「サイトのボリュームはどれくらいあればいいのだろうか？」などの成否の目安となる数値目標です。SEOアクセス解析ツールでは、各項目のコメントとして、どれくらいのレベルなのか、あるいはその改善点を挙げてくれます。

2 ● SEO TOOLSで効果を測定する

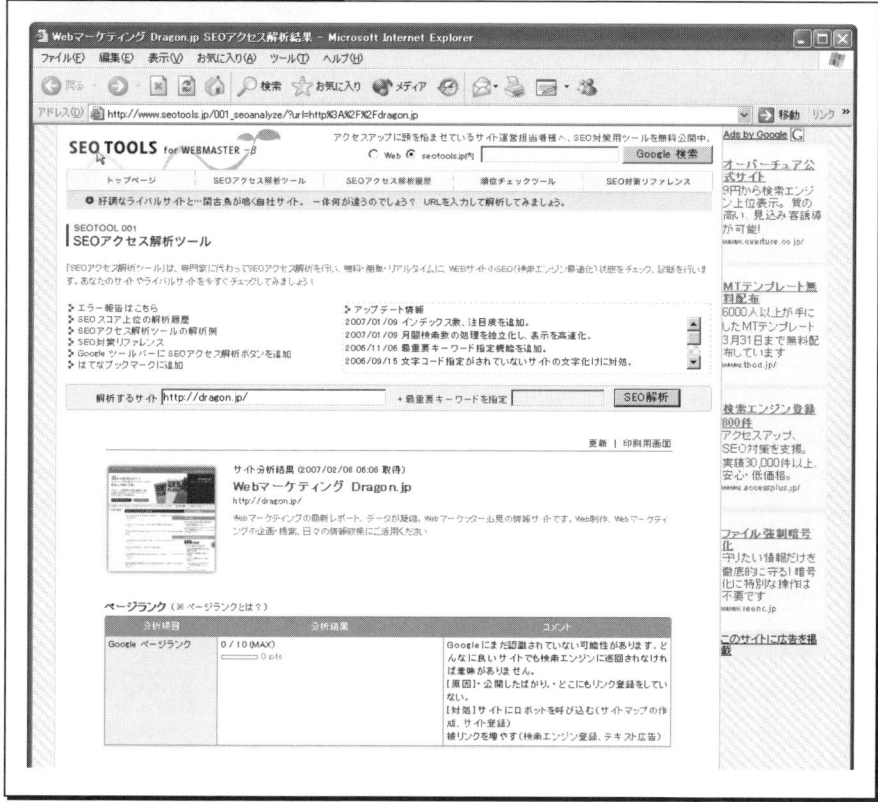

□SEOアクセス解析履歴

　SEOアクセス解析履歴では、先ほどのSEOアクセス解析ツールで総合評価「S」ランク「A」ランク「B」ランクの高評価サイトを、解析順に一覧紹介しています。ここに掲載されているのは、ほとんど大手企業です。

　自分のサイトと規模が違うから関係ないと思うのではなく、これら高評価サイトの中から同業サイトを探し出し、自分のサイトとどこが違うのか、自分のサイトのどの項目が弱いのか、ということを客観的に判断し、これからのサイト運営の目標に据えましょう。

順位チェックツール

　サイトのURLとキーワードを入力すると、そのキーワードにおけるサイトの検索順位を検索エンジンを横断して調べてくれます。SEOをするときに、あらかじめ設定したキーワードで、現在どれくらいの順位なのかを知るときには重宝します。何といっても、Google、Yahoo!、MSNの3大検索エンジンの検索順位が一覧表示されるのは便利です。

　また、一緒にそのキーワードの月間検索数も表示してくれますので、そもそも設定したキーワードがニッチキーワードなのかビッグキーワードなのかどうかも、ここで分かります。

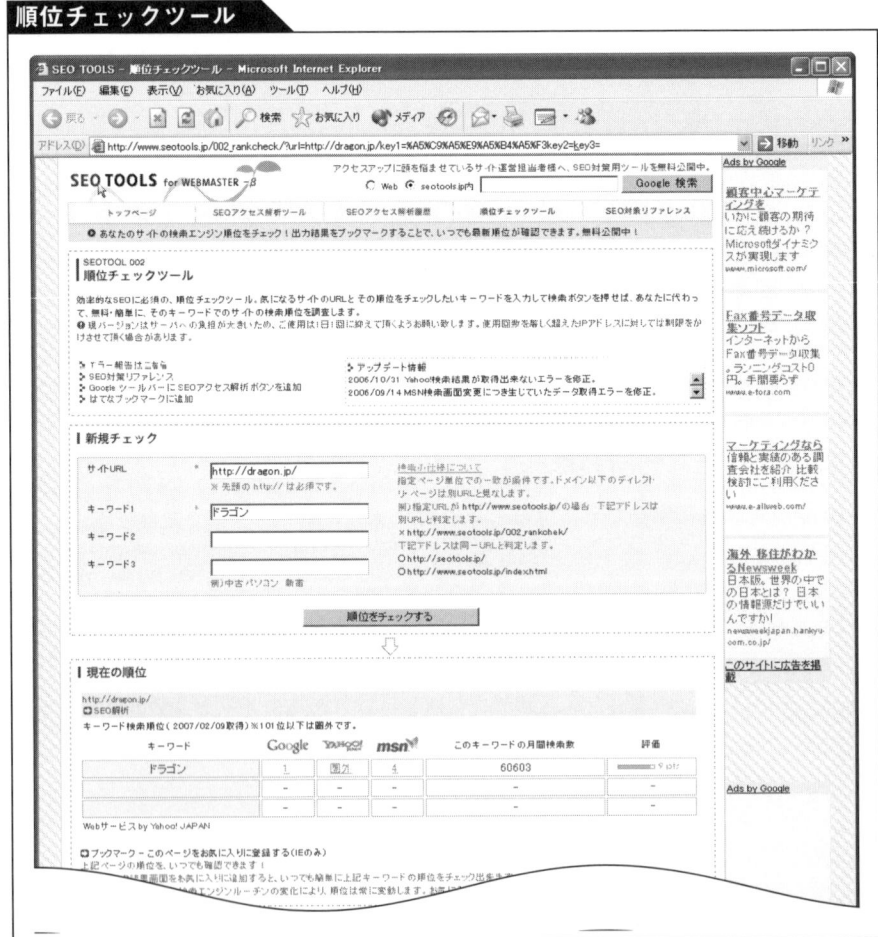
順位チェックツール

6.3 Google AdSenseで効果を測定する

□検索エンジンはキーワードを適切に判断しているか？

　ウェブページの内容を解析する技術を「セマンティック解析」といいます。これは単語単位ではなく文脈単位で内容を理解する技術で、この技術の使ったサービスがGoogle AdSenseです。このGoogle AdSense、ただ無闇に広告を表示するのではなく、ページの内容にふさわしい広告を表示します。

　ということは逆説的に、Google AdSenseに表示された広告から、Googleがそのページをどのようなページと認識しているのか分かるということです。

　例えば、Google AdSense表示枠に美白化粧品の広告が並べば、Googleはそのページが美白化粧品について書かれたページだと判断したということになります。もしそれがページの意図と異なっているようだったら、ページの文言を修正する必要があります。

　このように、Google AdSenseを使うことで、検索エンジンにどのように見られているのかを客観的に確認することができます。

　Google AdSenseを貼ることができないページの場合は、AffiliateSense.net（http://www.affiliatesense.net/about_adsense.htm）のサービスを使うことで簡単に確認することができます。

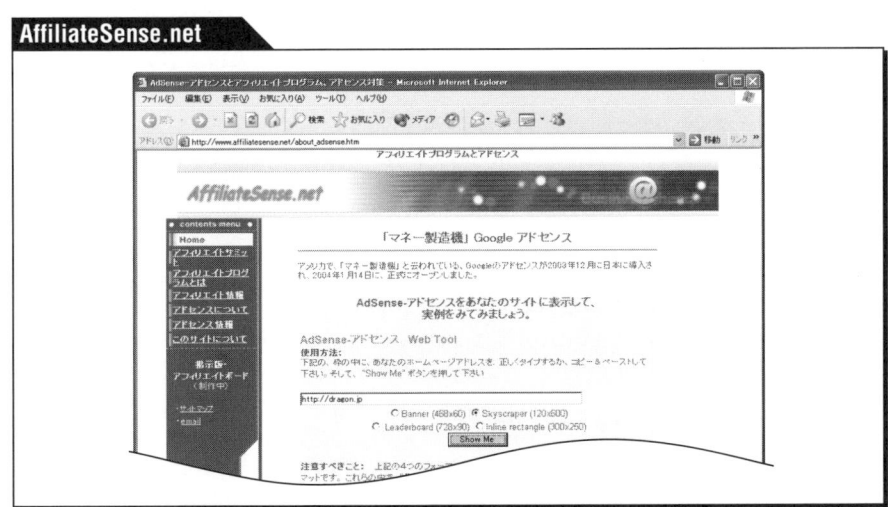

6.4 Google Analyticsでアクセスログを分析する

□アクセスログデータの4つのポイント

また、アクセスログを分析することで、大きく4つのことが分かります。

①ユーザーが多く流入してきているリンク元
②検索エンジンで使われるキーワード
③どのページに最初にユーザーが辿り着いているか。
④ユーザーがその後、どのような行動を取っているか。

アクセス解析ツール「Google Analytics」は、この4つのポイントを簡単に調べることができるツールです。

アクセスログから読み取れるキーワードは、実際にユーザーがサイトに訪れるために用いたキーワードです。その中でも頻出するキーワードに注目し、そのキーワードに最適化していくことで、この章の冒頭で出てきたPDCAのサイクルを回していきますので、「どのようなキーワードでどのページに辿り着いたのか」は常に把握しておく必要があります。

場合によっては、あなたが想定しているキーワードとは違うキーワードでユーザーが訪れてきているかもしれません。そんなユーザーが、あなたのサイト内をどのように巡回しているのか？ どんなコンテンツを探し求めていたのか？ これらを分析することによって、あなたのサイトの改善点が見えてきます。

具体的に、Google Analyticsの解析結果を見るポイントを説明しましょう。

①ユーザーが多く流入してきているリンク元
　リファラーを分析することでどういう経路でユーザーが自分のサイトにやってきたのか分かります。検索エンジン経由が大半だとしたら、もっと外部リンクを増やす必要があります。プレスリリース、メールマガジン、ソーシャルブックマークなどの被リンク獲得を前で挙げていますので（→P95参照）確認ください。

②検索エンジンで使われるキーワード
　使われた検索キーワードを上位から見ていき、大体の方向性がブレでいないか、確認します。想定していたキーワードが下位にあったときは、さらにそのキーワードに

力を入れたSEO（そのキーワードでの別コンテンツを設けるなど）を施す必要があります。

また下位に行くに従い、突拍子もないキーワードの割合が多くなります。実はこれらのキーワードの中に、自分のサイトとは相性が良いけれども、ウェブ全体で見たらニッチキーワードで、実は狙い目だった、ということが分かるかもしれません。

③どのページに最初にユーザーが辿り着いているか。

現在、トップページからやって来るのは全体の3割程度、後はすべてトップページ以外のページにやってきます。どのページに人がやってくるのかということを掴むと同時に、直帰率も計測します。高過ぎる直帰率は、何か問題があるのかもしれません。逆に問題がないから直帰率が高くなるということも考えられます。そのページで抱えている悩みが解決したので直帰したと言うわけです。その場合には回遊率を高めるための施策を取ります。

④ユーザーがその後、どのような行動を取っているか。

Google Analyticsでは、いわゆるコンバージョンレートも計測することができます。例えばメールマガジンの登録だったら、メールマガジンの紹介ページ、登録画面、登録後のサンクスページをそれぞれ指定して、「紹介ページ→登録画面→サンクスページ」という流れを計測できるのです。例えば、登録画面から直帰率が高いとしたら、どこかに不備があるのではないかと考えて、登録する情報量を削るなどの試行錯誤を行うことができます。

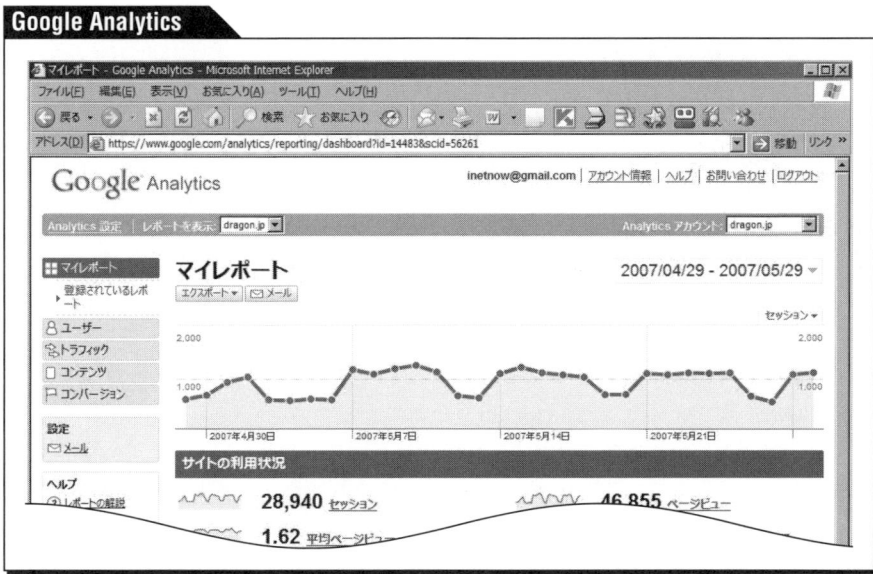

6.5 SEMの効果を測定する

☐ SEMではキーワード単位での効果測定が求められる

　SEMに取り組んでいる場合は、より効果測定が重要になってきます。

　SEMは広告費用が発生するものだけに、つい「掛けた費用に対して、どれだけのアクセスや成約があったか」ということだけを見てしまいがちです。もちろんそれは大切なことなのですが、その結果を次に繋げるためには、より細かな分析が必要になってきます。

　例えば、Google Adwordsでは広告料金の総額を決めることができます。設定した広告料金を消化したところで、すべての広告を表示しないということを決められるのです。しかし、それだと予算を消化したところで、成果を出しているキーワードも成果が上がっていないキーワードもすべて表示されなくなってしまいます。

　つまり、出稿しているキーワードごとに、成果を計った上で表示・非表示の選択をするなどの細かいケアが必要なのです。

　メリハリを付けた出稿プランでないと、広告料金がかさむばかりで成果がなかなか上げられない、ということになります。

☐ 自動ツールを活用しよう

　しかしながら、複数のキーワードでSEMを行っていると、なかなかそのような細かい対応は大変です。現在では1,000を超えるほどのキーワードに出稿することも珍しくないですから、そのような膨大な数のキーワードに対して、個々のキーワードの入札金額と表示順位を把握し、それぞれにふさわしい入札金額設定を施していったり、曜日や時間帯で集札金額の上限を決めていったりなどの広告管理を手作業で行うのは、現実的に不可能でしょう。

　そういった場合は、入札金額やタイミングを細かくカスタマイズできる自動入札ツールもありますので、これらを上手に活用していきたいところです。セプテーニの「BidMaster」やアイレップの「i-bidder」などが有名です。

　また、検索エンジン各社が提供するツールも洗練されてきています。まだ海外の一部サイトだけに提供されているサービスですが、Adwordsの管理画面の出稿キーワードの横に、「Great」「OK」「Poor」の評価が3段階で表示されるようになりました。これは費用対効果を表しています。「Poor」の評価が下ったキーワードに関しては、出

稿を取り止めるか、出稿し続けるのであればランディングページに修正を加えたり、あるいはそのページだけ極端に評価が低い場合には、リンク切れなどのページの不具合があるかもしれませんので、さらに年密な調査が必要になってきます。

☐ ウェブサイト オプティマイザーを使ったA/B スプリットテスト

さらに、キーワードの見直しだけでなく、そのキーワードから誘導されるページ自体の改善も、成約率向上には重要になってきます。

そこで、Googleは、Adwordsの広告主向けに「ウェブサイト オプティマイザー」というサービスを提供しています。このツールを使うことで、広告主は見出しや宣伝文句、画像などを変えて、どういったデザインのページがもっとも売上や契約締結などに繋がるかを試すことができます。

このように、広告文を変えた2つの広告を用意する、あるいは広告バナーの位置を変えた2タイプのデザインを用意して、どちらかが効果があったのかを調べる手法を、俗に「A/B スプリットテスト」といいます。あのAmazonも頻繁にこのスプリットテストを繰り返していると聞きますし、常に試行錯誤をしてベストプラクティスを導く努力は怠らないようにしておきたいものです。

Adwordsの管理画面

出典：Search Engine Roundtale

SEO「検索エンジン最適化」の教科書

第7章

ブログツールのSEO

検索エンジンとの相性をさらに高めるテクニック

7.1 SEOの視点から見たブログのメリット

□ブログと検索エンジンが好相性の理由

　総務省が2006年3月に発表したデータによると、868万人がブログを開設しているそうです。この数字は各ブログサービスのユーザー数の総計ですから、自前でブログを開設している人を含めれば、さらにユーザー数は膨らみます。アクティブユーザーはどれくらいいるのか、という疑問はあるものの、数字を額面通りに受け取るならば、ネットユーザーの10人に1人はブログを開設していることになります。

　すっかり市民権を獲得した感のあるブログですが、実は検索エンジンとの相性が良いという一面も持っています。一時期は検索エンジン結果上位をブログが占めるほど、高いSEO効果を示していました。もっとも今では検索エンジンもブログ対策を立てており、ブログだからといって無条件に検索上位に表示されることはありませんが、ブログが仕組みとして検索エンジンと相性が良いことは厳然とした事実です。

　なぜ、ブログと検索エンジンの相性が良いのでしょうか？　その理由を探ってみましょう。

□内部リンクが作りやすい

　いわゆる「ホームページ制作ソフト」を使ったことがある人なら理解できると思いますが、サイト内部のリンク設定は、かなり面倒な作業です。1ページ追加するだけで、トップページやサイドメニュー、他のページからのリンクなどすべてのリンクを貼り直す必要が発生します。しかも、ページ数に比例して作業量が等比級数的に増加しますので、記事を投稿するほど、更新頻度の低下やリンク切れなどのイージーミスの増加に繋がっていきます。

　しかし、ブログツールはそういったページ追加・作業時に発生するリンク設定問題から開放してくれます。ブログツールを使うと、最初にきちんとリンク設定さえできていれば、記事を投稿するごとに適切なリンクが貼られたウェブページが生成されるのです。しかも、トップページ、グローバルナビゲーション、サイドメニューと、内部リンクを縦横無尽に張り巡らせて導線を確保したサイトを構築することも可能です。

　またサイト構築後でも、ウェブページのひな型であるテンプレートデザインを修正して再構築するだけで、ほぼ全自動でリンク修正が完了します。

　さらには、プラグインの導入により、はてなキーワードのように、文中のキーワー

ドに対する内部リンクを生成することもできます（→P152参照）。
　このように、簡単にミスなく内部リンクを張り巡らせることは、SEOでは大きなメリットとなります。

□ 被リンクを得られやすい

　ブログでは記事を投稿すると、基本的に固有のURLによる静的ページが生成されます（ただし、WordPressのように、デフォルトで動的ページを生成するブログツールもあります）。この個別の記事ページに与えられたURLを「パーマリンク（Permalink）」といいますが、これは被リンクを獲得するためには最低限必要なものです。
　また、ブログは「トラックバック」という相互リンク生成機能を持っています。旧来の相互リンクと異なり、リンク対象は各ページになりますので、他のサイトやブログから関連性の高いページにユーザーを誘導することができます。
　このように、被リンクを獲得する点においても、ブログは秀でています。
　検索エンジンの多くは、被リンクの質と量をそのサイトの価値判断基準にしています。したがって、良質な被リンクを多く獲得することが、検索順位を上げるための最良の手段であることはいうまでもありません。

投稿フォームに記事を書くだけでページが生成される

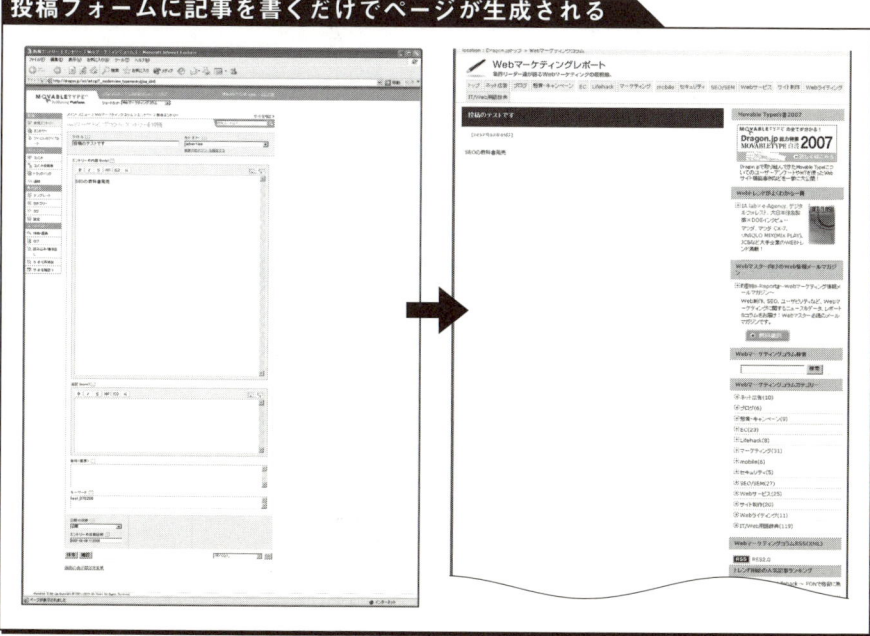

☐ CSSとhtmlの分離が実現されている

　SEOの基本として、html内のCSSとJavaScriptは外部化し、シンプルな<head>を目指すべき（→P73参照）という鉄則がありますが、ブログはデフォルトの状態でCSSとhtmlが分離した状態になっています。

　CSSだけではなくJavaScriptも外部化すれば、かなりシンプルな<head>が実現します。

☐ SEO対応のページが量産できるのがブログのメリット

　このように、ブログに特別なロジックが働いて検索エンジンと相性が良くなっているわけではなく、理由のひとつひとつはごく普通のSEO対策と重なってきます。つまり、特に意識しなくても、記事を投稿するだけで自動的にSEO対応のページが生成されるのが、ブログのメリットというわけです。したがって、今後ウェブサイトを構築するときは、ブログツール（ブログを構築するソフトウェア）を上手に取り入れることで、効率的にSEO対策を打つことができます。

　ここで再確認しておきたいことは、ブログを構築できるブログツールは、ブログだけではなくコーポレートサイトやECサイトなど一般的なウェブサイトの構築にも使えるということです。実際、ウェブサイトのコンテンツ更新にブログツールを導入しているケースは多数あります。

　ブログツールを取り込むことで、更新性に優れ、SEO効果も高いウェブサイトを構築しましょう。

ブログがSEOに有利な理由

内部リンクが作りやすい
ページを追加すると、自動的にリンクが貼り直されるので、作業ミスを気にすることなくリンクを張り巡らせることができる

被リンクを得られやすい
トラックバックを利用すればページ単位で相互リンクできる

CSSとJabascriptが分離している
ブログではデフォルトでCSSが分離している

7-2 どのブログツールを使うか？

□ サーバー設置型のMovable TypeかWordPressがお勧め

さて、サイト立ち上げにブログを使う場合、「どのブログツールを使えば、もっともSEOに効果があるのか」という問題があります。

現在日本で稼動しているブログは2種類あります。はてなダイアリー、ココログ、Livedoor blogなどのブログサービスを利用した「ASP型ブログ」と、ブログツールと呼ばれるソフトウェアをサーバーにインストールする「サーバー設置型ブログ」です。

ASP型は、既にサーバーにインストールされているブログツールを使うだけですので、開設が簡単で、しかも無料で提供されているケースも多いのが長所です。反面、決まったデザインしか利用できないといった自由度の低さや、ブログに広告が表示されることもある、などの短所があります。

サーバー設置型ブログとASP型ブログの比較

	サーバー設置型ブログ	ASP型ブログ
コスト	△ サーバー代＋ブログツールのライセンス料	◎ 無料～
拡張性	◎ プラグインで自由に拡張することができる	× プラグインによる機能拡張はほとんどできない
自由度	◎ ウェブサイト全体の体裁やディレクトリ構造を自由に変更できる	△ デザインをいじれる程度
導入の敷居	△ 最低限でもFTPの操作は必要	◎ ウェブメールを使えるくらいの知識で十分

一方、サーバー設置型ブログは自分でレンタルサーバーを借りて、そこにブログツールをインストールしなくてはならない初期設置の煩雑さが発生します。しかし、ブログツールを自由にカスタマイズできるという長所は代え難い魅力です。

このようにどちらにも一長一短ありますが、SEOを視野に入れたブログやサイトを設置したいのならば、ECサイトや企業サイトも構築できるほどの自由度を誇るサーバー設置型ブログを強くお勧めします。

特に本書では、日本でデファクトスタンダートとしてよく知られているシックスアパートの「Movable Type」と、海外では抜群の認知度を誇る「WordPress」をベースに話を進めます（他のサーバー設置型ブログツールでも押さえておくべきポイントは変わりませんので、十分応用可能です）。

なお、本書では、Movable Type 3.3X以降とWordPress ME 2.0.X以降を元に話を進めます。Movable Typeは他のバージョンと管理画面や設定項目など異なっている箇所も多いのですが、特に3.2からそれらが大幅に変更されました。もし旧バージョンユーザーでこの本に書かれていることをすべて実践したい方は、バージョンアップされることをお勧めします。

❑ Movable Typeの5つのメリット

Movable TypeとWordPressはそれぞれ異なった特徴を持っています。「どちらが優れているのか？」という問いに対して明確な答えは出ません。

ただし、その被ってくる優位性でも両者の間で微妙な差異がありますので、それを踏まえた上で、どちらが自分のサイトに向いているのか、ということを考えます。それぞれの特性を掴んだ上で、最適なブログツールを選択しましょう。

それでは、まず、Movable Typeのメリットから見ていきましょう。Movable Typeのメリットは、以下の通りです。

● コストパフォーマンスが高い

Movable Typeがこれほど支持された理由のひとつに、コストパフォーマンスの高さがあります。個人所有のサーバーやレンタルサーバーで個人的な日記等を書くためのライセンスである「個人ライセンス」は無償で提供されています。

個人ブロガーであっても営利目的の場合はライセンス料が発生しますが、それでも26,250円〜と他のCMSを比べ割安です。もちろん、何百万円、何千万円で提供されているCMSと比較すれば、機能に見劣りする側面もありますが、コストパフォーマンスの高さは比類ありません。

● ユーザーが多い

Movable Typeのメリットのふたつめは、日本人ユーザー数の多さです。

一般的に、ユーザーの数に比例して膨大な数のノウハウが共有されていきます。Movable Typeは書籍やネット上にも多くのノウハウが公開されていますので、困ったときにはトラブル内容で検索するとなんらかの解決策に辿り着く可能性が高いのです。

また、プラグインが数多く公開されているのも多くのユーザーがいる証で、もちろんそれらプラグインに対するノウハウも豊富に公開されていることはいうまでもありません。他のブログツールやCMSツールと比べ、導入とカスタマイズに関するノウハウの量は一歩抜きん出ています。

● 拡張性が高い

Movable Typeはプラグインを導入することにより機能拡張できます。世界中の有志が日々プラグインを制作し公開しているのです。この膨大なプラグイン群がMovable Typeをただのブログツールから、CMSツールへとクラスチェンジさせてくれます。逆にいえば、プラグインなしにMovable Typeを語ることはできないといっても過言ではありません。「こういう機能があったらいいのに」と切望する機能はたいてい、既存のプラグインで実現できるといって過言ではありません。SEOに効くプラグインも多数公開されていますので、これらの紹介や効果、使い方についても後のページで解説します。

● テンプレートでブログのデザインを簡単に変更できる

Movable Typeには、レイアウトデザインや装飾などページのテンプレートが世界中で公開されています。従来、デザイン設定などを行うにはスタイルシートの知識が要求されるため、Movable Typeのハードルは高かったのですが、Style Catcher機能を使うことで初心者でもブログのデザイン変更が簡単にできるようになりました。

公開されているテンプレートの中には、SEO効果を狙って組まれているものもありますので、それを利用するのも手です。

● デフォルトで静的なページを生成する

Movable Typeは基本的に静的ページを生成するので、検索エンジンと相性が良くなっています。

ただし、そのために、数千ページに及ぶような巨大サイトの場合は、全ページの構築に非常に時間が掛かることは覚えておきましょう。トップページの画像を差し替えるなどの大したことがない作業であっても、それが数千ページに及ぶ修正作業ともなれば、それなりの時間が掛かります。下手をするとサーバーの処理能力を超えてしまい、ページの生成途中でサーバーがダウンする可能性もあります。

したがって、「既に何千ページものコンテンツを抱えている」「一日に何本もの記事をアップする」あるいは「頻繁にデザインを修正する」といった特徴を持つサイトでは、WordPressのような動的ページを生成するブログツールが向いているかもしれま

せん。

■ WordPressの4つのメリット

続いて、WordPressを使うメリットを見てみましょう。WordPressのメリットは、以下の通りとなります。

● コストパフォーマンスが高い

CMSツールとしてMovable Typeのコストパフォーマンスは極めて高いのは先の述べた通りですが、とことんコストパフォーマンスにこだわりたい方には、WordPressがお勧めです。

こちらは営利目的であってもライセンス料金などの料金は一切不要です。

● デフォルトで動的ページを生成する

Dragon.jpサイトは、300近いコラムを掲載しています。これをMovable Typeで更新していますが、高い確率で再構築作業に失敗します。もちろんサーバーのポテンシャルに左右されるのですが、何百、何千というページの再構築では、サーバーに大きな負荷が掛かるのです。

こうした場合、ユーザーがアクセスする都度ページを生成する動的ページでは、再構築に関するサーバー負荷が抑えられます。サイトボリュームが大きいときや、頻繁にデザインやコンテンツ内容が変わるECサイトなどでは、動的ページが向いているといえるでしょう。

ただし、その反面、「動的ページはアクセスの増大には脆い」という弱点もあります（もっともそこまでのアクセスの集中は起きにくいのですが……）。

また動的ページには、検索エンジンに捕捉されにくいという側面がありますが、これはパーマリンク設定を変更することで対処できます。実際に検索結果によくヒットするAmazonも、動的ページと見せないような工夫を施した上で、動的ページを生成していますので、パーマリンク設定だけで十分SEOに対応できることが分かります。

● ユーザーが多い

まだまだ日本ではMovable Typeの知名度が勝っていますが、海外ではWordPressのシェアが高くなっています。このため、日本語でのノウハウの共有こそまだまだMobvable Typeにはかないませんが、世界規模で蓄積されたノウハウは莫大な量です。ほとんどが英語で書かれたものですが、そこにハードルを感じなければ、ぜひチャレンジしてみてください。

また、WordPress関連の書籍も日本国内で頻繁に出版されるようになってきますので、導入のハードルは低くなっています。

● デザイン変更が簡単

　Movable TypeはStylecatcherでデザインを変更することができますが、WordPressもThameの変更が簡単にできます。CSSのみが提供されるStylecatcherと異なり、テンプレートも含んでhtml部分もまるごと変更されます。

　ワンクリックでサイトのデザインを変更を簡単に変えられるため利便性は非常に高いのですが、テーマによっては<meta>タグに余計な情報が含まれていたり、おかしな記述がされているケースもありますので、導入後の確認と修正は必須です。特に、海外で制作されたテーマだと、手直しは避けられないと考えておきましょう。

Movable TypeとWordPressの比較

	Movable Type	Word Press
ユーザー数の多さ	日本ではデファクトスタンダード	海外ではシェアが高い
コストパフォーマンス	個人ライセンスなら無料	完全無料
デザイン変更	テンプレートが多数公開されている	テンプレートが多数公開されている
デフォルトで生成するページ	静的ページ	動的ページ
プラグインによる機能拡張	可能	可能

◻︎いずれもSEO仕様のチューニングは必至

なお、いずれのブログツールを選んだとしても、それをインストールした後に、さらにチューニングしていく必要があります。

ブログには「テンプレート」と呼ばれるページの雛形が用意されていて、記事を投稿すると、それらの情報をテンプレートにはめ込んで、ウェブページが生成されることになります。

ところが、検索エンジンと親和性の高いブログとはいえ、デフォルトのテンプレートをそのまま使っていてはSEO効果は半減します。あるいは、Movable TypeもWordPressも、他者が公開しているテンプレートデザインを簡単に自分のサイトに取り込むことができますが、テンプレートがSEOを考慮されていなかったり、海外仕様になっていることがあります。

そこで、ユーザーの手で、SEO仕様にブログのページ設定やテンプレートを変更する必要があるのです。

具体的には、テンプレート内で使われている「テンプレートタグ」の設定変更や、SEOに効果的なサイトレイアウトの採用、プラグインの導入などを行います。次節より、その詳しい方法を説明していきますので、参考にしてください。

テンプレートと生成されるhtmlソースの違い

テンプレート

```
<?xml version="1.0" encoding="<$MTPublishCharset$>"?>
<!DOCTYPE html PUBLIC "-//W3C//DTD XHTML 1.0 Transitional//EN"
 "http://www.w3.org/TR/xhtml1/DTD/xhtml1-transitional.dtd">
<html xmlns="http://www.w3.org/1999/xhtml" xml:lang="ja" lang="ja">
<head>
<meta http-equiv="Content-Type" content="text/html; charset=<$MTPublishCharset$>" />
<meta http-equiv="Content-Style-Type" content="text/css" />
<title><$MTBlogName$> Dragon.jp</title>
```

↓

実際に生成されるソース

```
<?xml version="1.0" encoding="UTF-8"?>
<!DOCTYPE html PUBLIC "-//W3C//DTD XHTML 1.0 Transitional//EN"
 "http://www.w3.org/TR/xhtml1/DTD/xhtml1-transitional.dtd">
<html xmlns="http://www.w3.org/1999/xhtml" xml:lang="ja" lang="ja">
<head>
<meta http-equiv="Content-Type" content="text/html; charset=UTF-8" />
<meta http-equiv="Content-Style-Type" content="text/css" />
<title>Webマーケティングコラム Dragon.jp</title>
```

7.3 <title>タグのチューニング

◻ 個別の記事タイトルを表示させる

　SEOを考えた場合、まず忘れてはいけないのが、<title>の設定です。

　例えば、Movable Typeのデフォルトの状態では、個々のページのテンプレートに<$MTBlogName$>と書かれていて、ページ生成時にその箇所にはブログの名前が入ってhtmlソースが生成されます。したがって、ブログの全ページが同じ名前になってしまいます。

　しかし、個別ページであっても、カテゴリーページであっても、サイト名しか表示されない<title>設定では不十分です。ユーザーはサイトのどこにいるかをタイトルから読み取ることもありますので、ページ内容にふさわしいタイトルが表示されるように、<title>を調整する必要があります。

　そのためには、個別の記事ページのタイトルは、「記事名 - ブログ（サイト）名」というのが一番自然なネーミングでしょう。Movable Typeなら、<$MTBlogName$>の代わりに<$MTEntryTitle$>と書けば、その箇所には記事タイトルが入ったhtmlソースが生成されることになります。なお、WordPressでの該当するテンプレートタグ名は<?php bloginfo('name'); ?>です。

　記事タイトルは検索ユーザーの目にもっとも留まりやすい要素ですので、ページごとにふさわしいページタイトルを付くように、きちんとカスタマイズしておきましょう。

<title>タグ部分のチューニング例

MovableType

- デフォルト： `<title><$MTBlogName encode_html="1"$></title>`
- 修正後： `<title><$MTEntryTitle$> - <$MTBlogName$></title>`

WordPress

- デフォルト： `<title><?php bloginfo('name'); ?> <?php if ( is_single() ) { ?> &raquo; Blog Archive <?php } ?> <?php wp_title(); ?></title>`
- 修正後： `<title><?php wp_title('');'-';<?php bloginfo('name'); ?></title>`

7.4 \<meta\>タグのチューニング

☐ \<keywords\>のチューニング

　Movable Type3.3からは、記事に対して複数の「タグ」を付与できるようになりました。これは、ひとつのページに対して複数の属性を付与することができる機能です。

　例えば、千代田区にあるお勧めのイタリア料理店の紹介ページを作ったとします。これをカテゴリーに納めようとすると、「千代田区」「イタリア料理」どのカテゴリーに入れていいのか思案のしどころです。しかしタグ機能を使って、このページに「千代田区」「お勧め」「イタリア料理」のタグを付加することで、「千代田区」「お勧め」「イタリア料理」のどのキーワードにも紐付けることができます。

　そして、このタグがページを示す属性を表しますので、タグをそのまま\<keywords\>に使うことで、ページごとのキーワード設定ができます。

　一方、WordPressのデフォルトのテンプレートには、タグの設定が入っていませんので、プラグインを使ってタグ機能を加えます。

★<keywords>のチューニング例

MovableType

- デフォルト　<keywords>の設定はない
- 修正後　`<MTEntryIfTagged><meta name="keywords" content="<MTEntryTags glue=","><$MTTag encode_html="1"$></MTEntryTags>" /></MTEntryIfTagged>`
（このソースを<meta>タグ内に埋めると、その記事で使われているタグが、<keywords>に反映される）

WordPress

- デフォルト　<keywords>の設定はない
- 修正後　プラグイン「Another Wordpress Meta Plugin」を導入すると、投稿画面に<description><keywords>の登録メニューが出現するので、keywordsをカンマで区切って入力する

☐ <description>のチューニング

　<meta>タグの<description>は、検索結果の説明文にも表示される重要なタグですが、ブログツールでは設定されていないことが多いタグでもあります。

　Movable Typeには、<meta>タグのために用意されているフォームはありませんので、別のフォームに記述されたテキスト情報を<meta>タグに適応させます。テンプレートの<discription>タグのところを書き換えれば、すべてのページに同じ<description>が適用できますが、SEO的には、やはりページごとに最適な<description>を設定したいところです。

　Movable Type・WordPress共に管理画面を活用すれば、個別の<description>情報を生成できます。

　Movable Typeの場合は、個別アーカイブのテンプレートの<meta>タグに、「`<meta name="description" content="<$MTEntryExcerpt encode_html="1"$> />`」を書き加えます。これでエントリー画面の「概要」のところに書き込んだ内容がそのままそのページの「description」に反映されるという寸法です。

　WordPressは、前出のプラグイン「Another Wordpress Meta Plugin」を導入すると、投稿画面に<description>の登録メニューが出現しますので、こちらに<description>の書き記せば反映されます。

◻ 検索エンジンに拾われないページを作る

その他、ページによっては、さらに追加しておいた方がいい\<meta\>タグもあります。

コンテンツが書かれていないページ（コメント確認ページ、トラックバック確認ページ、RSSフィード）は、検索結果に表示されても意味がありません。検索結果にRSSフィードがヒットした経験をお持ちの方ならお分かりいただけると思いますが、ユーザーにとって何の意味も持たないようなページが表示されて喜ぶでしょうか？

さらにいえば、カテゴリーアーカイブや月別アーカイブさえも、検索エンジンに捕捉されない方が好ましいのです。抜粋記事や記事目次だけが載っているカテゴリーアーカイブや月別アーカイブにいったん来て、そこから個別アーカイブに誘導させるよりも、直接個別アーカイブに誘導した方が、よりユーザー視点に立った施策といえるでしょう。

しかも、カテゴリーアーカイブや月別アーカイブは記事が更新される度に変わっていきます。そのため、検索エンジンのインデックス化する時期によっては、検索結果と異なるページ内容が出てきます。これに対して、個別アーカイブはパーマリンクなので、URLと内容に乖離が発生することはありません。ユーザー視点に立てば、直接個別アーカイブに誘導してあげる方がいいのです。

したがって、これらのページは、検索エンジンに補足されない方が好ましいといえます。そのために、\<meta name="robots" content="noindex,follow"\>を\<head\>部分に埋め込んでおきましょう。

なお、「必要な情報を見てそのまま直帰される」ということを回避して回遊率を上げるために、関連記事ページを表示させるなどの手段は用意すべきです。

◻ 不要な\<meta\>タグは削除しておこう

なお、提供されているテンプレートには、これら以外の\<meta\>タグの要素が含まれていることがあります。WordPressでは、\<meta name="generator" content="WordPress XXXX" /\>とバージョン情報が記載されています。

しかし、こうした要素はSEO的に必要ありませんので、削りましょう。不要な要素はhtmlからなるべく削り、シンプルなhtmlソースにすることが、検索エンジンに優しいページを作るポイントです。

7-5 <hX>タグのチューニング

☐ 見出しとして機能するようにしよう

　<body>内のタグもしっかり確認しておきましょう。<h1>や<h2>などは検索エンジンが重要視するために、ページタイトルやそのページの見出しに適用することが基本ですが、Movable Typeのデフォルトの状態では、<h2>は日付に割り当てられています。

　日付を強調する必要性はまったくありませんので、<h2>にはページタイトルやサイトタイトルが来るように、スタイルシートのテンプレートを修正しましょう。

　WordPressもテーマによっては、<h1>や<h2>がカレンダーに適用されていたりするので確認が必要です。

<hX>タグのチューニング例（MovableType）

- **デフォルト**: `<MTDateHeader><h2 class="date-header"><$MTEntryDate format="%x"$></h2></MTDateHeader>`
- **修正後**: `<MTDateHeader><div class="date-header"><$MTEntryDate format="%x"$></div></MTDateHeader>`

日付にh2が使われているので、divだけで対応するように修正した

パーマリンクの設定

□パーマリンクの重要性

　以前は1ページにつらつらと記事を書き足していくようなサイトが大半でしたが、そういうサイトではトップページのボリュームが増えてくると、古い記事だけを切り取って過去ログとして別ページに保管していました。そのような更新形態だと、トップページの記事を他人に紹介したいときには、URLを伝えた上で「このページの×月×日の記事」と言う他ありませんでした。しかも、過去ログに移動すれば、該当のURL自体が無効になってしまいました。

　しかし、ひとつのページにひとつの記事が割り振られていれば、そのURLだけを伝えるだけで済みますし、ページ自体が削除されない限りそのページはURLが変わることなく存在し続けます。先ほどから何度も出てきた「パーマリンク」のことです。

　現在ではパーマリンクの重要性は既に認知されていて、パーマリンクを前提としてウェブページにどういうファイル名を付けるのか、どのディレクトリにページを生成していくのかを考えることに軸足が移ってきています。

□Movable Typeでのパーマリンク設定

　基本的に静的ページを生成するMovable Typeでは、URL表記についてそれほど気にする必要はないのですが、注意すべき点があります。Movable Typeでのデフォルトの URL が、年月のディレクトリに連番が振られたhtmlファイルが生成されるように設定されている点です。つまり、デフォルトの状態で、記事を生成すると、http://hogehoge.jp/archive/07/01/00326.htmlといったURLになってしまいます。

　これでは、URLを見ても何についての記事か分かりにくく、しかも無駄に階層が深くなっているのもマイナスポイントです。ディレクトリ構造も、URL表記も、SEOをまったく考慮していないも同然です。ですから、設定を変更しておきましょう。

　また、長くなったカテゴリーアーカイブページを分割するために「MTPaginate」を使ったときは、ページ内に「？」「＝」を含む動的ページが生成されます。これらの文字や記号は検索エンジンと相性が悪いので、URLでは使わないことが望ましいのです。「MTPaginate」を使用しているからまったく検索エンジンに捕捉されないというわけではありませんが、代替のプラグインとして「Paged Categories Plugin」を使うことも選択肢に入れておきましょう。

個別アーカイブの生成設定（MovableType）

デフォルト　yyyy/mm/entry_basename.html
修正後　　　archives/entry_basename.html

□WordPressでのパーマリンク設定

　WordPressのような動的ページを生成するブログツールは、URL中に「？」「&」「％」「＝」「cgi-bin」「cgi」などの文字や記号を含む動的ページを生成します。先に述べた通り、これらの文字が含まれていると、検索エンジンに捕捉されにくくなりますので、これらを避けたURL設定が必要です。

　WordPressの管理画面でパーマリンク設定を見ると、デフォルトでは「http://hogehoge.com/?p=123」と生成されるように設定されていますので、それを変更します。「独自表記を以下の入力欄に記述」の欄にチェックを入れ、/archives/%postname%と入れることで、検索エンジンに嫌われないパーマリンク設定が完了します。

パーマリンクの設定（WordPress）

あるいは、裏技的な使い方ですが、/archives/%postname%.htmlと入れることで、静的ページとして印象付けることも可能です。SEOの効果としては、どちらでも変わりません。

また、投稿画面の投稿スラッグの欄に入力した英数字が%postname%として反映されますが、パーマリンクのURL名とページ内容はできるだけシンクロさせた方が好ましいといえます。適当に付けるのではなく、ある程度ページの内容に沿った名称を付けましょう。

なお、この投稿スラッグに日本語を入れると、英数字に変換されたURLが付けられます。検索結果には日本語名が付いたURLが表示されるので、誘導率の向上に繋がるかもしれません。もっとも、URL自体がとても長くなってしまい、覚えることが困難という弊害は起きます。

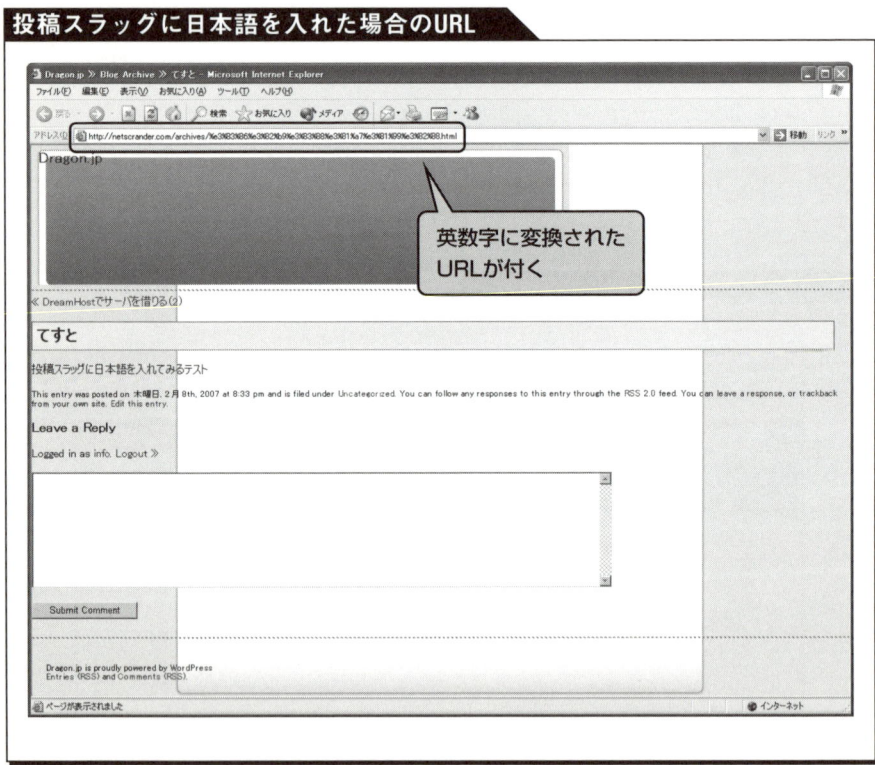

投稿スラッグに日本語を入れた場合のURL

英数字に変換されたURLが付く

7 パンくずリストを作ろう

☐ トップページ以外のページに来たユーザーに現在地を教える

　多くのユーザーが、検索エンジン経由で、トップページ以外のページにやってきます。つまり、どのページであっても、そのサイトの起点となり得るのです。

　例えば、dragon.jpサイトでいえば、トップページに来るユーザーは約25％ほどです。つまり、4人に3人はトップページではなく、その他のページに直接来ているということです。

　一般に、ある程度の規模のサイトであれば、トップページに直接来るユーザーは30％前後に落ち着くはずです。

　したがって、トップページ以外のページに来た70％のユーザーがそのまま直帰しないように、どのページにきても、そのページがサイトの大体どこに位置するのか分かりやすく提示してあげる必要があります。

　そのために、ぜひとも設置したいのが、パンくずリストです。パンくずリストを設置することで、階層構造などを伝えると共に、内部リンクと導線を確保することができます。

　このパンくずリストは、Movable Typeでは、テンプレートタグをうまく活用することで、簡単にパンくずリストが生成できます。また、WordPressでは、「Breadcrumb Nav XT」（http://sw-guide.de/wordpress/breadcrumb-nav-xt/）というプラグインを使うことで、簡単にパンくずリストを生成することができます。ぜひ設置しておきましょう。

パンくずリストのテンプレートタグ（Movable Type）

```
<a href="<$MTBlogURL$>">トップページ</a> &gt; <MTParentCategories glue=" &gt; "><a href="<$MTCategoryArchiveLink$>"><$MTCategoryLabel$></a></MTParentCategories>&gt; <$MTEntryTitle$>
```

「トップページ ＞ カテゴリー名 ＞ 個別アーカイブ名」という形でパンくずリストが表示される

78 RSSフィードの設定

□ 検索エンジンにもRSSを読んでもらおう

　ブログを生成すると、その更新された記事の見出しや概要が記述された「RSSフィード」と呼ばれるファイルも同時に生成されます。RSSリーダーは、このRSSフィードを定期的に巡回して、ブログが更新されたかどうかを判別します。そこで、きちんとhtml内の然るべき場所で、RSSフィードの場所を記しておく必要があります。

　ここで、<body>内で閲覧者にRSS登録を誘導する目的でRSSフィードへのリンクを貼っている人は多いのですが、SEOを考えるなら、それだけでは不十分です。検索エンジン向けに、<head>内でもRSSフィードへのリンク先を示しておきましょう。

□ RSSには概要だけ書くのがお勧め

　なお、現在、RSSリーダーでブログを購読しているユーザーは徐々に増えています。そういったユーザーに対して、どのようなRSSを配信すればいいのでしょうか？

　本文をすべて配信すべきかどうかということは議論の余地が残されていますが、個人的には全文を配信することはビジネスに直結しない可能性が高いのではないかと思います。RSSリーダー上で完結してしまいサイトには来てくれない可能性が高いのではないかと思うのです。

　ですから、RSSでは概要だけ配信して、全文はサイトに掲載するのをお勧めします。そして、概要では全文が気になる書き方をすることで、サイトに誘導するのです。例えば、「これだけはやっておきたいブログのSEO ベスト5」といった記事を書いて、RSSではその2までを配信すれば、高確率でサイトに誘導することができるでしょう。

RSSフィードへのリンク先を示すソースコード

```
<link rel="alternate" type="application/rss+xml" title="RSS" href="（RSSのURL）">
```

これを<head>に埋め込む

7-9 更新作業が終わった後にやること

□ PingサーバーにPingを打つ

　ブログの更新情報を記録する「Pingサーバー」にPingを送信することで、「Pingサイト」にブログの更新情報を告知することができます。Pingサイトに更新情報が掲載されれば、すなわち相互リンクが結ばれることになりますので、被リンクが確保されると共に、Pingサイトからユーザーを呼び込むことも期待できます（ただし、サイトによってはリンクに<nofollow>が付与されることもあります）。

　しかしブログツールや、ISP提供型ブログサービスもデフォルトでPing設定をしているところは少なく、多くの場合ブログ開設者自らが設定しなくてはいけません。

　Ping設定は、それほど難しいことではありません。Pingサーバーの一覧を見ていただけると分かるように、大手サイトが名前を連ねていますので、これらのサイトから被リンクを得られるように、Pingの送信をしておきましょう。

　なお、現在、国内外問わず、数多くのPingサーバーが存在します。これらをいちいち登録していくのも大変な作業です。また新規Pingサーバーを登録したり、削除したりといったメンテナンス作業も想像するだけでうんざりしてきます。

　ですから、Pingサーバーへの一斉配信サービスを提供しているサイトがあるので、そこに登録するといいでしょう。例えば「Pingoo!」（http://pingoo.jp/）では、そこへ登録するだけで他のPingサーバーへPing配信が完了します。

■Googleウェブマスターツールを使う

ここまで何度も出てきたGoogleウェブマスターツールですが、このツールを利用するためには、サイト構造を記したxmlファイルを用意する必要があります。

Movable Typeでは、RSSフィードのテンプレートをチューニングすることで、xmlファイルを自動生成することができますので、これを利用しましょう。また、記事を更新するタイミングで、検索エンジンに更新情報を自動で発信してくれる「MTGoogleSitemapsPing」(http://www.magicvox.net/archive/2006/05201647/) というプラグインもありますので、活用してください。

一方、WordPressには、Googleウェブマスターツール用に特化したxmlファイルを生成するプラグイン「Google Sitemap Generator for WordPress v2 Final」(http://www.arnebrachhold.de/2005/06/05/google-sitemaps-generator-v2-final) が用意されていますので、これを使います。なお、こちらは、sitemap.xmlの構築だけではなく、更新頻度や、トップページ、カテゴリーページ、記事ページなどの個別の優先順位設定などを行うことができます。これにより、あまり情報を拾ってもらいたくないページや、常に更新し続けているコンテンツなどをメリハリを付けて、検索エンジンに伝えることができます。

---

sitemap.xmlの例（Movable Type）

```
<?xml version="1.0" encoding="<$MTPublishCharset$>"?>
<urlset xmlns="http://www.google.com/schemas/sitemap/0.84">
<url>
<loc><$MTBlogURL encode_xml="1"$></loc>
<priority>1.0</priority>
</url>
<MTEntries lastn="9999">
<url>
<loc><$MTEntryPermalink encode_xml="1"$></loc>
<lastmod><$MTEntryModifiedDate utc="1" format="%Y-%m-%dT%H:%M:%SZ"$></lastmod>
</url>
</MTEntries>
</urlset>
```

①新しくテンプレートを作成します。（テンプレート名は任意）
②ファイル名はsitemap.xml。
③テンプレートフォームにxmlソースを書き加えます。
④Googleウェブマスターツール登録ページに、そのsitemap.xmlを置いたURLを記入します。

※引用元：http://blog.creamu.com/mt/2006/05/movabletypegoogle.html

□ソーシャルブックマークしてもらう

　ソーシャルブックマークサービス（SBM）は、オンラインブックマークサービスのひとつで、自分を含め様々な人とブックマーク情報を共有することができます。ブックマークされた総数でランキングされたり、他ユーザーのブックマーク動向を確認したりなど、有益な情報を探る手段のひとつとして認知度が上がっています。

　代表的なサービスとして、日本でははてなブックマーク、海外ではdel.icio.us（デリシャス）やdigg（ディグ）が人気です。

　SBMが起点となってブレイクした記事も最近ではよく見かけるようになり、どれだけSBMに登録されるかが良質な記事の基準にまでなっています。SBMにブックマークされると、露出の拡大という集客効果やブックマークサービスからリンクを貼られることによる被リンクの獲得が期待できます（del.icio.usなど一部のSBMでは、<nofollow>タグが付与されます）。

　記事内容としては「まとめ」系コンテンツや、「TIPS・裏技」系コンテンツがブックマークされやすいなどの傾向がありますが、その他にもブックマークされやすいウェブページの条件がいくつかあります。

　ひとつは、パーマリンクであること。SBMでは、記事のURLを登録していきますので、記事ページがパーマリンクであることがブックマークされる上での最低限の仕様といえます。

また、記事ページに「この記事をブックマークする」ボタンが付いていることも条件です。記事ページに、「このエントリーを（SBMの名称）に追加」ボタンが付いていると、それを読んだユーザーはボタンを押すだけでブックマークできるので、当然ブックマークされやすくなります。日経BPやasahi.comの記事ページの一部にも、「このエントリーをはてなブックマークに追加」ボタンが付いています。

　下図に、「このエントリーをはてなブックマークに追加」のリンクを作るソースを掲載しておきますので、ぜひ活用してください。また、WordPressには、このボタンを記事に自動付与する「wp-hatena」（http://hiromasa.zone.ne.jp/blog/archives/446/）というプラグインがありますので、これを活用するのもいいでしょう。

　さらに、MovableTypeには「AddToHatenaBookmark」（http://code.as-is.net/wiki/AddToHatenaBookmark_Plugin.ja_JP）という、記事を公開するごとに自動的にはてなブックマークの自分のアカウントに登録してくれるプラグインもあります（要はてなアカウント）。

SBMへのリンクを作るソース（MT/WP）

はてなブックマーク

文字でのリンク

```
<a href="http://b.hatena.ne.jp/append?<$MTEntryPermalink archive_type="Individual"$>">はてなブックマークに追加</a>
```

画像を使ってボタンらしく見せる場合

```
<a href="http://b.hatena.ne.jp/append?<$MTEntryPermalink encode_url="1"$>"><img src="画像のURL" alt="このエントリーをはてなブックマークに追加" title="このエントリーをはてなブックマークに追加" width="画像の横幅" height="画像の高さ" border="画像を囲む枠の太さ"></a>
```

del.icio.us

文字でのリンク

```
<a href="http://del.icio.us/1?url=<$MTEntryPermalink archive_type="Individual"$>">del.icio.usに追加</a>
```

画像を使ってボタンらしく見せる場合

```
<a href="http://del.icio.us/1?url=<$MTEntryPermalink archive_type="Individual"$>"><img src="画像のURL" alt="このエントリーをdel.icio.usに追加" title="このエントリーをdel.icio.usに追加" width="画像の横幅" height="画像の高さ" border="画像を囲む枠の太さ"></a>
```

7-10 プラグインでSEO仕様にパワーアップさせる

☐ SEOに有効なプラグインはたくさんある

　Movable TypeやWordPressはプラグインによって機能を拡張できますが、副次的な効果として意外とSEOに効くプラグインが多いのです。そこで、ここでは、そういったSEOに有効なプラグインを紹介していきます。これらのプラグインを使って、SEOが効いたサイトを構築していきましょう。

　なお、プラグインを使うにあたって、使用料金の有無、ライセンス形態など様々な利用規定が設けられているので、使用前にはその確認を忘れずにしましょう。

☐ 画像アップロード時に<alt>属性を追加するプラグイン

　SEOでは、画像ファイルには、<alt>属性を付けることが鉄則です（→P63参照）。ところが、Movable Typeでは画像をアップロードするのは比較的に簡単なのですが、これに<alt>属性を付けることは結構面倒な作業でした。

　しかし、「imagealt」を利用すれば、アップロード時に<alt>属性を入力するフォームが出てきますので、ここに最適な文言を入れるだけで、<alt>属性が付いた画像をアップロードすることができます。

☐ 関連記事を表示するプラグイン

　サイトの課題のひとつに、「いかに回遊率を上げていくか」があります。興味のある記事をひとつだけ読んでそのまま直帰されてしまっては、そこからなかなかビジネスに発展させていくことはできません。

　自分のサイトのファンになってもらうためには、検索エンジンユーザーに少しでも多くのコンテンツに触れてもらうことが重要です。そこで、記事の末尾にその記事に関連する（あるいは方向性が近しい）記事へのリンクを貼り、芋づる的にユーザーが記事を読んでくれるようにしておきましょう。

　MTには、「Related Entries」、WPには「Related Posts Link」というほぼ同一機能を持つプラグインが用意されていて、記事を投稿するときに関連性がありそうな記事を選択することで、関連記事として表示させることができます。

　また、MovableTypeには、「UTW mod Related Post」という、半自動的に関連記事

を掲載できるプラグインもあります。このプラグインは「UltimateTagWarrior (UTW)」というタグ機能プラグインを併用するのですが、これにより、UTWで付けられたタグ情報を分析して、近しいと判断される記事を関連記事として表示させることができます。何百、何千もの記事の中から、関連記事を手作業で紐付けていくのは大変ですので、多少精度が悪くても、こういったプラグインを使うこともありです。

❏ 自動的に文中リンクするプラグイン

　内部リンクを増やすためには、はてなキーワードやWikipediaのような用語集コンテンツを用意しておくのが効果的です。

　その効果はふたつあって、ひとつは回遊率の改善です。Wikipediaで芋づる式に記事を読んだ経験がある人は想像しやすいと思いますが、内部リンクの充実によりユーザーの直帰率を下げることができます。

　もうひとつは、内部リンクの充実による被リンクの獲得です。Wikipediaでは記事中の用語にはリンクが貼られていて、その飛び先はやはりWikipediaの該当の項目です。Wikipedia内で内部リンクが密接に構築されているわけです。内部リンクは外部リンクほど重要視されませんが、「ちりも積もれば山となる」の例え通り、地道な積み重ねが検索順位に影響を与えることは少なくありません。特に激戦区のキーワードなら、こういった積み重ねがより重要になってきます。

　ただ、こういった用語集コンテンツを完全手作業で行うのは大変です。そこで、半自動で行ってくれるプラグインを活用します。

　MovableTypeで、文中リンクを自動的に貼ってくれるプラグインが「MTSakuinPlugin」です。MTSakuinPluginは、あらかじめ設定しておいたキーワードが記事中に出てくると、自動的にサイト内リンクを貼ってくれます。もちろん受け皿になるページをあらかじめ作っておく必要があります。

　WordPressの場合は、「Lexicon Wordpress Plugin」が自動的に文中リンクを生成してくれるプラグインです。なお、用語集ページも生成してくれますが、Wikipediaのように用語ごとにページが用意されるわけではなく、1ページにまとまった状態で生成されるので、ロングテール効果はあまり期待できません。

　ただし、こういったプラグインはサーバーへの負荷が高いので、サーバー環境が貧弱な場合、再構築に時間が掛かったり、あるいは失敗する可能性もあります。導入の際には一気に用語集コンテンツを作るのではなく、様子を見ながら徐々に立ち上げていきましょう。なお、Movable Typeの場合は、再構築するページ単位を少なくすることで、サーバーへの負荷を抑えることができます。

　また、サイト内に用語集やヘルプを設ける手間が掛けられない場合には、Wikipediaの該当項目や検索結果へリンクを貼ることもできます。

　Movable Type用の「dosearch」とWordPress用の「wikipedia linker」は、共に指定

した文中のキーワードに対して、Google・Yahoo!の検索結果、並びにWikipediaの該当項目にリンクを貼ります。文中に「seo」というキーワードがあった場合は、WikipediaのSEO項目へのリンクや、GoogleやYahoo!で「SEO」を検索した結果ページへのリンクを貼ることができます。

ただし、ユーザーがそこから流出してしまい、回遊率の向上は見込めません。そういった効果を度外視して、ユーザーにより良いコンテンツを提供したいときに用いたい選択肢のひとつです。

❏ コンテンツを拡充するプラグイン

外部の情報を色んな形でサイトに取り込むことで、コンテンツの拡充を計ることができます。サイトに彩を加えるようなブログパーツではなくて、サイトの回遊率や利便性に寄与するものが多数ありますし、もちろんSEOにプラスに働くものもあります。

例えば、地図情報はコンテンツの中に不可欠な要素となりました。その牽引となったのが、Google Mapsで、サイト内に自由に表示させることができるようになりました（地図データを商用目的するような使用は要相談）。このGoogle Mapを組み込むためのプラグインがあります。

Movable Type用の「Mapper Plugin」はテンプレートタグ内に、住所を指定するだけでその場所のGoogle Mapか、ALPSLAB clipを表示させることができます（選択可能）。WordPress用の「WP-SimpleGmaps」は 経度や緯度の座標指定を入れなくても、記事投稿画面のGoogleMapsから目的の場所を探して生成されたコードを貼り付けるだけで、記事内にGoogleMapsを表示することができます。

また、最近、RSSを使って情報を発信するサイトが増えてきましたが、これらのRSSの情報を拾ってきて、自分のブログ内に表示させるプラグインもあります。これを利用すると、例えば天気情報や、はてなブックマークの人気エントリー一覧を、自分のサイトにほぼリアルタイムで表示させたりすることができます。

ただ気を付けなくてはいけないことはそれをメインコンテンツにしないことです。RSSで引っ張ってきた情報だけで、ウェブサイトのコンテンツを成立させることができますが、これはスパログ（スパムブログ）と呼ばれる行為です。あくまでもサイトのコンテンツに＋αを加える目的でのみ使いましょう。

❏ スパム対策するプラグイン

アンカーテキストである<a>タグは、<nofollow>属性を指定することで、リンク先のページランクに影響を与えることを阻止できます。この仕組みは、多くのサイトからリンクされているサイトは良いサイトである、という検索エンジンのアルゴリズムを逆手に取り、ありとあらゆるサイトにトラックバックを貼りまくるというトラック

バック対策として採用されました。

　Movable Typeには3.3以降に標準搭載された、<nofollow> Pluginを使うことで、トラックバックやコメントに含まれるリンクに<nofollow>属性を自動的に付加してくれます。もちろん3.3以前のユーザーもプラグインを導入することはできます。

　また、WordPressにはトラックバックスパム対策プラグインとして「Akismet」が標準搭載されています。高機能と誉れが高いこの「Akismet」を実はMovable Typeでも使うことができます。

SEOに有用なプラグイン

画像に<alt>属性を追加する
(MT) imagealt……http://www.luckypines.com/mt/2006/07/alttransformer.html

関連記事を表示する
(MT) Related Entries……http://www.kalsey.com/2002/07/related_entries_plugin/
(MT) UTW mod Related Post……http://aoina.com/archives/65
(WP) Related Posts Link……http://erwin.terong.com/2005/09/24/wp-plugin-related-posts-link/

自動的に文中リンクする
(MT) MTSakuinPlugin……http://www.ideamans.com/tool/mtsakuinplugin.php
(WP) Lexicon Wordpress Plugin……http://www.shamusyoung.com/twentysidedtale/?p=413

自動的に文中リンクする（Googleへのリンク）
(MT) dosearch……http://www.bayashi.net/archives/entry/2006/000286.html
(WP) wikipedia linker……http://www.naviwave.com/blog_w/?p=77

Google Mapを表示する
(MT) Mapper Plugin.ja……http://code.as-is.net/wiki/Mapper_Plugin.ja_JP
(WP) WP-SimpleGmaps……http://aoina.com/archives/45

RSSを表示する
(MT) Feeds.App……http://code.appnel.com/feeds-app
(WP) mcRSSlist Plugin……http://matopc.myvnc.com/archives/2005/05/03/mcrsslist/

スパム対策
(MT) <nofollow> plugin……3.3以降に標準搭載
(WP) Akismet……標準搭載

※(MT)：Movable Type　(WP)：WordPress

☐ テキスト要素のデザイン性を崩さずにSEO対策をするツール

　検索エンジンは基本的にテキスト情報を収集しますので、デザイン重視のサイトだと、デザインとSEOの狭間で悩むことが少なからず出てきます。

　例えば、ページの見出しを表現するとき、デザイン性を優先するなら見出しのテキストを画像で表示させることになり、SEO優先なら画像で<h1>タグで見出し情報を表現することになります。画像でテキストを表現すれば、たとえ<alt>属性で画像に代替テキスト情報を付けたとしても、見かけのインパクトほど検索エンジンは評価しないのです。デザインを優先して画像で表現すべきか、そのままテキストとしてSEOを優先すべきか、悩ましい問題です。

　そこで、テキストでありながらデザイン性を確保する手段として、「Beautiful Japanese」というツールがあります。

　これはテキストをFlashを使ったフォントに置換して表示してくれるツールです。もともとはテキストとしてhtmlに記述されており、ページが表示される際にFlashフォントに置換しているだけですので、htmlの構造を崩すことなく、しかもSEOやユーザビリティも同時に成立させることができます。

　SEOが効果的なサイトといえば、無味乾燥なテキストサイトのイメージが強いのですが、このようなツールを使うことにより、デザイン性を損なうことなくSEOが効いたサイトを構築することもできます。

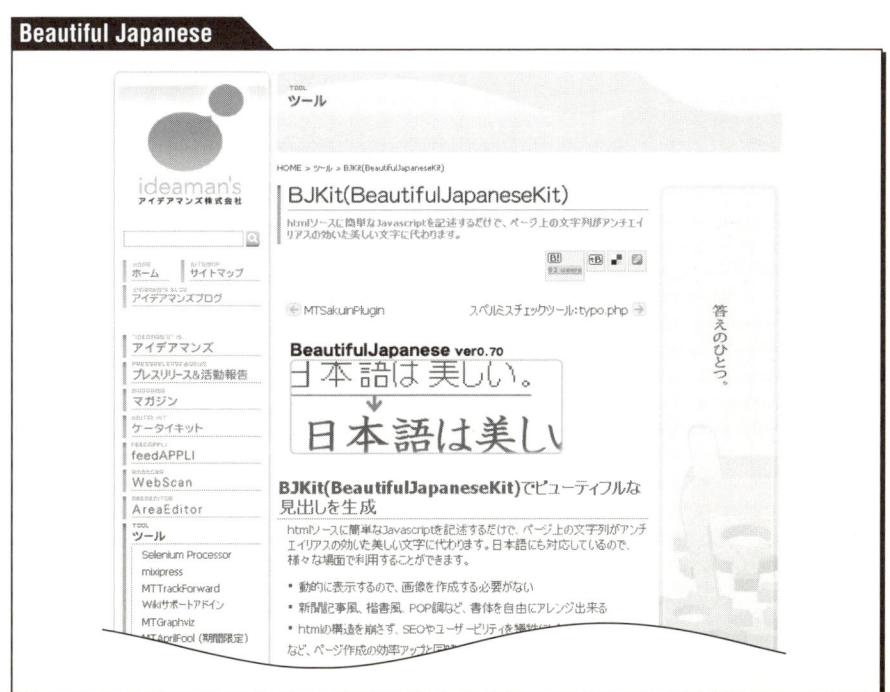

あとがき

□本書を全面的に書き下ろした理由

『SEO「検索エンジン最適化」の教科書』、いかがでしたでしょうか？

この本は、改訂版の枠を超えて、ほとんど書き下ろしとなりました。

これは、私自身の苦い思い出に起因します。

ある実用書を買いました。人生にいくばくかの影響を与えるほどの名著でした。

それから5年後、続編が発売されるというので、期待に胸を膨らませて購入したのですが、タイトルは変わっているものの中身はほとんど前著と一緒で、ラストの1章だけが新たに追加されているだけでした。全体の10%しか新しい内容ではなかったのです。残りの90%の内容にしても、挙げている例が最新の事例に差し変わっていれば印象が違ったのでしょうが、そういったこともなく、しかし価格は前著よりも高くなっていて、これほどがっかりした買い物はありませんでした。

期待外れでがっかりした思い出といえば、検索結果からスパログ（スパムブログ）に行ったときも同様です。スパログとは、WikipediaやAmazonから情報を引っ張ってきてページを生成しているブログのことで、プログラムによって自動生成されるウェブ2.0的手法を濫用したブログといえるでしょう。

情報を求めて検索をしたときに、スパログにぶつかったときの徒労感は例えようもありません。それらしい内容に見せて、その実、色んなサイトから情報を引っ張ってきて合成しているだけなのです。目新しい情報や新発見があるはずありません。見るだけ無駄なのです。

公開されている情報を組み合わせて表現する、いわゆるマッシュアップの手法は否定しませんし、それにより優れたサービスを実現しているサイトも数多く知っています。ただし、そこにはオリジナリティの要素が不可欠だと考えています。

焼き直しの再編集本とスパログ、共通することは「オリジナリティの欠如」です。借り物やあり物だけで完結しているようなコンテンツに、どのような魅力があるでしょうか？

そこで、この本は前著を手にした人でもがっかりすることがないように、ほとんど書き下ろしとなりました。オリジナリティ全開です。

もっともSEOのテクニックなどは前著から抜粋している部分も若干ありますが、コンパクトに再編集しています。前著をお読みくださった方にとっても、SEOの新しい教科書として、必要にして十分な情報をご紹介できたと思っております。

❏ SEOとオリコンチャートの類似点

さて、最後に、ひとつ注意をしておきましょう。

本書を読むことで、あなたはSEOの基本を身に付けることができました。しかし、これで満足してしまってはいけません。あなたには、まだまだやるべきことがたくさんあります。

例えば、こう考えてみてください。

あなたには、トップアーティストになってオリコンCDチャート1位を飾る夢があります。そのためには、まずCDデビューのチャンスを掴まなければなりません。

この場合、最短経路はオーディションで優勝を勝ち取ることでしょう。それも地方都市の主催する小さなオーディションではなく、大手音楽事務所やテレビ局が主催するオーディションならばCDデビューはほぼ確実です。

しかし、そこで歌やパフォーマンスが審査員に認められて、並みいるライバルの中から優勝を勝ち取ったとしても、デビューのチャンスが巡ってきただけで、デビュー曲がヒットするとは限りません。「メディアへの露出を増やす」「楽曲を一般受けしそうなものにする」「タイアップ」「ライブハウスを回る」といった地道な活動を通して、CDのセールスを伸ばしていきます。そして、オリコン1位を目指すのです。

さて、ここで問題です。「オリコン1位を飾る」を「Googleの検索結果1位になる」に置き換えると、「SEOを施す」ことはトップアーティストになるためのどのプロセスにあたるでしょうか？

オーディションでグランプリを勝ち取ることでしょうか？

CDデビューを果たすことでしょうか？

CDセールスを伸ばすために地道な活動をすることでしょうか？

──正解は「オーディションに応募する」ことです。SEOをすることは「オーディションに応募する」という意味しか持たないのです。SEOをやったらそれで終わり、と思っている人は、オーディションに書類を送っただけでとんとん拍子でデビューできて、あまつさえデビュー曲がオリコン1位を約束されたと信じてやまない夢想家でしかありません。SEOは魔法のツールではないのです。

Google検索結果1位になっても、それが成果に繋がらなければ何の意味も持ちません。"検索結果1位になる＝ビジネスチャンスを増やした"ということでしかないのです。同時並行で考えなくてはいけないことは、他にもあります。

検索エンジン経由でやって来たユーザーがそのまま検索結果に戻ってしまう、あるいは必要な情報だけ取得してすぐに帰ってしまう、いわゆる「直帰率」を下げること、サイト内に少しでも長くいてもらうために「回遊率」を向上させること、またサイトに来たユーザーに資料請求や購買に繋げる「コンバージョンレート」、この3つは気に掛けておかねばなりません。

検索上位表示を目指しつつ、直帰率を下げ、回遊率とコンバージョンレートを上げ

ることがワンセットでSEOといっても過言ではありません。成果を出すサイトを作っていくためには、これらの要素も疎かにしてはいけないのです。

　SEOに捕らわれて、検索エンジン結果に一喜一憂することよりも、検索エンジンの向こう側にいるユーザーを意識してみてください。それによっては、SEOよりもむしろSEMに予算を割いた方が効果的な場合もあるでしょうし、試行錯誤と分析は常に怠らないようにしましょう。

　厳しい言い方になってしまいましたが、SEOはあくまでも手段でしかない、ということを今一度認識してください。

　もっとも、SEOを意識せずにGoogle検索結果1位を目指すのは、路上ライブから見出されてアーティストになってオリコン1位を飾ることと同じです。よほど実力があれば実現できなくもありませんが、あまりにも偶然性に頼り過ぎています。趣味でやっている分にはいいのでしょうが、ビジネスとしてやっていくにはあまりにも無計画過ぎます。

　要は、「SEOはやって当然、そこから先が勝負のポイント」ということです。

◻︎支えてくれた人に感謝を込めて

　なお、この本を書くにあたり社内外の方より多くの助言をいただきました。この場をお借りして御礼申し上げます。

　また、数多くのサイトやブログでの情報も本を書く上でのヒントにさせていただきました。そしてソースコードやデータの一部を引用させていただきました。重ねて御礼申し上げます。

　比類なき遅筆のため、前著に引き続き、秀和システムの担当者様にはご迷惑をお掛けしました。幾度となく心が折れそうになりながらも、その都度支えていただき無事発行の運びとなりました。

　そして執筆が追い込みになるにつれ、会社に泊り込む機会も多々ありましたが、その間しっかり家庭を支えてくれた妻に最大限の感謝の気持ちを送ります。

　ありがとう。

2007年3月

　　　　　　　　　　　　　　　　　　ドラゴンフィールド株式会社　吉村　正春

【著者紹介】
吉村　正春（よしむら・まさはる）

1970年生。日刊メールマガジン「InternetNOW!」に編集スタッフとして参加して以降、ウェブライターとしてウェブ業界に関わり続ける。ドラゴンフィールド株式会社所属。ウェブ業界専門誌「WEB FLASH」（毎偶数月発行）、およびウェブマーケティングメールマガジン「週刊e‐Report」編集長。

SEO「検索エンジン最適化」の教科書

| 発行日 | 2007年　3月　9日 | 第1版第1刷 |
| | 2009年　2月 20日 | 第1版第5刷 |

著　者　吉村　正春

発行者　斉藤　和邦
発行所　株式会社　秀和システム
　　　　〒107-0062　東京都港区南青山1-26-1 寿光ビル5F
　　　　Tel 03-3470-4947（販売）
　　　　Fax 03-3405-7538
印刷所　株式会社平河工業社

Printed in Japan

ISBN978-4-7980-1597-2 C3055

定価はカバーに表示してあります。
乱丁本・落丁本はお取りかえいたします。
本書に関するご質問については、ご質問の内容と住所、氏名、電話番号を明記のうえ、当社編集部宛FAXまたは書面にてお送りください。お電話によるご質問は受け付けておりませんのであらかじめご了承ください。

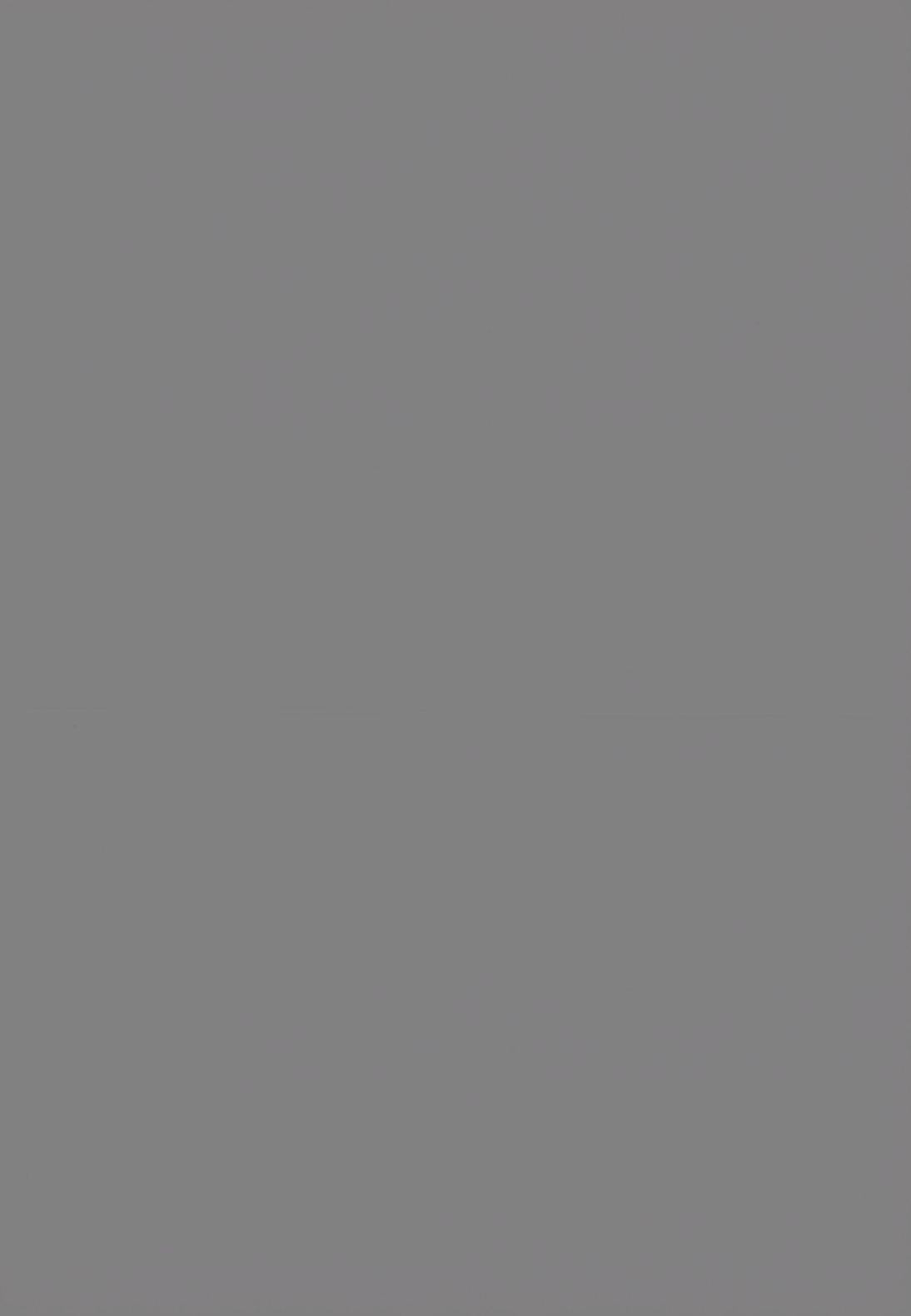